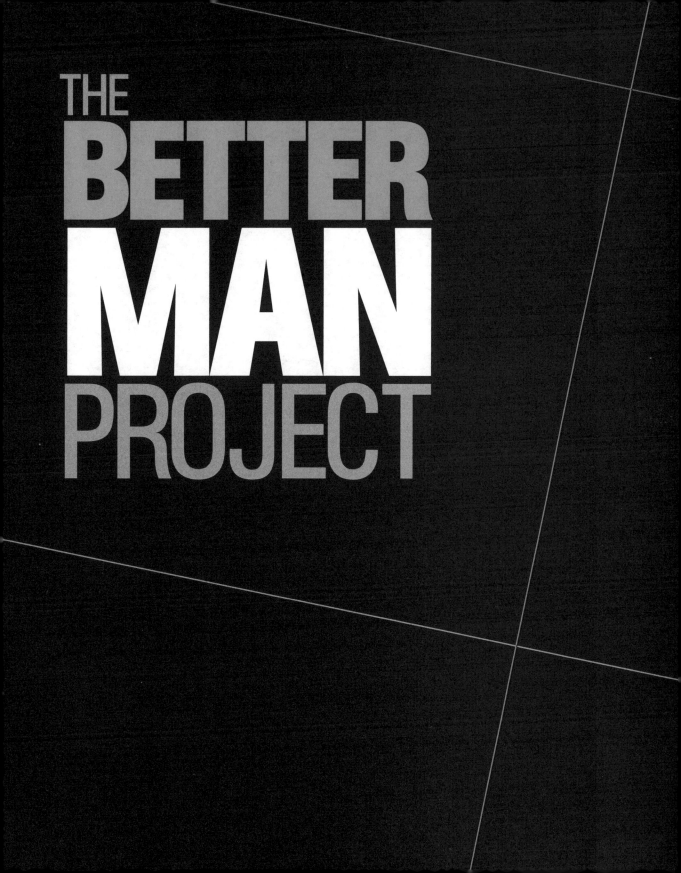

THE
BETTER
MAN
PROJECT

THE BETTER MAN PROJECT

2,476 TIPS AND TECHNIQUES THAT WILL FLATTEN YOUR BELLY, SHARPEN YOUR MIND, AND KEEP YOU HEALTHY AND HAPPY FOR LIFE!

35 DIY PLANS TO MAKE YOU AMAZING!

BILL PHILLIPS, EDITOR-IN-CHIEF, **AND THE EDITORS OF Men'sHealth**

RODALE

To the loves of my life: Robin, Lindsay, and Taylor
I may never be perfect, but I will always try to be better

Conte

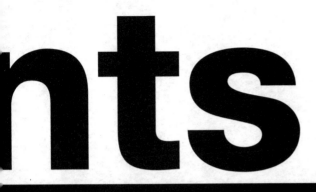

nts

Foreword

I hear this disturbing refrain all the time—from the media, from health care providers, and even from guys I know: "Muscle mass, testosterone, energy, strength, all start declining in our 20s and 30s. It's not my fault that I'm rolling downhill faster than a Schwinn with worn brake pads."

As a guy (and doctor) who just turned 43, I say: Bullshit!

Okay, I'll admit that this isn't such good bedside manner for an E.R. doc, but I'm genuinely disheartened by the excuses I hear. Come on guys! Our lives don't have to be a sad story of inevitable decline! Don't give up when the game is just beginning; this is the game of your life, and you can win it.

You see, because I've been fortunate to learn that my health doesn't need to decline as I age, I feel like I'm roaring out of the locker room after half-time in my game of life. And I'm fired up! The coach has just given me a rousing pep talk, and I have great strategies for success. Exactly the kinds of motivation and information you'll find in *The Better Man Project*, in fact. Don't worry, you don't need to run a marathon, quit drinking beer, or live solely on seaweed to stay strong and healthy. You don't have to go on some complicated regimen of supplements or join a monastery.

But you do need to *start paying attention*. To your activity levels. To the ways you spend your free time. To your methods of handling stress. To the foods you eat. To the ways you interact with loved ones. Sound difficult? Only if you let it be, because doing all of those things are your keys to a better, more enjoyable, more passionate way of living! You're not going to let the downward pull of aging dictate who you are. You're going to seize control of that process and control the action going forward, and upward.

To do that, you just need sound strategies and a willingness to stay on the field of battle. Yes, you're going to feel the changes, especially at first. But that's the point, right? Change you can feel and appreciate?

I acknowledge that I have a few more aches and pains now when I first get out of bed in the AM, but it's a small price to pay for all the benefits I get for living an engaged life. I feel as vibrant and healthy as ever. Maybe even more vibrant and healthy, especially when you compare it to my early days working in the consulting industry, when I was letting my career dictate my activity levels and also using stress and time constraints as an excuse to live on the slacker diet—beer, frozen pizza, repeat. But it didn't make me feel great then, and it would be a disaster now.

Trust me, I still have plenty of stress in my "grown-up" life as a physician and as the host of the television show, *The Doctors*. Yet I can honestly say that what brings me the most sense of satisfaction has nothing to do with being on TV or having an exciting career, but rather maintaining my ability to do as many push-ups and pull-ups as when I was 20 years old.

And because I maintain my fitness level, I have been blessed *in my 40s* to ride the Leadville 100—a mountain bike race that traverses 100 miles and begins at 11,000 feet!—and to will myself and my bicycle up the classic climbs of the Tour de France as I did on a recent trip. It isn't the usual kind of R&R that I'm after, but rather I'm looking for Renewal and Rejuvenation. Physical activity, and the pure fuel that energizes it, gives me that. When I hop in my kayak in the mountains of Colorado and paddle the challenging whitewater of the beautiful Arkansas River, I realize: *This is living*. My heart pounds, my senses are alert, my muscles are pushing—and suddenly age 43 feels like the best year of my life.

And I'm confident that 44, 45, and beyond will be even better.

Is that the way you look at it, too? I hope so. But for many guys, the "middle ages" feel like the time of life when you give things up. No more backpacking trips with their buddies, no more pickup basketball, no more pounding it on the double black diamond ski runs. It's the premature end of their vision of themselves as active guys, as guys who can take on new skills, as guys who can get better every year, every day, every minute. But the only reason that would be true is if *you allowed it to be*—if you gave up before the game was half over.

There's plenty of time left on the clock for you to rally and win.

You just need a good coach and some proven strategies. The kind you'll find in the pages of *The Better Man Project*. You could open this to almost any page and get to work on one thing you find there, and it will open you up to a whole new way of living and help propel you to a personal victory in the second half.

How will you do that? By making health your primary hobby. If that sounds difficult, it shouldn't. Because by investing in health—your body, your mind, your spirit—you lay the groundwork for enjoying everything in your life more. Health is the spark that ignites your personal drive to succeed in your career, your active pursuits, and your relationships. Not only will you live better and usually longer, you'll become a better coworker, friend, spouse, father...you name it.

You also can inspire others in their own pursuit of good health. And in a world where the obesity rate has quadrupled among adolescents in the last 30 years, the nation's kids are in need of some serious inspiration! So is your buddy, who let an injury derail him a decade ago. So is your boss, who might see you as a leader if you launch a self-improvement campaign. So is your wife, who wants to feel that your life together is still moving forward—in the bedroom and out of it. By setting an example as someone who's pushing hard for success, you can help those around you to personal victories as well. When you succeed, your whole team succeeds.

Those are all great reasons for you to commit to the many lessons in *The Better Man Project*. In my own life, I don't just want to live long, I want to live great, and this book provides the know-how and inspiration to do just that.

And the end game of this beautiful journey is not *just* more sex at an older age (but that *is* awesome by the way), not *just* a top-10 age group finish in your first triathlon or mud run (though you can absolutely accomplish that if you try), not *just* a waistline that shrinks to fit into your college jeans (just do us a favor and replace those bellbottoms, okay?), but rather, it's the feeling that you've seized the initiative in life once again. Suddenly you're dictating the action in the second half of the game, and you're going to win it on your own terms. This doesn't mean you'll be immortal, but it does mean you'll pack more enjoyment into every waking minute of the time you have left.

Your end game WILL BE a better and longer life. Why not live it now? The first step is simple: Just turn the page.

TRAVIS STORK, M.D.

DR. STORK is an Emmy-nominated host of the talk show, *The Doctors*, and a board-certified emergency medicine physician. He is author of *The Doctor's Diet* and *The Lean Belly Prescription* and is a member of the *Men's Health* medical advisory board.

Read This Page First!

Hey! Thanks for buying this book!

What's that? You didn't buy it? Somebody gave it to you hoping you'll take better care of yourself?

Then thank them for me. And before you think about using it for kindling or calf raises, read this page. I think it will convince you that you don't have to overhaul your life to improve your health. In fact, that's the whole point of this book: My goal is to show you that it doesn't take a lot of work to be better. Just make a few small adjustments and you'll get thinner, stronger, smarter, healthier, and live longer. You'll become a better man, and maybe even earn that promotion—or have more sex as a result. It'll take just a minute or two. The reading, I mean.

—BILL PHILLIPS

DO THIS!	GAIN THIS!
Replace your ham sandwich with tuna twice a week.	**Lower your risk of heart disease 25 percent.**
Drink red wine from Chile instead of France.	**Reduce your risk of cancer.** Chilean cabernet sauvignon is 38 percent higher than French red in flavonols, antioxidants that plunder cancer-causing free radicals.
Position your rearview mirror 2 inches higher than normal.	**You'll immediately sit up taller,** improving your posture and reducing your chances of a backache.
Eat two apples a day.	**Lose 10 pounds in a year.** The big dose of fiber promotes weight loss. And you'll swallow about a gazillion natural anti-cancer compounds.
Eat two potassium-rich bananas a day.	**Lower your risk of stroke** by about 20 percent.
Leave something on your plate.	**Live about 7 years longer, you ape.** In a study at the University of Wisconsin at Madison, primates that ate 30 percent less as adults lived 9 percent longer on average than those who didn't restrict their calories. The researchers say calorie restriction leads to long-term weight loss and helps to delay the effects of aging in monkeys–and possibly men, too.

DO THIS!	GAIN THIS!
Have more frequent orgasms.	**Improve your resting heart rate variability** (HRV), a new method for assessing the health of your heart. HRV refers to the beat-to-beat alterations in heart rate. Although it sounds counterintuitive, you want variability versus metronome-like consistency between beats. High HRV suggests dominance of your parasympathetic nervous system, the side that promotes relaxation, digestion, and sleep. Sex strengthens your parasympathetic nervous system, allowing it to better counter your sympathetic nervous system, which is the fight-or-flight side of the nervous system connected to stress.
Swallow some bacteria, specifically *L. acidophilus* and *B. lactis*.	**Poop more regularly.** Populating your gut with probiotics from yogurt and kefir helped constipation sufferers improve their symptoms by 62 percent.
Be more like a caveman.	**Improve your sex appeal.** A University of Alaska study showed that men who tackled "caveman challenges like handling fire or swimming in moving water were more sexually alluring to women than those who took modern risks like riding a motorcycle without a helmet." It seems primal natural dangers let you flaunt your evolutionary fitness. May we suggest whitewater kayaking or rock climbing with your date?
Focus on your lower molars.	**Have fewer cavities.** People spend 62 percent less time brushing the inner surfaces of their teeth as they do the outer surfaces. Give all sides equal time.
Take 10.	**Remember more.** Resting quietly for 10 minutes after learning something new could help you retain 20 percent more, according to Scottish researchers.
Bulk up on roughage.	**Stay alive.** A Korean study found that men who ate the most fiber were 27 percent less likely to die over an 11-year period than men who ate the least. Aim for 38 grams a day to fight the inflammation linked to type 2 diabetes and stroke.
Turn up the heat and stretch.	**Fry 459 calories.** That's the average number of calories a man incinerates in a 90-minute session of Bikram (hot) yoga.
Take the stairs.	**Find fewer germs on your index finger.** In a study, researchers found that 61 percent of elevator buttons in hospitals were crawling with bacteria compared to 43 percent of toilet flush handles. Plus, stairs burn 10 calories every minute.
Shift your perspective.	**Boost your performance.** Men can generate more force and bang out more reps by focusing on external cues (for example, shoving the ground away during a pushup), according to a review of studies in the *Strength and Conditioning Journal*.
Sweat more.	**Improve your fertility.** Harvard researchers found that men who worked out the most had a 33 percent higher sperm count than those who exercised the least.
Read the rest of this book.	**Make yourself a lot more successful** and live at least 10 years longer, if not way more. A landmark 8-decade study found that better than average men (that is, men who worked hard to achieve career success) lived about a decade longer and were less likely to get sick than less successful men.

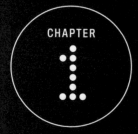

Your Latest DIY Project:
YOU

Do you want to live forever? I don't.

Actually, who am I kidding? I'd love to live forever, but only if I could look good, stay healthy, and still do all the things I love. (I'd also like Eternity to have a Starbucks.) I bet you feel the same way. When you feel strong and healthy, when you're confident about your work, when you're stoked about waking up in the morning and attacking your day, when you're impressed with who's staring back at you in the mirror . . . well, life is pretty awesome. That's the kind of longevity we're after.

■
Better
INSTANTLY
↓
Adopt this mindset: I will get a little bit better every day. The cumulative effect of that one change will transform your entire life.

For as long as men have walked the planet, we've been fascinated by the idea of living forever. In the 5th century B.C., the Greek dude Herodotus first wrote about the fountain of youth. Simply bathe in its waters, he proclaimed, and your youth will be restored. In 1513, an aging Ponce de León left Puerto Rico and went looking for such a magical fountain of agelessness—and found Florida instead. How's that for irony?

Part of our fascination is easy to explain, as expressed in German painter Lucas Cranach the Elder's 1546 work titled *The Fountain of Youth* (clear is the old clever) shown below. The painting depicts a simple rectangular pool filled with 2 feet of water and two dozen naked women, all preening for attention. The meaning is clear: Where there is youth and water, there's the possibility of skinny-dipping. No wonder Ponce was gone so long.

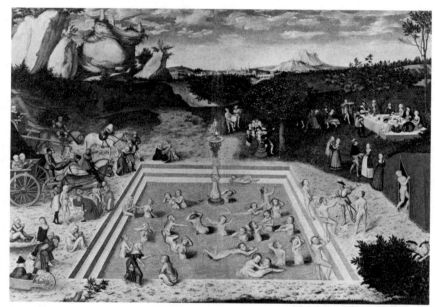

SPRING BREAK CIRCA 1546

These days, thanks to modern science, the whole fountain of youth concept doesn't pass our sniff test. Still, we're not ready to completely abandon the fantasy of eternal good looks, strength, health, and vitality. Exhibit A: the ever-regenerating Wolverine from *X-Men*.

Of course, when trying to achieve Wolverine-level physicality, it helps if you look like Hugh Jackman. Think about this: Hugh has graced the cover of *Men's Health* magazine multiple times. As that magazine's editor-in-chief, I can tell you firsthand not only that he is a gentleman—which immediately makes him a "better man" than most—but also that he has the fitness and training discipline of an elite athlete. And the guy is well on his way to the big 5-0. He's a shining example of what's possible for you and me.

While nobody has figured out a path to immortality, and it's not exactly on the horizon, I think most guys would gladly accept the next best thing: having a body and mind that look good and work great all the way up until the moment we kick the bucket many decades from now. In a way, we'd like to live like . . . a seagull. That's right, the enviable thing about some seabirds is that even old ones act as strong and virile as they did in their youth, until one day they just drop into the bay and become fish food.

How's that for a goal? Live as healthy and strong as you are today until the end of your life at 90, 100, or beyond.

"Seabirds tend to be very long-lived, and there is evidence in some species—like common terns, which are related to gulls—that they don't show many signs of aging before their death," says Mark Haussmann, Ph.D., an associate professor of biology at Bucknell University in Lewisburg, Pennsylvania, who studies animal physiology. His research shows that some of the longest-living birds seem to protect their cells— and what's inside those cells—better than mammals do. They have higher levels of helpful antioxidants, and they also do a better job at protecting the ends of their DNA, called telomeres, from damage, he says. "Telomeres shorten with aging, and in wild animals and humans, telomere shortening rates are a predictor of life span." That's because they're an indicator of cell damage. "In these long-lived birds, telomeres shorten very, very slowly, suggesting that their cells and their DNA experience less damage than some other animals'."

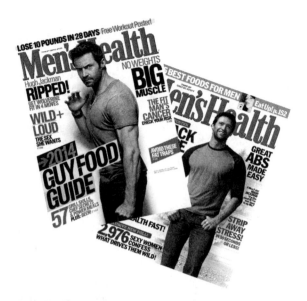

TRY THIS!

Pop Before You Drop

Scientists in the Netherlands say taking 100 milligrams of aspirin at night can reduce the odds of a blood clot forming in the morning. Men tend to have a higher risk of heart attacks in the morning, so this strategy may prevent the danger, says *Men's Health* cardiology advisor John Elefteriades, M.D. Just check with your doctor before you start aspirin therapy.

Your telomeres are under constant attack, but you can toughen them up. We'll show you how. Of course, the very genes you start with matter, too. Research shows that some people hit the genetic jackpot and enter the world with a leg up when it comes to health, vitality, and longevity. There's no good way to assess whether you carry these hearty genes, so err on the safe side. "For most of us, there's an interaction between our genes and the environment," says Nir Barzilai, M.D., director of the Institute for Aging Research at Yeshiva University's Albert Einstein College of Medicine in the Bronx, New York. "When we stress the environment with things like smoking and obesity, we live shorter lives."

And the flip side is also true: There are so-called bad genes, but having them doesn't necessarily mean you're doomed, says Alexander Kulminski, Ph.D., a senior research scientist at the Population Research Institute at Duke University. "Contrary to common expectations—that genes can unconditionally affect risk of certain health traits—it appears in many cases that this is not true," he says. "The effect of genes can be different in different conditions, in different ages, and different genders."

I sure hope he's right. There's an angry gene on my dad's side of the family that causes CADASIL, a disease that leads to dementia and stroke at a young age. My dad had it, and it likely contributed to his death from a fall at the age of 59. I'm surely doing my damnedest to keep it calm, even if that means kale on my plate.

The truth is, there are a lot of people—with good genes and bad—who live very long lives. And they stay healthy well into their years. One study from Boston University showed that the average person spends 18 percent of his life living with at least one disease, but supercentenarians—people who live to 110 or older—only spend 5 percent of their lives sick. Imagine staying healthy until you're 104. Think what you could do with all those years. That's my kind of definition of free time.

So how do you guarantee yourself a seagull's life as you move forward? How do you ensure that you'll operate at the same or a higher level as you are today, both physically and mentally? Answer: You get *better* every day.

Better takes effort, of course. If you choose instead to lie back and eat and drink like you did when you were 25, exercise when the mood strikes you, put in 60-hour workweeks, drive too fast, avoid broccoli and quinoa and rectal exams (the kind your doctor gives), then better isn't in your cards. More likely, you'll be sitting in a nursing home with pureed peas on your chin at 90 instead of skydiving like George H.W. Bush.

Getting better is always better than the alternative.

I love the word "better" because it's loaded with potential. "Better" is *achievable*. Any man can get better. Better health, better fitness, better career, better sex, and on and on all the way out to the best "better" of all: better life.

Our mission at *Men's Health* is to help each reader get better each day. That formula works so well—our readers tell us so—because it's bottom-line, no-excuses *doable*. Any man can get a little bit better each day. If you adopt that mindset, even if that's the only adjustment you make today, you're better already.

I want this book to help you make your health and fitness better as effortlessly as possible. That's why you'll see many different features sprinkled throughout, like "Better INSTANTLY," super-quick bits that you can apply to your life immediately. Grab 'em and go. In later chapters, you'll see even more transformative tips and expert advice, all of them easy to apply to your life.

Now here's what happens as you make all these small changes: The cumulative effect of daily better begins to add up and multiply over days, weeks, and months. You start to change. First, a little. Then, a lot. It's profound. The weight seems to just melt away. You can't wait till your next workout. You can't imagine ever eating another Oreo.

Meanwhile, you begin to see yourself differently. So do your girlfriend and your boss. You walk taller. You're more confident in meetings. Cute strangers on the street hold eye contact a split second longer. Did she just smile at you? Yes, she did.

Simple truth: Once you realize that you can change your body, you feel like you can do anything. I know: *Men's Health* readers do it every day and share their stories of transformation with us. You can do it too.

Now it's your turn. You're about to launch Project: You, an effort to become a little bit better every day. Don't worry—I'm here to help (feel free to hit me up on Twitter @MHBetterMan with questions). So let's talk about how your reinvention project will play out.

What to Expect

Any successful journey starts with a first step. To know where you're going, you have to know where you've been. Maybe you're reading this because you know you have improvements to make. Perhaps you have a clean bill of health and just want to keep things that way. Either way, I want you to assess whether you're really on the right track—or veering into the danger zone. We'll do that in the next chapter with a series of simple self-tests. No doc, no waiting, no co-pay.

After your reality check, I'll give you the tools to improve those results so you can live a healthier, fuller life. At *Men's Health,* we have connections with the top researchers and doctors in the world. Here's what they've told us: If you know your body and take care of it, you'll keep it humming like a well-tuned vintage muscle car. If you don't, then you'll cough, wheeze, and backfire to the finish line.

Better INSTANTLY

↓

Consuming two glasses of water or a cup of soup to begin a meal can reduce your total calorie intake by up to 20 percent because it makes you feel full.

Low-Tech Life Extension

Try these five longevity strategies, no cryogenics necessary!

+1 YEAR
SWALLOW A BITTER PILL

Make that a piece of dark chocolate. Harvard research showed that people who ate dark chocolate just once a month lived longer than people who didn't eat it or ate milk chocolate. It may have something to do with the antioxidants in dark chocolate. When choosing a dark bar, look for the percentage of cacao; the higher the number, the more antioxidants inside. Bitterness also increases with cacao content, so you may need to work up to the heavy-duty stuff.

+2 YEARS
KEEP SWINGING

Join an organized team sport like softball or basketball, but not pub darts. A Japanese study found that men who were still involved in sports at age 65 outlived their inactive counterparts. Researchers believe it had to do with the combination of exercise and social interaction. The peer pressure to hustle out to left field or cut to the basket may keep you from rotting in a rocking chair.

+2 YEARS
STOP THE HAND-WRINGING

Really now, has worrying ever gotten you anywhere? Then can it. You'll enjoy life more and have more life to enjoy. A study of more than 6,000 Chicago residents by the Rush Institute for Healthy Aging determined that those who were the least anxious on a day-to-day basis lived the longest. Why? A constant state of stress has been shown to undermine the immune system. Go for a run. Play basketball. Distract your one-track mind with a brain game like Suduko or, hell, even a video game like *Halo*. Got a DVD player? A *Three Stooges* marathon is better than Xanax to the worried male mind.

+3 YEARS
TAKE THEE TO CHURCH

Or to the synagogue, or to the sweat lodge, wherever you might worship. University of Pittsburgh researchers say that weekly attendance at religious services may add years to a person's expiration date, an increase equal to that seen with using cholesterol-lowering medicines. Not religious? Commit to a weekly group activity that feels like a spiritual experience—like, say, watching football.

+8 YEARS
BELIEVE IN DR. YOU

Believing that you are in control of your health can be a self-fulfilling prophecy. According to a Canadian study of healthy elderly people, study participants who predicted that they would live 8 more years actually did, while those who foresaw an early funeral got exactly that. Beliefs may well beget actions, negative and positive.

The average man only lives to 76, but I want you to live much longer and better than other guys who manage to make it that far. I want to help you spend zero of those years in a wheelchair. Or impotent. Or incontinent. I want you to live like a seabird with a hard-on. And this book is going to help.

After Chapter 2's self-test, Chapter 3 will introduce the Seven Horsemen of the Apocalypse—the top seven causes of death in men. I've broken them down by age group so you can identify the biggest threats you face right now. It's easy to worry about plane crashes, shark attacks, and Ebola, but this fact-check will show you the bogeymen you really need to fear. Then, I'll share the bad habits that accelerate aging and leave you vulnerable to common killers. This chapter isn't trying to scare anybody; it's about giving guys who may think nothing bad will ever happen to them the data to convince them they can easily become a statistic without a little self-care.

Chapter 4 will be the start of your journey to being a better man. We'll begin by upgrading your food habits. And we'll make it easy—eating right doesn't have to be a miserable slog. It can be simple and delicious! Most of the chapters start with the "Fast Five"—a handful of easy steps to get you started immediately. Later, if you've got the gumption, you can take on more advanced challenges to get even better than better.

In Chapter 5, we'll help you shape up. Whether you're a CrossFit junkie or a couch surfer, it doesn't matter. We'll show you how to build strength, power, and stamina while reducing your risk of injuries. The payoff? You'll look better, feel more energetic, and come out healthier.

Chapters 6 and 7 will focus on taking charge of your health by getting you to know your body as well as you do your investment portfolio. This is crucial for all men, mostly because so many men blow it off. While you're ultimately in charge of your own body, good doctors can also catch problems before they become bigger problems. We'll show you how to recruit the best M.D., P.T., and more and tip you off to the essential diagnostic tests that can provide you with the knowledge to take lifesaving steps.

In Chapter 8, we'll say good night to insomnia, sleep apnea, and other slumber saboteurs. You will be amazed by what a few improved Z's can do.

Chapter 9 will focus on your mind. The latest data from the American Psychological Association show that the average guy lives with a stress level of 4.6 out of 10—higher than the level that the experts consider healthy (3.6). We'll help you lower your score. Plus, we'll show you how to vanquish other mental saboteurs, including depression, anger, and dementia.

Chapter 10 is all about your favorite subject—sex! To be a better man, you may need to be a better lover. To be a better lover, you may need to be a better man—that is, a more patient and understanding man who listens to her more and tries to fix less. Fortunately, there are people who study this stuff, so we can show you the best ways to have better sex and more of it.

Chapter 11 is all about troubleshooting. From minor annoyances like colds to serious struggles like kidney stones, we'll show you the best ways to stay in peak condition when surprising symptoms strike.

Finally, in Chapter 12, we'll tackle DIY projects to help you patch up your weak spots. Need to lose that beer belly? Check. Annihilate back pain? Check. Make your body the strongest it's ever been? We'll break down 35 important goals into easy steps.

Throughout the book you'll notice a collection of quick hits designed to make you better fast:

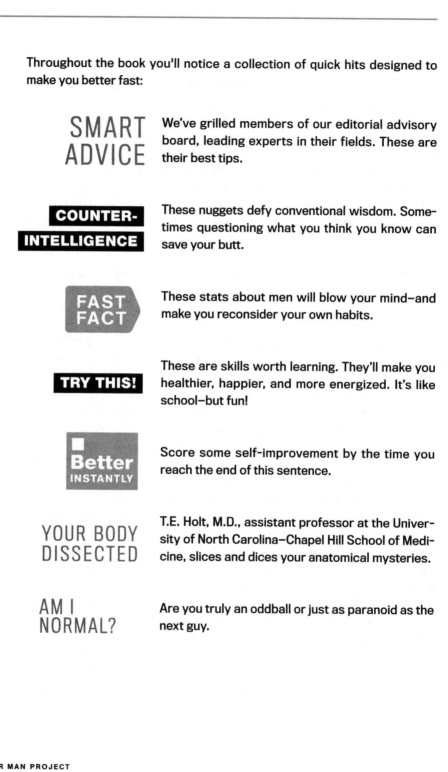

SMART ADVICE

We've grilled members of our editorial advisory board, leading experts in their fields. These are their best tips.

COUNTER-INTELLIGENCE

These nuggets defy conventional wisdom. Sometimes questioning what you think you know can save your butt.

FAST FACT

These stats about men will blow your mind—and make you reconsider your own habits.

TRY THIS!

These are skills worth learning. They'll make you healthier, happier, and more energized. It's like school—but fun!

Better INSTANTLY

Score some self-improvement by the time you reach the end of this sentence.

YOUR BODY DISSECTED

T.E. Holt, M.D., assistant professor at the University of North Carolina–Chapel Hill School of Medicine, slices and dices your anatomical mysteries.

AM I NORMAL?

Are you truly an oddball or just as paranoid as the next guy.

One of Life's Great Secrets

You've got a powerful set of tools in your hands right now. The info in this book, mixed with your simple decision to get a little bit better each day, is nothing less than a life-transforming formula. You'll be different. You'll feel different. People around you will notice the change. You'll be happier. More energetic. Excited to make more improvements. Your success will feed additional success. I've seen this formula work time and again. It's no joke, but it brings a hell of a lot of smiles.

Oh, and not to be outdone by any late-night infomercial: *Wait, there's more.* As a bonus, while you read this book, you'll come to understand one of the great secrets of life. Normally, great secrets of life only come in a fever dream brought on by eating the worm at the bottom of a mescal bottle. But I believe in saving you time and a hangover. I'll tell you this secret right here, up front, no waiting. I learned it by spending many years editing hundreds of health and fitness stories; you can't work this closely with that material and not learn a couple of things. Even if you refuse to believe this secret right now, I predict you'll become a true believer as you read on. It's inevitable.

Okay, are you ready? Here's one of the great secrets of life: Even if you do everything right already—eat off the food pyramid, exercise every day, outperform every goal you set at home and at work—you can be a better man. You can still make today a little bit better than yesterday.

Now that's a code to live by. Let's get started!

Better
INSTANTLY
↓
Learn to use wit instead of sarcasm and skepticism instead of cynicism, and you're ahead of most men.

How to Be Better Than Average in Less Than 5 Minutes!

This book is loaded with so much useful information, I can bust a gut just thinking about it. Before we get to the heavy lifting, though, here's a quick warmup that'll help you start becoming better than the average American man almost instantly.

Health

THE AVERAGE MAN gets two or three colds a year, and the average upper respiratory infection lasts 7 to 10 days.

BE BETTER THAN AVERAGE: Don't try to blow out a cold. Blowing your nose vigorously could make your cold last longer. Using CT scans, researchers at the University of Virginia discovered that nose blowing actually forces some mucus backward, propelling bacteria and viruses directly into your sinuses and triggering reactions that can make your cold worse. Limit your honking and take decongestants as soon as symptoms appear.

THE AVERAGE MAN has a one-in-three chance of having high blood pressure (a systolic, the top number, reading of 140 mmHg or over; and a diastolic, the bottom number, reading of 90 mmHg or over).

BE BETTER THAN AVERAGE:

→   Lose 4 pounds. The Framingham Heart Study found that overweight men who lost as little as a pound a year for 4 years cut their risk of developing high blood pressure by as much as 30 percent.

→   Have more sex. In a 2006 study at the University of Paisley, Scotland, people who had sex at least once in a 2-week period had lower blood pressure than those who engaged in no sexual activity, and their blood vessels responded better to stress.

THE AVERAGE MAN is more than twice as likely to die in an auto accident as the average woman.

BE BETTER THAN AVERAGE:

→   Look both ways at green lights. Running a red light causes more than 75,000 fatal accidents a year, and with the increase in distracted driving caused by texting, these side-impact crashes are on the rise.

→ Flare out your mirrors. Many people have their side mirrors adjusted incorrectly. When you can see the back corner of your car after leaning toward the mirror, it's adjusted correctly, according to the American Automobile Association.

Nutrition

THE AVERAGE MAN gets no nutrition counseling when he goes to his doctor for a checkup.

BE BETTER THAN AVERAGE: Snack on this no-co-pay nutrition advice: Eat a handful of nuts every day. A study in the *American Journal of Clinical Nutrition* found that people who ate an ounce of mixed nuts—specifically almonds, walnuts, and cashews—five or more times per week slashed their heart disease risk by 29 percent. The mono- and polyunsaturated fat content may reduce LDL cholesterol, says Harvard researcher Frank Hu, M.D., Ph.D.

THE AVERAGE PERSON eats three servings of vegetables or fruits a day, not the seven that are recommended for good health.

BE BETTER THAN AVERAGE: Never say no to an apple. Bring baby carrots to munch on at work. Broccoli and dip, anyone? Eating at least seven servings a day is associated with a 42 percent lower risk of death from any cause.

Fitness

THE AVERAGE MAN in his 30s or 40s has a body fat percentage of 26.

BE BETTER THAN AVERAGE: Get it down to 20 or below by building more muscle. Lift heavier weights for fewer reps. If you're currently doing 3 sets of 12, work your way to 5 or 6 sets of 4 reps of big muscle exercises.

Morality

THE AVERAGE MAN thinks it's okay to lust after his daughter's hot college friends.

BE BETTER THAN AVERAGE: Think about how you would feel if your daughter's hot college friends' fathers were lusting after *your* daughter. Then, practice virtue. Exercise it like a muscle. "People who exercise virtue know that when they get in a certain situation, they hardly have to think about it because they know how they will act," says Christian Smith, Ph.D., a professor of sociology at Notre Dame.

THE AVERAGE MAN has lied to his wife or girlfriend about where he went; 50 percent of men say they have lied to get a woman into bed.

BE BETTER THAN AVERAGE: Think selfishly before you lie. Lying breeds more lies, and harboring these secrets can be so stressful it can compromise your immune system, scientists say. On the flip side, telling the truth is good for body and soul. In a study at Notre Dame, researchers asked one group of subjects to avoid telling major and minor lies for 10 weeks. A control group received no such instruction. The researchers monitored the subjects' health and checked on their truthfulness using polygraph machines. At the end of the study, the researchers found that truth telling correlated with better health. The subjects in the group that told fewer lies reported improved relationships, better sleep, less tension, and fewer headaches and sore throats.

Sex

THE AVERAGE MAN doesn't think he lasts long enough during intercourse.
BE BETTER THAN AVERAGE: Work with her. Women have difficulty focusing on sexual sensation, so they need high arousal to reach orgasm, according to sex researcher Cindy Meston, Ph.D., the author of *Why Women Have Sex*. Trade your goal-oriented approach for a more pleasure-oriented one. "Think of sex as a circle, not a staircase."

→ Women are attracted to men who know how to fix things, so tightening a few screws might just loosen her inhibitions. "DIY skills prove you can care for her," says Vinita Mehta, Ph.D., a Washington, D.C., psychologist who writes about relationships. It also shows you're confident. "When a man says, 'I got this,' it's music to our ears," says Amy Matthews, host of HGTV's *Renovation Raiders*.

Work

THE AVERAGE MAN says he's more stressed by work than his father was and regularly beats himself up over making mistakes.
BE BETTER THAN AVERAGE: Put your pride aside. Remember that you are human, and humans are fallible. If you screw up, fess up. Apologizing is still the best and most disarming rehab step. Then learn from your bollix and move on.

Wealth

THE AVERAGE MAN'S salary plateaus at age 45.
BE BETTER THAN AVERAGE: Use that figure to shock yourself out of mid-career complacency. The secret to breaking through the salary plateau is self-promotion. Think of your career as an ongoing political campaign. Besides doing your job well, continually demonstrate your value to people who can help you, and build a network of colleagues who rely on you. Also, next time you receive a compliment or thank-you, ask, "Would you mind putting that in a quick note to my supervisor?"

THE AVERAGE MAN has saved less than 3 months' worth of living expenses for emergencies.

BE BETTER THAN AVERAGE: Save 9 months' worth to be safe. The old rule used to be 3 months, but that's not enough. In recent years, an out-of-work American needed nearly 5 months to find a new job. To start building up, stash away a minimum of $100 a month. You can save that by reviewing your monthly contracts for cellphone, cable TV, and other services. New deals are always available, and all you have to do is ask for them.

Life Satisfaction

THE AVERAGE MAN rarely expresses gratitude. And yet, there's at least a decade's worth of proof from scientific studies showing its power to improve three key aspects of your life: your health, your marriage, and your job.

BE BETTER THAN AVERAGE: Count your blessings. Write down a list of what you are grateful for and count them up. "That seemingly simple practice produces almost immediate results," says Robert A. Emmons, Ph.D., a professor of psychology at UC Davis who has conducted more than a dozen studies on the power of gratitude.

→ Thank her. A study in the journal *Emotion* found that expressing gratitude twice a week boosted positive perception of a mate by 19 percent.

→ Thank your dad. If "I love you" wasn't a common phrase around your house growing up, it can be hard to say it out loud to your pop. So don't bother. "Instead, show your love by noting a specific connection," says Scott Haltzman, M.D., a psychiatrist and author of *The Secrets of Happy Families*. Pick a recent event as a springboard and say, for instance, "Now that I'm a father, I'm grateful for what you taught me. You were a great model." That's what every father wants to hear—assurance that he had a positive impact.

The *MH* Self-Check

So, How Are You Doing?

I love cars. Before my *Men's Health* gig, I worked at *Popular Science* magazine. One of my responsibilities: Test-driving new cars—as many as I could every year. During that time, I grew to love . . . well, every new car. Let's just say there are worse gigs.

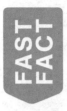

75

**Approximate
percentage of
your body
weight you lift
when you do a
standard
pushup**

Source: Journal of Strength
and Conditioning Research

I'm especially partial to BMWs. That love affair started in my teens, after the neighbors bought a used 5 Series. I grew up in a small western Pennsylvania town; there weren't a lot of German luxury sedans around town. I was immediately taken by the sleek design, the purr of the engine, the ass-kick off the line, the precision steering. You can almost picture the steel and aluminum working together in unison like an orchestra of red-hot metal.

Your body is like a car. You've surely heard that one before. The comparison is common for a reason: Men understand it instantly. Cars and bodies have moving parts and circulatory systems, they require fuel, and so on. And more important, we appreciate what it takes to care for a car.

The question is, Do you treat your body as well as you do your car? You take your car for a yearly inspection, right? And in between, you check the tires, change the oil, and address any other problems that could slow down your ride.

Do you think about your body in the same way? You should. Regular inspections—doctor's appointments—can help you catch problems before they break you down. In between, you can spot-check on your own. Would you ignore a big scratch in your paint job? A squeaky sound every time you hit the brakes? Probably not. If you want your body to rock strong for the equivalent of 200,000 miles, then kick your tires and check your fluids—take stock of your health and fitness. Subtle problems eventually progress to major ones, our experts tell us, so don't wait for your doc to find them.

This chapter is a collection of easy self-tests you can do to establish where you are right now. It's tough to get better if you don't have a baseline so you can tell what needs improving. How healthy are you, really? Even if you exercise regularly, how fit are you? Are you fit by *Men's Health* standards (which are a little higher than most)? You'll find out by the time you finish this chapter. Grab a number 2 pencil. Your body check begins . . . now.

The *MH* Take-at-Home Test

How Healthy Are You?
The Morning Session

Set your alarm clock for 15 minutes earlier so you can kick your tires before you head off to work, or do this at-home test on the weekend. These 11 self-checks will give you a good snapshot of your overall health. We'll gauge your fitness level in the afternoon session, starting on page 24.

 CHECK #1 *Did you wake up with an erection?*
___YES ___NO

When your eyes open in the morning, your penis should be standing at attention. Apologies for starting off so personally, but this is important. If you don't usually have morning wood, you could have low testosterone—especially if you have other symptoms like fatigue and a reduced sex drive, says Charles Walker, M.D., an assistant professor of urology at the Yale University School of Medicine. That's a problem because low T increases your risks of heart disease, osteoporosis, and other diseases. It can also leave you feeling sluggish and just crappy in general. There could be another reason your flag hasn't risen to meet the dawn: An arterial problem that's preventing blood-flow, he says. Because the arteries that feed your penis with blood are so small, arteriosclerosis (hardening of the arteries) often shows up there first, causing weak erections. This could be an early sign of heart disease. Don't mess around here. See your primary-care physician or a cardiologist. Meanwhile, check out Chapter 6 for erection-saving advice.

 CHECK #2 *What time is it?*
CHECK THE CLOCK. HOW LONG DID YOU SLEEP LAST NIGHT? _____ THE NIGHT BEFORE? _____

If you tend to log fewer than 7 hours, you invite illness into your life. Studies link sleep deficits with higher risks of obesity and heart disease. If you don't sleep soundly, go to bed 15 minutes later the next night. If you sleep great but feel groggy in the a.m., go to bed 15 minutes earlier. Repeat to find your ideal amount. Need advanced help? See Chapter 8 for more ways to improve your slumber number.

CHECK #3 *The walnut test*

The apt comparison for your prostate gland, size-wise, is a walnut. And your walnut gets bigger as you get older; it's a fact of life. When the enlarged gland presses against your urethra, you may find yourself urinating by nightlight. Did you get up to pee in the middle of the night? More than once? Often this is caused by benign prostatic hyperplasia—BPH—the technical term for an enlarged prostate. But this can also be triggered by an infection or even prostate or bladder cancer. Don't worry: It's far more likely to be BPH, but here's an easy way to do a quickie prostate exam yourself that has nothing to do with bending over.

ANSWER ON A SCALE OF ZERO TO 3, ZERO BEING "NOT AT ALL" AND 3 BEING "ALMOST ALWAYS." IN THE LAST MONTH, HOW OFTEN HAVE YOU . . .

. . . had a sensation of not having emptied your bladder completely after you've finished urinating?

⓪ ① ② ③

. . . found it difficult to postpone urination?

⓪ ① ② ③

. . . needed to wake up to urinate between bedtime and the time you got up in the morning?

⓪ ① ② ③

. . . had a weak urinary stream?

⓪ ① ② ③

Now add up your score: It should be lower than 4. If it's higher—or if your score changes the next time you take this test—see your doctor so he or she can, er, put a finger on the problem. (See page 106 for the complete poop on digital rectal exams.)

CHECK #4 *Clock your resting ticker*

___ BEATS PER MINUTE

The ubiquitous doctor's stethoscope is not always the most reliable way to check your heart health. While resting heart rate speaks volumes about your ticker, you are rarely resting calmly when you are sitting on the edge of an exam table with a cold scope pressed against your chest. Your heart should be checked first thing in the morning—difficult for your doctor to do unless you two are sleeping together—so do this instead: While still lying in bed, place your index and middle fingers on the inside of your wrist or the side of your neck. Count the beats for 15 seconds. Multiply that number by four to get your beats per minute. Your typical tempo before getting out of bed should be between 60 and 100 beats a minute. If you're sub-60, are you a runner? Do a lot of cardiovascular activity? You're probably fitter than most. A faster rate may indicate an infection or dehydration. Even just 1 point above 100 could suggest you are at risk for a life-threatening electrical dysfunction like atrial fibrillation, says Robert Wergin, M.D., president of the American Academy of Family Physicians.

Do You Smoke?

If so—epic fail, dude. Fifty years after the surgeon general first warned of the hazards of lighting up, smoking is still considered America's number one preventable killer. But if you still smoke and you don't think quitting is in the cards, consider a few new strategies. For one, recent research from the University of Georgia found that joining an online support group made smokers more confident that they could quit, raising their odds of success. Participation is key, and the researchers recommend using WhyQuit.com's Turkeyville group on Facebook. Or check out the 1-800-QUIT-NOW hotline for access to many services.

CHECK #5	**Are you crooked?**
	__YES __NO

This test determines if you fall into the bad-posture club—about 60 percent of men do, says Fábio Araújo, M.Sc., who researches posture at the Institute of Public Health at the University of Porto in Portugal. To see if you're in that majority, take a good look at yourself after you step out of the shower. If you drew horizontal lines across your body, would the lines across your shoulders, hips, nipples, pelvis, knees, and ankles be parallel? If so, you're in good alignment, which means you probably sit up straight and stand correctly. Next, put your back against the wall and stand straight, looking straight ahead. Is there extra space behind your neck and shoulders? If the distance is greater than 5 inches, your neck muscles might be stiff or your shoulders may be rolling forward. Is your lower back attached to the wall without any free space? If so, you probably lack muscle extensibility. Men are particularly susceptible to having a flat spine, which can cause chronic back pain, he says. Finally, bend forward at your hips. Repeat to the right, the left, and back and fully rotate your back for both sides. If you have pain or feel stiffness, you may need to improve your posture.

If you failed any of these posture tests, take the more comprehensive DIY test in Chapter 12, starting on page 294. It pinpoints key problem areas and offers at-home remedies to try. In the meantime, try this posture-improving exercise: Lie on your back on the floor with your knees bent, feet flat, and arms perpendicular to your torso. Your hands should be in loose fists, palms up. Slowly rotate your arms until your fists are palms down while lifting your

Urine Trouble
Four signs that you might be pissing away your health

Cloudy. The forecast: bacterial infection, especially if there's a foul smell or burning sensation. The cloudiness is a byproduct of white blood cells working to fight germs.

Bloody. Blood can signal an enlarged prostate or kidney stone or even cancer. Have it checked out right away.

Frothy or foamy. There's too much protein in your pee, which means your kidneys aren't doing their job of filtering it out. This could signal the start of diabetes or kidney disease.

Brown or rusty. Rust-hued urine can be a bacterial calling card. Blood sometimes looks brown. The same color change can also be caused by bilirubin, a liver byproduct that can signal liver disease.

* If you notice any of these in your pee, say something to your doctor or urologist.

shoulders and head slightly. Reverse the arm roll, raising your hips a few inches. Complete 10 to 15 reps, moving as effortlessly as you can. If this feels too gentle, you're doing it just right.

 CHECK #6   *Did you spit pink into the sink?*
___YES ___NO

When you brush your teeth, your gums shouldn't bleed. Bleeding gums could signal anything from gum disease, which is serious in its own right, to a cancer, says Mark Wolff, D.D.S., Ph.D., professor and chair of the department of cariology and comprehensive care at the New York University College of Dentistry. Have your dentist check it out. You go twice a year, right? And between checkups, about once a month, gape in front of a mirror to examine your yapper for any unusual bumps, red or white patches, swelling, or bleeding. Then feel for any unusual lumps on either side of your neck. Anything odd that persists for 2 weeks should be checked out by a dentist. M.D.'s feel they are less proficient than dentists at identifying cancerous lesions in the mouth, according to a study in the *Journal of the American Dental Association*. Oral cancer is highly treatable if found early.

 CHECK #7   *Gut check*
The quick: Wrap a tape measure around your waist, halfway between your ribs and your hips. Divide that number by your height in inches; the ratio should be 0.5 or lower. Studies have shown that this ratio is a better predictor of developing heart disease or diabetes than body mass index (BMI) or waist-to-hip ratio, two other commonly used fatness indicators.

And the dead: The newest tool, called A Body Shape Index (ABSI), is even more useful, though it requires a computer and a few more measurements. A 2014 *PLOS One* study found that people with the highest ABSIs had a 61 percent higher risk of dying from any cause than those with the lowest, even if their BMIs were considered normal. ABSI factors in your age and height and waist circumference numbers. Take the test by entering your measurements and age into the ABSI calculator at absi.nl.eu.org. If your number is 1, your risk of premature death is about average. Are your numbers in either test too high? Pay close attention in Chapter 6. The belly is a key barometer of your overall health. "A lot of inflammation in the body is derived from fat tissue in the belly," warns *Men's Health* advisor Eric J. Topol, M.D., a cardiologist and pioneer of cardiovascular medicine research.

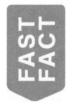

Age at which the average person's brain starts to slowly decrease in size

Source: Proceedings of the National Academy of Sciences

CHECK #8 ### *The ugly duckling*

Once a month, take off all of your clothing and examine every inch of your body. Don't rely on a screening with a dermatologist, because it may not happen. Fifty-seven percent of men say they are unlikely to schedule a screening. But people who perform regular skin self-exams are twice as likely to find melanoma as those who don't inspect, according to Dartmouth College researchers. Check for "the ugly duckling," a mark that looks odd or has changed appearance (shape or color). For examples of ugly ducks, check out preventcancer.org/skin/know-your-abcdes. If you happen to be exceptionally furry, have your mate check after you come out of the shower—it's easier to see skin (and moles) through hair when it's wet.

CHECK #9 ### *Count your breaths*

_____ PER MINUTE

Sometimes breathing fast is normal—at the gym, in bed, when your neighbor's dog chases you down the street. But rapid breathing can also signal a respiratory infection, asthma, or being way out of shape. Count each time your chest rises and falls—up and down counts as 1—in a minute. The average is 10 to 18 breaths. Yours?

CHECK #10 ### *Your eyesight, hearing, and memory*

Eyes: Hold this page out at arm's length. If you're over 40 and need to strain to read it, you may have presbyopia, a condition resulting from the loss of elasticity in your eyes' lenses. See an eye doctor for reading glasses.

Ears: Think back to the conversations you've had in the last week. Did you think that people you were speaking with were mumbling? The high frequencies that sharpen speech drop out first, so people with hearing loss tend to think others aren't speaking clearly. Other high-frequency sounds to watch: The inflection at the end of a question and the chatter of children. See an audiologist if you suspect problems. Pop in earplugs when mowing the lawn.

Brain: Your brain runs on electrical signals, so you should check for faulty wiring once in a while. Have you recently forgotten events or appointments? Do you have trouble coming up with lists of examples—for instance, breeds of dogs or actresses you like (Natalie Portman cannot be forgotten)? These can be early signs of cognitive impairment, says Douglas Scharre, M.D., director of the division of cognitive neurology at Ohio State University's Wexner Medical Center in Columbus. Chapter 9 offers lots of ways you can protect your brain and make it stronger.

CHECK #11 *How many hours do you spend sitting per day?*
_____ HOURS

Sentenced to the chair? Even if you work out every day, that's no guarantee that you spend enough time movin' and shakin'. Studies have shown that people who spend 6 or more hours a day with their butts parked in a chair have a higher risk of a variety of health problems—including heart disease, colon cancer, mental distress, and even an early death. Guesstimate how many total hours you spend on your ass. If you work from a chair, get a stand-up desk or computer stand. I have one, and it's a life changer.

No budget for a standup desk? Then make a habit of standing whenever you talk on the phone or do any work that doesn't involve typing. And build some body weight exercises that you can do in your office into your day. Check out Project 12: Build a Workout You Can Do Anywhere on page 261 for ideas. It's based on bodyweight exercise routines that truckers do when they can't get to a gym.

Check Your *Oh*-dometer
Frequency of sex suggests good physical and mental health

How often do you do it? There's no right answer—it should be as much as you and your partner want to. "Just like eating and sleeping, sex is a basic, fundamental part of being human," says Lisa Diamond, Ph.D., a professor of psychology at the University of Utah in Salt Lake City. And as such, your coital count signals both your physical and mental health. If your libido's in the tank, an underlying cause could be clinical depression. Erectile dysfunction happens to most guys once in a while, but if it's a regular occurrence—even during masturbation—run to the doctor. Flip to Chapter 10 for a plan to upgrade your sex life. Just in case you're curious, here's how often other guys are getting it on, according to the Kinsey Institute.

AGE	25–29	30–39	40–49	50–59
SINGLE GUYS				
Not in the past year	47%	40%	49%	68%
A few times per year to monthly	22%	24%	18%	15%
A few times per month to weekly	27%	23%	22%	12%
2 or more times per week	4%	7%	10%	6%
PARTNERED GUYS				
Not in the last year	21%	16%	30%	34%
A few times per year to monthly	10%	7%	9%	11%
A few times per month to weekly	36%	33%	24%	32%
2 or more times per week	33%	46%	37%	24%
MARRIED GUYS				
Not in the last year	2%	5%	9%	21%
A few times per year to monthly	9%	16%	16%	25%
A few times per month to weekly	46%	47%	51%	38%
2 or more times per week	43%	33%	24%	16%

* Percentages rounded to the nearest whole number. Percentages may not add up to 100 due to rounding.

How Fit Are You?
The Afternoon Session

Even a neuroscientist will tell you: How well or poorly you age is determined by more than your DNA. Your lifestyle plays a significant role. Consider your activity level. The amount and quality of your exercise can actually delay and reverse aging's impact on your heart, brain, muscles, and even your skin. Do you think you get enough exercise? Are your muscles standing up to sarcopenia (age-related muscle and strength decline)? For an honest assessment, put on your workout clothes and run through these fitness checks. Your performance will be obvious to you, but if you want to know how you measure up against other guys, we've consulted some of the smartest fitness experts in the world to come up with a battery of tests that reveal just how much work you've done, and what's still left to do. There's "in pretty good shape" and there's *Men's Health* fit. Find out where you stand.

CHECK #1 *Is your core weak?*

Even if you don't have an ounce of fat, you could be soft in the middle. This test will tell. Lie facedown on the floor and place your hands shoulder-width apart on the floor with your thumbs in line with the top of your forehead. Lift your elbows off the floor and position your feet the way they would be in a pushup with your ankles flexed. This is the starting position (a). Now, push yourself off the floor while maintaining a straight, stiff plank position from your shoulders to your heels (b). If your hips dip lower than your torso, your core is weak. Try the test again with your hands repositioned at chin level. If you still can't keep your hips from sagging, you need even more core work.

THE MH FIT STANDARD: Hold a stiff arms-extended plank for 10 seconds.

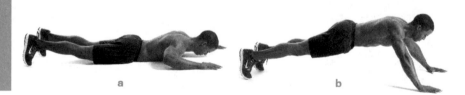

a   b

You: By the Numbers

The self-tests in this chapter reveal a lot about your overall health and fitness level. But here's what they won't reveal: blood pressure, cholesterol, fasting blood sugar, liver function, vitamin D level, and that you might be developing a hernia. Yes, I'm recommending that you schedule a physical with your doctor. In Chapter 6, I'll review all the basic (and some not so basic) diagnostic tests that our experts say men should have based on their age and family health history. Knowing your vitals is vital, especially if it's been a long time between doctor visits. Having all your numbers on hand shows you a baseline for—you guessed it—*getting better.* Rare is the man who doesn't have room for improvement in, say, his LDL score or his diastolic blood pressure. To continue the car analogy, not having an annual physical is like never checking a single fluid level, ever. Sooner or later, you're calling a tow truck.

 ## Lower-body power

Vertical leap is a solid measure of explosive leg power, and it peaks during your 20s, as the chart below sadly indicates. Stand flat-footed next to a wall and, holding a piece of chalk in your hand, reach up to mark your standing reach height. Next, take a step away from the wall. Bend your legs and, swinging both arms to propel you, jump off both feet and reach as high as you can, marking the highest point of the jump with the chalk. Make three attempts to get your best performance. Measure the distance between the standing reach mark and the jumping reach height and compare to the average man.

THE AVERAGE GUY'S VERTICAL LEAP

AGE	LEAP HEIGHT
20-29	19.7 inches
30-39	16.9 inches
40-49	13.8 inches
50-59	11.0 inches

THE MH FIT STANDARD: 22 inches

Optional Check #2a: Standing broad jump

The standing broad jump is another great test (especially if you don't want to mark up a wall). This evaluation is used by strength coaches and drill sergeants to gauge raw leg power because it requires several muscle groups throughout the body to fire at once. Stand with your toes on a line and your feet shoulder-width apart. Dip your knees, swing your arms, and jump as far as you can. Have a buddy measure the distance from the starting line to the backs of your heels.

THE MH FIT STANDARD: 8 feet

CHECK #3 *Anaerobic endurance*

You'll have fun with this one. Performing the squat, biceps curl, and push press exercises with dumbbells as a single compound move is an accurate measure of your anaerobic endurance, or your ability to work at near-max intensity in bursts of 20 to 60 seconds. Anaerobic endurance reflects the stamina of your fast-twitch (type II) muscle fibers, which generate energy in the absence of oxygen (i.e., when you're sucking wind). How to do it: Use dumbbells that together total roughly 30 percent of your body weight (that's a pair of 30-pounders if you weigh 200) and hold them at your sides with your feet shoulder-width apart. Keeping your back naturally arched, push your hips back and lower your body until your thighs are parallel to the floor. As you stand up, curl the dumbbells to shoulder height using a neutral (or hammer) grip (palms facing) and then press them straight overhead, using your legs in the effort. Return to the starting position and repeat the compound move for 1 minute.

THE MH FIT STANDARD: 20 reps in a minute

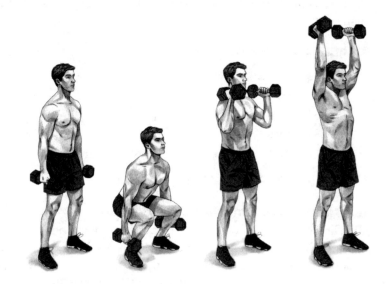

Mobility

Mobility is a quality great athletes hone, but most regular guys ignore. The more mobile you are, the less likely you are to injure your joints. See how you do with the wall squat check. A lot of people fail this test because they have a rounded back or inflexible ankles. Stand facing a wall with your feet shoulder-width apart and toes 2 inches from the baseboard and turned slightly out. Keeping your feet flat, chest up, and back naturally arched, see how far you can lower your body without touching the wall or falling backward.

THE MH FIT STANDARD: A full squat—that is, when your hamstrings touch your calves, in control

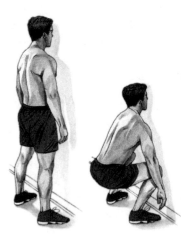

The Beep Test

Cardiovascular endurance isn't just a sign of your 10K potential or how long you'll last in a 48-minute game of basketball. People with solid aerobic health tend to have a longer life expectancy than those who lack it, according to a German study review. The Beep Test or 20-meter shuttle run is a classic measure of aerobic fitness. Easiest way to do it is to download the Beep Test app for your iPhone (Beep Test Solo, $1) or Android device (Beep Test, free). Place two cones 20 meters (about 65 feet) apart on a track or field, hit the start button on the app, and run from one cone to

Better
INSTANTLY
↓
Before your next snack, review your previous meal. Research shows that remembering what you've already eaten makes you less likely to overindulge.

the other. When you hear the beep, run back. Continue until you can't reach the opposite cone before the next beep sounds. (The time between beeps will shorten as you progress through the test.) Then hit the RECORD SCORE button.

THE MH FIT STANDARD: Level 12

 ### Upper-body power

A powerful upper body doesn't just look good shirtless, it also helps transfer force to the world around you. The clapping pushup—which requires explosiveness as well as strength—is an old-school move that many still consider the ultimate test of upper-body pushing power (thanks in no small part to Sly Stallone's *Rocky*). Get into a pushup position, with your body straight from head to ankles. Lower yourself until your chest is 3 inches from the floor. Push yourself back up explosively so your hands leave the floor. Maintain a straight body as you clap in midair and land back in the starting position.

THE MH FIT STANDARD: 10 clapping pushups without stopping

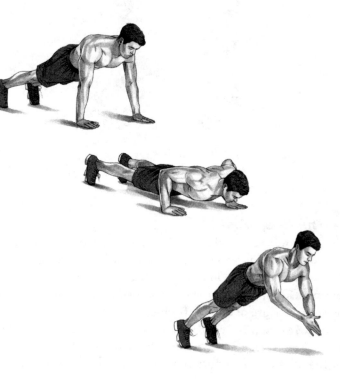

The Go-Muscle Test

The muscles of your posterior chain provide the power behind many of the most important skills in sports; consider them your "go" muscles. These include your lower back, glutes, hamstrings, and calves—lots of muscles that may not be visible in the mirror but are vital to overall fitness. And no exercise hits them harder than the deadlift does. Load a barbell with the maximum amount of weight you think you can lift once, and roll the bar on the floor until it's close to your shins. Bend at your hips and knees and grab the bar using an overhand grip that's just beyond shoulder width. Keeping your lower back naturally arched, pull your torso back and up, squeeze your glutes, thrust your hips forward, and stand up with the barbell. Reverse the movement to lower the bar to the floor, keeping it as close to your body as possible.

THE MH FIT STANDARD: 1.75 times your body weight

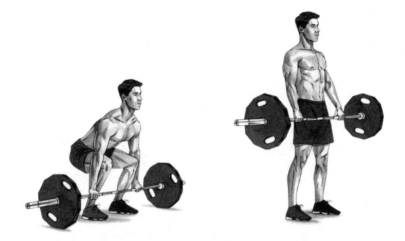

FAST FACT

41

Percentage reduction in risk of dying of cancer over 12 years among men who got fit, versus those who stayed out of shape

Source: Medicine and Science in Sports and Exercise

CHECK
#8

Flexibility

The sit-and-reach check is a time-tested measure of flexibility in the lower back and hamstrings, two areas that are often super tight in men, especially those who sit in a chair at work. Tightness in these muscles is a major cause of back and knee pain. Check it out: Place a yardstick or cloth measuring tape on the floor and put a footlong piece of masking tape across the 15-inch mark. Take off your shoes and sit down with your legs out in front of you and your heels at the edge of the tape, one on each side of the yardstick. Keep both knees locked and pressed flat against the floor. (You can have a helper hold your knees down.) Now straighten your arms forward and place one palm over the back of the other hand. Bend forward, reaching as far as you can with your fingers while making sure that neither hand is reaching farther than the other. Take a few practice reaches, then hold the reach for 2 seconds while your partner records your distance.

THE MH FIT STANDARD: 17 inches

THE AVERAGE GUY'S SIT-AND-REACH SCORE

AGE	REACH
20-29	15-17 inches
30-39	15 inches
40-49	13-15 inches
50-59	11-13 inches

The 60-Second Health Screen

Don't want to do all the tests in this chapter? Boooo. Okay, then at least do this one. It'll just take a minute and it'll give you a better picture of your health and fitness than even standing on a weight scale. It's a chinup test. Since chinups involve literally pulling your own weight, they reveal your weight relative to your strength. That's something the scale can't reveal, since it can't tell you whether any gains or losses you have came from fat or muscle. Do chinups at the same time every day and write down how many you can complete. That way you'll be able to track changes over time. *Men's Health* weight-loss advisor David Katz, M.D., M.P.H., the founding director of Yale University's Prevention Research Center, does this routinely: "If little by little I'm finding that I can do 1 less this week than last week and 1 less the next week, then either I'm getting weaker—which isn't good—or I'm getting fatter, which isn't good." The average healthy guy should be able to pull himself up 5 to 10 times. "For guys who are just sort of big and beefy, the assumption can be that you're big and strong," says Dr. Katz. But if you can't pull that weight up, you're not brawny—you're just too heavy.

So . . . What Does It All Mean?

Picture a team of number crunchers at, say, Google or Facebook or Amazon. They report to work every day and parse a brand-new set of data showing what happened in their business in the last 24 hours. Those numbers tell the managers of that business what's happening and how to react. Data drives every decision they make.

Now imagine the data crunchers show up to work tomorrow and no data has been collected. What are they supposed to do? Play foosball all day? (I love foosball, but my 12-year-old kicks my ass every time. Drives me nuts.) *I need data*, especially in my job as editor of a magazine. If I don't know how our readers react to each issue, or how many issues we've sold, and where, and all the other pieces of the business puzzle, I can't make a decision. Or I have to make a decision based on gut instinct, which is fine and can even work—except I'd never know it because I have no data for comparison.

Back to you: If you don't have any data about your health and fitness, how can you possibly make informed decisions on your eating, workouts, and everything else you'll tweak to improve? You can't. But now that you've done all these self-tests—and also had a complete physical, I hope—you have the data you need. And when it comes time to check it all again down the line, you'll have even more information that reveals trends. Hopefully, after reading this book, positive trends.

Are you getting better? Can you get even better than better?

As the Who sang, you better bet your life.

Life Snatchers and Age Accelerators

What would you do if someone offered you the exact details of your death?

Date, time, location, cause. Would you want to know? How would you handle the information? I bet I could predict your behavior, depending on how much time you had left. If you had 6 months before a semi took you out, I'd see a trip to Vegas in your near future.

If you had 5 years before some form of cancer got you, I'd predict an immediate change in how you value each day. But if you had, say, 53 years before having a heart attack in your sleep, I'd bet you wouldn't be fazed at all. You might even be comforted: Fifty-three years is a long stretch, and Pink Floyd always said life is long and there is time to kill today.

It's all amusing speculation. But what if some of it had basis in fact? What if science could give you a betting line? Guess what: Data strikes again.

In this chapter, we'll drill down into the most common causes of death, and then take on other health problems that move your aging rate into the fast lane. It's disturbing, but in this case there's no such thing as too much information.

Life Snatchers

This chart, brought to you by millions of dead people, shows what's most likely to kill you by age, according to the Centers for Disease Control and Prevention (CDC). Do I have your attention now? Find prevention tips on the following pages.

TOP SEVEN MAN KILLERS BY AGE GROUP

	AGES 25–29	30–34	35–39	40–44	45–49	50–54	55–59	60–64	65–69
#1	Accident	Accident	Accident	Accident	Heart disease	Cancer	Cancer	Cancer	Cancer
#2	Suicide	Suicide	Heart disease	Heart disease	Cancer	Heart disease	Heart disease	Heart disease	Heart disease
#3	Murder	Murder	Suicide	Cancer	Accident	Accident	Accident	Chronic lung diseases	Chronic lung diseases
#4	Heart disease	Heart disease	Cancer	Suicide	Suicide	Chronic liver diseases	Chronic liver diseases	Accident	Diabetes
#5	Cancer	Cancer	Murder	Chronic liver diseases	Chronic liver diseases	Suicide	Diabetes	Diabetes	Stroke
#6	HIV	HIV	Chronic liver diseases	Murder	Diabetes	Diabetes	Chronic lung diseases	Stroke	Accident
#7	Flu/Pneumonia	Diabetes	Diabetes	Diabetes	Stroke	Stroke	Suicide	Chronic liver diseases	Chronic liver diseases

Accidents

Sometimes men are their own worst enemies. Okay, not sometimes—often, as the data show. Our penchant for risk taking can land us in big trouble, and I'm not just talking about Evel Knievel stuff. In the age groups shown in the chart on the opposite page, more than three-quarters of accidental deaths come from two causes. Number one is poisoning. You can reduce your risk by avoiding religious cults, and staying in control when you drink—see page 204 for more on that. Then make sure you always read the labels carefully on prescription and over-the-counter drugs. Overdoses from prescription painkillers, in particular, are on the rise.

The number two cause behind accidental deaths? You guessed it—car crashes. We could write a whole separate book on driving safety, but let's start with the most obvious. To reduce your risk, don't drive after drinking. Period. Refusing to drink and drive doesn't make you less of a man—it makes you the better man. People with a blood alcohol concentration of just 0.01 percent, well below the 0.08 legal limit, are 46 percent more likely to be officially and solely blamed by accident investigators than are the sober drivers they collide with, a University of California at San Diego study reveals. For many men, it only takes one drink to hit that level. Before getting behind the wheel after a few drinks, consider the impact of a DUI arrest on the Four Fs: Family, Friends, Future, and Finances. The first three are obvious, but did you know that a DUI in some states can cost you between $6,000 and $19,000? Visit drinkinganddriving.org for more ways to avoid a costly mistake.

Next, put down the damn phone. Dialing triples your risk of crashing. Texting also increases your chances by three times, according to the Virginia Tech Transportation Institute, making it pretty much the stupidest thing you can do while driving, short of having an orgy while blindfolded.

Also, when you're tired, pull off the road. Sleepiness is a contributing factor in about a quarter of all crashes and near-crashes. If pulling over isn't an option, drop the cabin temperature by 15°F. Researchers in Sweden found that lowering and raising the temperature at random intervals lasting 5 to 8 minutes increases alertness. Rest also increases alertness. Take one.

Of course, even when you're sober, the road can bring on surprises, so get smarter about how you handle them. Start by losing the attitude—72 percent of drivers think they're more skilled than the next guy. This cockiness gets us in trouble when the unexpected happens. Exhibit A: When researchers at Clemson University used computer simulation to test the way people drove in fog, they found that most went too fast and would have hit an obstacle. When a crash seems inevitable, you can stay alive by taking the actions on page 36.

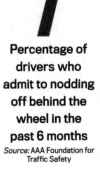

FAST FACT

7

Percentage of drivers who admit to nodding off behind the wheel in the past 6 months

Source: AAA Foundation for Traffic Safety

You Veer Off the Road

YOUR INSTINCT Swerve back onto the road
THE RIGHT RESPONSE Lift off the accelerator

"Gently straighten up your car and scan ahead for obstacles," says Paul Gerrard, the director of global training at the Audi Sportscar Experience in Sonoma, California. "If you swerve back right away, you will likely overcorrect, careen across the road, and lose control." Maintain your composure and look for a smooth transition where you can reenter the road. If you're straddling a high curb, slow to 25 mph before attempting to drive over it.

Your Tire Blows

YOUR INSTINCT Stomp on the brakes
THE RIGHT RESPONSE Don't touch the brakes

Instead, take your foot off the gas, hold the wheel firmly, and gently countersteer to overcome any pulling or fishtailing the blowout has caused, says Debbie Prudhomme, the cofounder of Training Wheels driving school in Minnesota. Let the weight of the car slow it down, and when you feel in control, lightly apply the brakes, signal, and pull off onto the shoulder.

You See a Deer Ahead

YOUR INSTINCT Swerve
THE RIGHT RESPONSE Hit it

Animal impacts account for only 0.6 percent of fatal crashes, but if you swerve, you could end up in a head-on collision with a car or tree, says Jeff Payne, the founder of Driver's Edge, a nonprofit performance-driving school. And don't slam on the brakes, either: You'll cause the front of your car to dip, making it more likely that the deer will slide up the hood and crash through the windshield. Instead, aim for the deer's butt. Deer don't generally go in reverse, says Payne, and if you're lucky, it will jump out of the way.

You're About to Rear-End the Car in Front of You

YOUR INSTINCT Brake hard
THE RIGHT RESPONSE Brake even harder

"Push the brake to the floor," says Gerrard. "This sounds obvious, but statistics show that people who think they're braking hard are using only about half the car's braking power." Note: If you've never jammed on your brakes, Gerrard recommends practicing in an empty parking lot so you're familiar with the amount of pedal pressure needed. A BMW new-car salesman once had me do this during a test-drive. I was happy to because it wasn't my car—and I was shocked by how quickly it stopped. Which reminds me: Don't ever buy a demo car.

You Hit Black Ice

YOUR INSTINCT Turn away from the slide, and hit the brakes
THE RIGHT RESPONSE Wait a split second

"You have to decide quickly: Will I regain traction before I lose control and/or hit something?" says Payne. "If you think you will, then keep your foot off both the gas and brake until your tires grab again." At the same time, point your car in the direction you want it to go. Sliding out of control? Slam on the brakes, says Payne. Your car will slide in one direction, which will at least make it easier for other drivers to avoid hitting you.

Cancer

The top cancer killers for men strike the lungs, prostate, colon, and pancreas. The easiest way to dodge lung cancer is to quit smoking (or avoid smokers)—see page 280 for more on that. Then pay attention on page 290, where we'll show you how to check the radon level in your home. The poison gas, which can lurk in bedrock and sneak through your foundation, is the number two cause of lung cancer. To protect your body from prostate and colon cancers, flip to page 106.

Pancreatic cancer is a special case—it's relatively rare but extremely deadly (that's what got Steve Jobs). You might be able to reduce the (harsh) odds by keeping your weight under control. Research suggests that people who are overweight or have diabetes are more likely to develop pancreatic cancer. One more thing you can do? Eat less smoky, salty meats like ham and bacon. A study review in the *British Journal of Cancer* concluded that for every 1.8 ounces of processed meat people ate per day, their pancreatic cancer risk increased by 19 percent. One theory? Because processed meats are preserved with nitrite, they may contain *N*-nitroso compounds, which can reach your pancreas through your bloodstream and possibly induce cancer, the researchers say.

Of course, not every man who develops a cancer will die from it. If you detect tumors early, you can improve your chances of survival and minimize complications. Here's another case where our gender raises our risk: A study

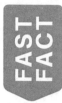

21

Percent of people with certain types of cancer who waited more than 3 months to see an M.D. after noticing a symptom, throwing away valuable treatment time and potentially lowering their survival odds. Why the lag? The top reasons were embarrassment, worry, feeling too busy, and uncertainty about how serious the symptoms were.

Source: British Journal of Cancer

in the *Journal of Urology* showed that among men and women with the same types of cancer, men were 13 percent more likely to die. Studies also suggest that women go to doctors more often and pay closer attention to their bodies than men do. Put two and two together, and the explanation could be that when women have cancer, they detect it earlier, when their chances of recovery are higher. The screening tests on page 106 will help you catch suspicious problems before they turn into total-body nightmares. It's also smart to watch for the common symptoms below, according to the American Cancer Society. Many of them could also indicate health problems other than cancer, but they're still worth investigating.

→ Unexplained weight loss
→ Fever
→ Fatigue
→ Pain in the head or back
→ Darkened, red, yellowed, or itchy skin
→ Change in bowel habits or blood in your bowel movements
→ Pain when urinating or blood in urine or change in how often you go
→ Excessive hair growth
→ Sores that don't heal
→ White patches inside your mouth
→ Unusual bleeding or discharge
→ Coughing up blood
→ Lumps
→ Indigestion or trouble swallowing
→ Changes in warts or moles
→ Nagging cough or hoarseness

Chronic Liver Diseases

You probably learned as a kid that if you cut off a salamander's leg, it will grow back (hopefully you never tried it on your cat). The human body may be no match for this amphibian, but one organ in particular does have amazing regenerative abilities: your liver. It constantly repairs itself—but if you continually abuse it, your liver won't be able to catch up. Unfortunately, plenty of guys are falling behind. The most obvious cause of chronic liver trouble is alcoholism, but you don't have to booze to lose: A study recently published in the *American Journal of Epidemiology* estimated that 19 percent of Americans have nonalcoholic fatty liver disease (NAFLD), with men ages 30 and older disproportionately represented. The condition is associated with diabetes, insulin resistance in pre-diabetic people, and obesity, one likely explanation for why NAFLD diagnoses have risen in the past decade. Left unchecked, the condition can eventually progress to a stage known as nonalcoholic steatohepatitis, which can lead to extensive scarring and ultimately liver failure. In NAFLD's early stages, virtually no symptoms exist. You usually feel fine. Often the only indicator is the elevated levels of liver enzymes in your blood—that serves as a clue that healthy cells have been replaced by fat ones. When your doctor checks your cholesterol, ask him to add a liver enzyme test.

If you have NAFLD, losing as little as 5 percent of your body weight could lead to measurable improvements in liver function. Many doctors advise patients to follow low-carb diets that cut down on the refined kind, such as white flour and sugar. (The liver converts excess sugars to fat.) You'll want to fill up on nuts, seeds, green vegetables, and fatty fish: In a South Korean study, men who ate the most nuts and seeds and foods rich in vitamin K, folate, and omega-3 fatty acids had the lowest risk of NAFLD. Exercise is also critical—one study published in the journal *Gut* reports that adhering to a regimen of resistance exercise three times a week for 8 weeks can reduce liver fat by 13 percent, perhaps by increasing blood sugar sensitivity and burning fat. Other studies suggest that cardio exercise has similar effects too. And watch what you pop: A little acetaminophen can erase aches, but too much can wipe out your liver. (Your body makes toxic byproducts as it breaks down the drug.) In fact, acetaminophen overdoses are a top cause of acute liver failure, the FDA reports. Stay under 4,000 milligrams in a single day. Remember that acetaminophen lurks in more than just OTC painkillers—it's an ingredient in more than 600 medications—so accidentally ingesting too much can be easy to do.

Chronic Lung Diseases

These ailments can literally suck the life out of you. Now, the first step to keeping your lungs clear is a no-brainer: If you smoke cigarettes, your chance of chronic obstructive pulmonary disease (COPD), one of the most common lung diseases, nearly triples. COPD can leave your airways irritated and inflamed, leaving you breathless. But even if you've never touched a cigarette, your lungs are still aging. By your mid-30s, your alveoli—the tiny air sacs in your lungs that allow oxygen to cross into your bloodstream and carbon dioxide to exit—begin to lose surface area, say scientists at Georgetown University. This makes your lungs less efficient at transporting oxygen.

One way to protect your lungs is to work them with exercise—more on that in Chapter 5. You might also want to hit the dairy aisle. A study published in the *Journal of the American College of Nutrition* found that people who consistently downed two daily servings of low-fat dairy, such as reduced-fat milk, yogurt, and cottage cheese, showed fewer signs of disease-related lung damage. Credit the vitamin D in fortified dairy products: This nutrient may help improve lung function, the scientists say. In addition, milk is loaded with vitamin A, which is thought to switch on genes involved in the production of new lung tissue. Aim to eat two or three servings of fortified dairy a day, and you'll be taking in up to 10 micrograms of vitamin D and up to 455 micrograms of vitamin A.

Diabetes

If you have type 1 diabetes, you probably already know it. The biggest threat for the rest of us is type 2 diabetes, which interferes with your body's ability to produce insulin, a hormone that regulates blood sugar metabolism. As a result, your blood sugar can skyrocket. A lot of people don't realize that glucose is corrosive to your body's tissues. That's why your body spikes insulin so quickly to help remove glucose. But if your body starts to resist insulin? Trouble. Obesity is the biggest risk factor for this disease, but you don't have to be tubby to have it—there are plenty of normal-weight people developing diabetes. (Tom Hanks is one of them.) And you could be next: The CDC estimates that eight million Americans have undiagnosed diabetes. If you have symptoms such as frequent urination, feeling thirsty or hungry even though you're eating, fatigue, blurred vision, slow healing of wounds, or tingling or numbness in your hands and feet, see a doctor. On page 260, we'll tell you more about how to avoid the big D.

Flu/Pneumonia

Despite what you might think, the flu wasn't deadly only back in the 1800s. Maybe you knew it killed people in this century, but thought they were probably all elderly people or babies. Wrong again. The flu and pneumonia are cause-of-death number seven in the 25-to-29 age group, and they also crack the top 10 in several others. For goodness' sake, will you start getting a flu shot every fall? People who had their yearly flu shot had a 60 percent lower chance of having to go to the doctor because of the flu during the 2013 to 2014 flu season, the most recent data available before this book went to print. As soon as September hits, visit your doctor or local pharmacy to get pricked. Even better, show up well rested. If you consistently log enough shut-eye, your flu shot may be more effective because sleep helps maintain levels of B cells and T cells, which trigger the immune response when you receive the vaccine.

After the vaccine, your best bet to evade the flu (and other nasty viruses) is to avoid touching your eyes, nose, and mouth, where germs can enter your body. And always wash your hands the way epidemiologists do: Scrub with warm, soapy water as long as it takes you to sing "Happy Birthday," wipe your hands with a paper towel, and then use it to turn the tap off. Throw the towel away, grab another, and finish drying. Use that paper towel to open the door to exit.

Another good strategy? Take your meditation: Calming your mind can help fend off the flu, according to a study from the University of Wisconsin at Madison. People who completed 8 weeks of meditation training were 35 percent less likely to develop a cold or the flu than those who didn't take a daily dose of *om*. Meditation helps reduce stress, which may improve immune function. Try a class in mindfulness-based meditation. To find one near you, visit http://locator.apa.org.

If you still catch the bug, see page 223 for tips to treat it. But if you start to develop symptoms of pneumonia, such as a bad cough, fever, shaking chills, shortness of breath, chest pain, headache, sweating and clammy skin, loss of appetite, low energy, fatigue, or confusion, see a doctor. If you have underlying health problems, take special care—you have a higher risk of flu complications. In a study by the California Department of Public Health, about 80 percent of people in their 20s, 30s, 40s, 50s, and 60s who died from the flu had underlying metabolic diseases; one in three had a chronic lung disease, and about 27 percent had chronic heart disease.

Heart Disease

It's the deadliest disease in the world. No doubt you've heard the PSAs and seen the "wear red" campaigns. But do you know what heart disease really is? It's an umbrella term for the myriad things that can go wrong with your ticker. A valve can leak or tear, leaving you fatigued. Your heart rhythms, run by electrical signals, can short-circuit, stopping your heart cold. But scientists say the most common culprits behind heart attacks are clogged arteries, the result of cholesterol buildup in your artery walls. Oxidized particles of LDL (bad) cholesterol are infiltrating your artery walls all the time. They drop off lipids that are required for your cells to function—but sometimes they deposit too much. Small amounts of LDL cholesterol inside your artery walls are removed by HDL particles, but if the HDL can't keep up, the LDL causes your arteries to narrow and stiffen. Then, white blood cells enter your artery wall to gobble up excess cholesterol, but they become engorged and turn into foam cells. This triggers inflammation, causing more repair cells to show up, creating more plaque. A cap forms over your damaged artery wall. If the cap ruptures, the plaque may ooze out and trigger the formation of a blood clot, which could block your artery. Result: heart attack. If you experience sudden faintness, nausea, or sweating, and it's accompanied by chest pain (especially if the pain radiates to your back, jaw, or either arm), call 911.

Pretty scary, right? But the fact that heart disease is so common has led to a silver lining—scientists have studied it extensively. They know a lot that can help you prevent The Big One. And I plan to share it with you. First, the tests on page 102 will reveal clues about your risk. If you have certain risk factors, you may need to see a heart doctor—we'll show you how to find one on page 124. Then, we'll show you how to reduce your risk on pages 242 and 262.

HIV

Treatments for this virus have improved vastly since the 1980s. Still, once it progresses to AIDS, it's a bona fide killer. The vast majority of new cases come from sexual contact, according to CDC data, so get tested, and ask your partner to do the same. Remember that you can be infected for a decade without any symptoms. And always wear condoms if you're not monogamous.

Murder

We can't help too much with this one. But I do know this—men are more likely than women to commit this crime and to be victims of it. Here's one idea: Encourage your legislators to support stronger gun laws. That's not a political opinion; researchers have found a correlation. A study in the *Journal of Urban Health,* for example, discovered that after the state of Missouri relaxed a law requiring gun buyers to obtain a permit before buying firearms, gun-related homicides increased by 25 percent.

Stroke

This is one that I worry about—strokes run on my dad's side of the family. Many of the same risk factors that cause heart disease can increase your risk of a stroke as well. After all, it all comes down to bloodflow. Strokes occur when your arteries have to stretch more than they should, often as a result of high blood pressure. Under that stress, microscopic tears form in the innermost layer of your arteries. Your body tries to repair the damage by churning out clot-forming platelets. Meanwhile, other molecules, including LDL (bad) cholesterol, cellular debris, and calcium, become trapped inside the artery wall, forming plaque. Your immune system deploys specialized white blood cells to break down the plaque, but those cells can't break it down. Instead,

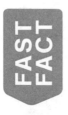

15

Number of developed countries that have lower rates than the United States of men dying prematurely from preventable causes like heart disease, certain cancers, and diabetes
Source: Health Policy

they combine into foam cells, which spur inflammation. Your arteries' smooth muscle cells form a hard cover over the mixture, stiffening your arterial walls. This pushes your blood pressure even higher. As blood flows past the buildup, pieces of plaque break loose and float through your bloodstream and toward your brain, where a clot can become stuck in a tiny cerebral artery. Blood and its precious cargo, oxygen, cannot reach the brain cells fed by that artery, causing an ischemic stroke. Without oxygen, your brain cells start to die off within minutes. Depending on the brain region and number of cells affected, symptoms and complications can range from dizziness and hellacious headaches to paralysis, coma, and even death.

Keeping your BP under control is one way to avoid a stroke—more on that on page 242. Another thing to watch for? An abnormal heart rhythm. One variety called atrial fibrillation is a common cause of strokes. "This kind of irregular heart rhythm, which is extremely common, causes clots to form in the heart and then be launched up into your brain," says David Liebeskind, M.D., a *Men's Health* brain health advisor. "This can cause anything from lack of symptoms to devastating disabling stroke." If you feel like your heart skips a beat sometimes, and it's not just the pitter-patter of excitement, see your doctor. Plenty of treatments can make a-fib less dangerous.

For good measure, avoid benders. In a 16-year study from Finland, men who had one or more hangovers a year were 2.3 times as likely to experience a stroke as those who'd never been hungover. As you process excess booze, your blood pressure spikes, raising your risk of a brain attack, the researchers say.

Suicide

Tragically, some men end their own lives. In fact, one in six men seriously considers ending it all at least once in their lives. And CDC data show that suicide is rising in middle-aged people. While suicide carries a stigma, researchers know the truth: It's just like dying from any other disease, and the ailment is a mental illness. Don't be embarrassed about seeking help if you're struggling. Some major warning signs that you—or a friend—are in trouble? Poor sleep, sudden changes in behavior, loss of interest in favorite activities, feelings of hopelessness, and collecting weapons or pills or other means to hurt oneself. An overnight attitude shift from negative to positive is one of the biggest red flags, because it may signal that the person has come up with a plan to escape the pain through death. If you need help, call the National Suicide Prevention Lifeline at 1-800-273-TALK (8255). Then consider talking things out with a therapist.

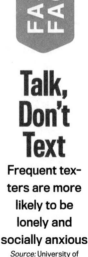

FAST FACT

Talk, Don't Text

Frequent texters are more likely to be lonely and socially anxious
Source: University of Missouri

The Age Accelerators

If you can dodge an early death, don't you want to spend your extra years feeling good? We probably all know a 90-year-old who still runs and drives, and we know 50-year-olds who can barely move. We've all seen classic cars that run like new, and new vehicles that sound like they need to vomit. To increase your odds of being the former, avoid things that speed up the aging process. Start with these seven.

Bad Food Choices

Whether you eat all the wrong foods or too much of everything, a poor diet is almost a surefire guarantee that you'll age faster than your DNA intended. That's especially true if your choices lead to weight gain. Scientists used to think that fat was just unsightly. Now they know that body fat functions like an organ—except unlike other organs that help your body, excess body fat releases chemical byproducts that slow down your metabolism and speed up the aging process. To limit calories and take in more nutrients, aim to eat foods that are still close to the condition they were harvested in—fruits, vegetables, whole grains, meats, for example. Limit processed foods, which are packed with salt, sugar, and additives and preservatives you just don't need.

Another consequence of consuming sugary, high-processed foods that jack up blood sugar is a something aptly known as AGEs, which stands for advanced glycation end products. Chronic high blood sugar due to a poor diet causes your red blood cells to get coated—or glycated—and stick together. When these glycated cells clump together, they produce AGEs, substances that lead to many of the symptoms of aging, including diabetes, Alzheimer's disease, heart disease, and skin damage. The answer is replacing sugary, processed foods with whole foods.

See Chapter 4 for more on the foods that will keep you healthy for life. And remember this: Being overweight is one of the prime drivers of premature aging. Losing weight is one of the best things you can do to look, feel, and be younger in body and mind.

Poor Sleep

If you don't sleep soundly or enough, your whole body will suffer. Many of the doctors I've talked to, in all specialties, say sleep is one of the most critical components of a healthy, happy, productive life. Sleep helps your brain forge new connections. It also recharges your body's systems. For instance, while you're in dreamland, you produce less of the stress hormone cortisol, but you produce more growth hormone. This hormone-balancing act helps to keep your immune system in check. That could be why skimping on sleep has been shown to increase your risk of weight gain, cancer, and basically any health problem you can possibly imagine. It might sound like an exaggeration, but decades of medical literature can't be wrong. To improve your sleep, turn on *The View*. Or, better yet, flip to Chapter 8.

Stress

Occasional stress is good for you. It's motivating. Without stress, I never would have finished writing this book! A little jolt of stress gets you going by triggering the release of hormones like adrenaline—it's the old evolutionary fight-or-flight response. You've heard of it. However, unlike our ancient ancestors, modern men aren't (usually) running away from predators. For us, stress and its subsequent rush of hormones can cause us a lot of headache and heartache. Over time, chronic stress can make you look and feel older and contribute to a whole bunch of problems, including several of the deadly diseases described earlier in this chapter. Squash stress—and other emotional saboteurs—with the strategies in Chapter 9. Meanwhile, try these simple Jedi Mind Tricks for banishing stress in...

60 SECONDS: Set a timer for a minute, closes your eyes, and focus on breathing deeply and on observing your thoughts, suggests Michael Irwin, M.D., a professor of psychiatry at UCLA.

15 MINUTES: Stretch while seated: Lean forward, back, and to each side, and stretch your arms above your head. Hold each pose for six slow breaths, and then sit and breathe deeply with your eyes closed.

30 MINUTES: Exercise. Just 30 minutes of sweating can reduce anxiety, and it may even help you handle future stressors.

Addiction

If you can avoid boozing, smoking, and doing drugs, you'll do your body a big favor. These vices cause damage faster than you think: It only takes 15 minutes for cigarette smoking to harm your DNA, according to a study published in *Chemical Research in Toxicology*. Fifteen minutes. And over a lifetime, that stuff adds up. Guys who drink excessively or smoke have about triple the risk of dying during a given time period compared to those who don't use, according to studies published in *Addiction* and the *New England Journal of Medicine*. See page 204 for more on alcohol addiction and page 280 for tips on how to quit smoking. If these or harder drugs have you in their clutches, visit the American Psychological Association's website (locator.apa.org) to find a therapist who specializes in addictions and substance abuse.

Inactivity

Sloth is one of the seven deadly sins, and not even a fun one. And research suggests you should take the "deadly" part literally. Researchers in Sweden found that the people who move the most every day—whether they work out or not—are less likely to die over 12 years than those who are slugs outside of their regular exercise. Other studies have shown that people who spend 6 or more hours a day with their butts parked in a chair have a higher risk of a variety of health problems—including heart disease, colon cancer, and mental distress. That's because sitting deactivates the skeletal muscles in your lower body, ushering in negative metabolic consequences. It's never too late to change: A study published in the *British Journal of Sports Medicine* showed that people who reduced their sitting time actually lengthened their telomeres, protective pieces of DNA that are linked to aging. So what's a desk jockey to do? Get up more often. Stand up at your desk. Schedule walking meetings. Move around during conference calls. Then check Chapter 5 for workout advice. And for your favorite exercise of all, check Chapter 10. Finally, find more ways to protect and lengthen your telomeres on page 282.

Toxins

You wouldn't swallow something poisonous on purpose, but you may slowly be poisoning yourself. Scientists have long known that exposure to large amounts of toxins—like lead, mercury, or arsenic—can kill you. But now, research also suggests that chronic exposure to relatively low quantities of toxic chemicals can wreak havoc on your health. These substances may build up in your blood, body fat, or other tissues, where they can disrupt your

Better
INSTANTLY
↓

If you sit for more than 6 hours a day, make a new rule: Stand anytime you talk on the phone—at home and at the office.

SMART ADVICE

FROM *MEN'S HEALTH* FAMILY MEDICINE ADVISOR **TED EPPERLY, M.D.,**
PRESIDENT AND CEO OF THE FAMILY MEDICINE RESIDENCY OF IDAHO

"It may sound harsh, but a lot of men are pretty dumb about their health. A man's body is like a finely tuned machine that needs to have attention paid to it early instead of late so that they can have a better quality of life downstream. In the late teens to probably 29, I see what I call the young immortals. They don't recognize that too much alcohol, too much sex, too much smoking, too much bad behavior is going to catch up with them. Men should know that how they treat themselves now will have echoing effects throughout their lives. From 30 to 50, men tend to have a growing recognition of their vulnerability and mortality and that they now need to pay attention. Sadly, sometimes bad behaviors are already too far along to easily correct, such as smoking or obesity. Other behaviors may be easier to change, such as driving too fast, not using a seatbelt, not wearing a helmet when they use a bike or motorcycle. Men who do these things start to realize they're playing with fire. From 51 to 70, men start to pay attention. They keep their weight under control, take medicines appropriately, and more, but by then so much water has already passed under the bridge. It's not a losing battle, but it's a battle that's harder to win in terms of going back to peak health. Then of course from 71 on, men are survivors. They've already done the right things, and that's why they're still alive. Most of the men that haven't done these things—who've been the young, foolish, impervious types—they've died."

hormones and other body systems. Check page 290 for a DIY project that will help you reduce the toxins in your life.

Ignoring Risk Factors

If high blood pressure, high blood sugar, or high cholesterol go undetected, they will wreck your body. Trouble is, sometimes men don't know they even have these problems until they have a heart attack or a stroke—and by then, it might be too late. Ask your doctor about screening tests, and keep an eye out for signs of trouble yourself. In one study, researchers at the University of Wisconsin found that physicians failed to diagnose hypertension in 67 percent of young adults during 4 years of office visits, possibly because they chalked up high readings to white coat hypertension, a stress-related BP spike. See Chapter 6 for a list of tests to ask for and the results that should raise an eyebrow.

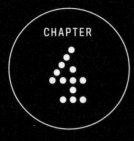

CHAPTER

4

Upgrade Your Diet

Want to feel better?
Perform better?
Then EAT better.

Food is different than it used to be.

When I was a kid, I knew fruits and vegetables were good for me, and McDonald's fries were deliciously bad. That's about it. Cholesterol was just becoming a household word, but my mom was unfairly blaming eggs. We didn't know about partially hydrogenated anything, let alone trans fats.

■

Better
INSTANTLY

↓

Remember: The fewer ingredients in your food, the fewer pounds you'll gain.

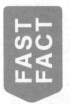
Omega-3 might as well have been a model of a Tandy computer, and quinoa a traditional Mongolian greeting. High protein, low carb, gluten free, organic—none of these terms meant anything to anyone. If someone asked you to name a celebrity chef, you'd come up with Julia Child and maybe, *maybe* James Beard if you were a foodie (another term that didn't exist). Today you could probably rattle off half-a-dozen Iron Chefs without thinking about it much.

My point: The Information Age has done to food what it's done to everything else—caused information overload. Covering it all like a lumpy, cold gravy are the food industry, which engineers flavors to make us want more of what they're selling, and the restaurant industry, which manages to shoehorn a day's worth of calories into one cheeseburger.

You want to eat better, but how do you sift through all the noise and temptation to gain *control* over your diet? It's not about willpower. It's about sanity. It's about slowing everything down so you can process what your body truly needs and separate it from what your pleasure center wants. Here, in one chapter, is what I consider to be the best food knowledge a man can use. It answers the three most important questions.

→   *What should I eat?* I'll give you scores of examples.

→   *How should I prepare it?* Lots of great ideas here.

→   *How do I know which foods provide what benefits?* I'll spell it out for you.

Think of this chapter as a supermarket of knowledge: amazing information all in one place, but organized for easy selection, consumption, and digestion. And no junk-food aisle! Here you'll learn what to eat, when to eat it, and how to make sure your active life stays properly fueled for maximum performance.

Don't have time to read this whole chapter? For a quick jump start that'll immediately improve your health, make these fast five simple changes . . . and come back later for seconds.

The Fast Five for Food

Simple stuff you can do right now.

1 **Eat more foods from the produce aisle.**

You're a smart guy, so you already know that it's important to eat your vegetables. What you might not know is just how powerful a diet rich in fresh produce can really be. Recent research published in the *Journal of Epidemiology and Community Health* showed that people who ate at least seven servings of fruits and vegetables per day were 42 percent less likely to die during a 1-year period than those who ate less than one serving. Produce is packed with important vitamins, antioxidants, minerals, and filling fiber. Try stirring spinach leaves into soups or omelets, piling vegetables on sandwiches, and snacking on fruit with yogurt.

2 **Eat some protein at every meal.**

Think of protein-rich foods as powerfoods for your body. Consuming 30 grams of protein at each meal can help turbocharge your body's muscle builders, according to research in the *Journal of Nutrition*. When study participants ate that amount, their protein synthesis level—the key to muscle growth—was 25 percent higher than that of people who skewed their consumption by loading their protein at

TRY THIS!

Reclaim a Lost Weekend

You shouldn't plan to overdo it with wings and beer on the weekend, but if it happens, compensate: A study from Finland shows that slim people eat less on weekdays to counteract piggish weekends. People who lost weight were often heavier on Sundays or Mondays. Buy a scale that links to an app so you can track weight fluctuations over the long term. If your weight is creeping up week after week, it's time to make bigger changes. And pay attention: You're likely to overeat after your favorite football team loses, a study in *Psychological Science* shows. People ate an average of 10 percent more calories, especially from sugary and fatty foods, on Mondays after their city's NFL team lost. One theory: You may take the team's failure personally and turn to comfort foods to cope, the researchers say. To avoid this, think about the positive parts of your life, such as your family or good health. Or focus on another of your favorite teams (in MLB, say) that's having better luck.

dinner, as most Americans do. Spiking your protein synthesis levels a few times a day gives your body more opportunity to add muscle. Power up on protein four times a day to aid your workout gains and build more lean mass. Even if you're looking to lose weight, eating protein can help by keeping you full and preserving your muscles so you lose fat, not strength. Consider this daily plan from *Men's Health* nutrition advisor Mike Roussell, Ph.D.

BREAKFAST: Scramble 3 whole eggs with 4 whites. Eat with ⅔ cup of oatmeal.
PROTEIN PAYOFF: 36 grams

LUNCH: Have 5 ounces of chicken breast, ⅔ cup of quinoa, and ½ cup of sauerkraut.
PROTEIN PAYOFF: 48 grams

DINNER: Have 5 ounces of steak or fish with a baked potato.
PROTEIN PAYOFF: 44 grams

SNACK: Have 1 cup of low-fat cottage cheese, ¼ cup of walnuts, and ½ cup of blueberries.
PROTEIN PAYOFF: 31 grams

* *Note*: Too much meat and dairy for your taste? Then sub in some of the terrific vegetarian sources of protein, like legumes, nuts, and seeds.

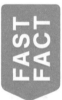

3 Replace processed grains with whole grains.

Compared with their refined and processed cousins, whole grains are rich in fiber and nutrients, and they've been linked to a variety of health benefits. One recent study from Norway suggested that eating three servings of whole grains a day reduces type 2 diabetes risk by 32 percent. We'll show you our favorite whole grains on page 67. If you buy products like bread and cereal, choose whole-grain varieties. Look for products that say "100% Whole Grain" or have less than a 10-to-1 ratio of carbohydrates to fiber.

4 Break up with sugar.

Think of sugar as a crazy girlfriend who is great in bed. *Not. Worth. It.* Just by eating and drinking a typical American diet, we suck down about 23 teaspoons a day of added sugar—that is, sugar not occurring naturally in food. That's 367 calories' worth, for a weekly total of 2,569 calories. That's the equivalent of a whole extra day of eating, *and it's nothing but sugar*. The American Heart Association recommends that men limit their daily intake of added sugars to 9 teaspoons a day, or 144 calories' worth, on average. The reason? Too much sugar is toxic; I mentioned earlier what glucose does to your body's tissues. But you may not know the following: Table sugar—sucrose—is made of glucose and fructose. Glucose is absorbed by your intestines and makes its way into your bloodstream; there, a hormone called insulin helps shuttle it to your cells, where it's used as fuel. Any extra is stored as glycogen in your liver and muscles. Fructose, on the other hand, bypasses the insulin step and goes straight to your liver, where it's mostly converted to fat. (Start reading food and drink labels, if you haven't already, and put down stuff containing high-fructose corn syrup.) Here's the scary part—studies have linked consumption of excess sugar to not only weight gain, but also diabetes and heart disease.

Our bodies crave sugar, but fruit can help you wean yourself off it. Most fruits contain fructose and glucose in roughly equal proportions, but the sugar is naturally occurring, and fruits also have fiber and nutrients. And fruit is self-regulating: You'd have to eat more than four small apples to take in the 65 grams of sugar you'd guzzle from a 20-ounce bottle of pop. Speaking of soda, the average American quaffs one-third of their daily added sugars in drink form. I used to be one of them. I quit not long after I started at *Men's Health* and, not coincidentally, dropped 12 pounds over the following few months. It wasn't that hard. There's nothing nutritionally redeeming about sugary drinks, especially soda. (Besides its high sugar content, the preservatives, dyes, and other additives might be harmful, too.) One study from Japan showed that men who drank one or more sugar-sweetened beverages per day were 35 percent more likely to develop type 2 diabetes than those who rarely or never consumed the drinks. That's just one reason you should give them up.

5 Drink more water.

It keeps you hydrated without calories. And since your body sometimes misinterprets thirst as hunger, drinking a glass of water can help you eat less. Plus, H_2O has health benefits of its own. Staying hydrated can help you fend off diabetes, according to French researchers. In a 9-year study, people who downed 17 to 34 ounces of water daily were 36 percent less likely to develop high blood sugar or diabetes than those who drank less. When you're dehydrated, your brain pumps out more vasopressin, a hormone that tells your liver to produce glucose. Water is especially important when you exercise: A dehydrated athlete not only runs slower than a hydrated one, but may also be in a worse mood and feel less energized afterward, according to University of South Florida research. To gauge your fluid requirements, weigh yourself before and after an event. If you lost weight, you may need to drink more on your next race day.

FAST FACT

12

Number of tea-spoons of sugar found in some carbonated beverages

The *Men's Health* Food Pyramid

The U.S. government's traditional food pyramid, updated in 2011 to MyPlate, is well intentioned, but it doesn't include enough protein and fats for the better man—that is, the active man. That's why *Men's Health* nutrition advisor Alan Aragon, M.S., created this pyramid.

Need help meeting these requirements? What follows is a breakdown of the most beneficial powerfoods out there, grouped by category. You simply cannot lose with any of them (except your belly, of course).

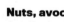

5 **Starchy foods:**
2 to 4 servings

1 serving = 2 slices bread; 1 cup rice, pasta, beans, or corn; 1 cup cereal (like Total Whole Grain or Cheerios); 1 small potato (guys who are extremely active or struggling to add muscle can double up on these.)

1 **Nuts, avocado:**
1 to 2 servings

1 serving = ¼ cup nuts, 2 Tbsp nut butter, ½ avocado

2 **Fats, oils:**
2 to 4 servings

1 serving = 1 tsp olive oil or other oil, 1 pat butter

3 **Dairy:**
2 to 4 servings

1 serving = 1 cup milk, 6 oz yogurt, 1 oz hard cheese, ⅓ cup cottage cheese

4 **Fruit:**
2 to 4 servings

1 serving = 1 medium whole fruit, ¼ cup dried fruit, 1½ cups fresh fruit

6 **Low-starch vegetables:**
3+ servings

1 serving = 1 cup, raw, of any vegetable besides potato or corn

7 **High-protein foods:**
4 to 8 servings

1 serving = 3 oz meat, 1 scoop protein powder, 3 eggs

70 Powerfoods

Leafy Greens

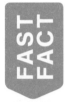
Iceberg is fine, but you can do better. The deeper the color of your greens, the more phytonutrients and antioxidants they contain. These nutrients pack a powerful punch: An increase of 1.15 servings per day of leafy green vegetables may lower your risk of type 2 diabetes by 14 percent, notes a study review in the *British Medical Journal*. That's because their antioxidants may help ward off the oxidative stress that can lead to diabetes and other chronic diseases. Try these high-powered greens:

BABY SPINACH. Three cups of raw spinach serves up about a quarter of the amount of iron men need each day, plus a hit of bone-building calcium. Toss with slices of a blood orange, walnuts, and balsamic vinegar. Shopping tip: Buy spinach from the front of the display, where it's more exposed to the light. Exposing greens to artificial light may help make them more nutritious. In a USDA study, spinach stored under fluorescent light (as it is in a store's produce section) had more folate and vitamins C, E, and K_1 than spinach stored in darkness.

RADICCHIO. This spicy, red-leaf chicory is popular in Mediterranean salads. It's rich in lutein (for eye health) and vitamin K (for bone strength). Toss it with freshly boiled pasta, olive oil, and Parmesan.

PURSLANE. A lemony-tasting green, purslane is packed with the hormone melatonin, which can function as an antioxidant. It has at least 14 times the melatonin found in any other vegetable tested by researchers at the University of Texas at San Antonio.

ARUGULA. It's a peppery salad green, although younger leaves have less of a bite than mature ones do. Arugula has vitamin A (for vision), vitamin C (for immune function), and vitamin K (for blood clotting). In addition, it contains heart-protecting compounds known as flavanols. Toss arugula into cooked rigatoni; add a drizzle of olive oil along with some roasted cherry tomatoes and shaved Parmesan. Or use it instead of lettuce on a burger or sandwich.

DANDELION GREENS. Don't mow down these weeds. Dandelion leaves can nicely counterbalance heavier grilling fare. (Perfect lawn? Buy the greens by the bunch at a grocery store.) A cup of raw greens yields 2 grams of gut-filling fiber and more than triple the calcium of the same amount of raw spinach. To help balance their bitterness, add a glug of white wine to the sautéed greens after they wilt, then cook for another minute. They pair well with steak.

Cruciferous Vegetables

These guys have powerful nutrition benefits: One Italian study found that eating cruciferous vegetables at least once a week may decrease your risk of multiple cancers compared with eating them occasionally or not at all. Cruciferous vegetables contain compounds called glucosinolates that can help block tumor growth. Consider these:

KALE. When it comes to nutrition, kale is king. These greens may lower your risk of diabetes and cardiovascular disease. Dump baby kale into pasta, soup, or salad.

BROCCOLI. These florets contain an active form of an enzyme that may help your body extract beneficial compounds called isothiocyanates, which help fend off cancer. Eat your broccoli raw or lightly cooked; heat reduces the enzyme's activity. Try broccoli sprouts instead of lettuce in a sandwich, or mix broccoli into coleslaw.

CAULIFLOWER. Think of it as "white broccoli"—nutritionally, that is. Cauliflower contains indole-3-carbinol, a compound that may help thwart cancer and repair your DNA. Break a head of cauliflower into florets. Toss with oil and then with 1 tablespoon of curry powder. Roast in a 425°F oven until browned and tender.

BROCCOLI RABE. A relative of cabbage and turnips, broccoli rabe also goes by the moniker rapini. It has edible leaves and stalks that are a little

COUNTER-INTELLIGENCE

Are You Sabotaging Your Salads?

Low-fat dressings may inhibit your body's ability to absorb nutrients. In a Purdue University study, people who ate salads dressed with a moderate amount of an oil that's rich in monounsaturated fat (such as canola oil) absorbed more disease-fighting carotenoids than those whose salads were drizzled with a small amount. Carotenoids are fat soluble, so their absorption may be boosted by dressings that contain more mono fats, the scientists say.

For the ultimate salad dressing, shake up these ingredients in a jar. Store any extra in the fridge for up to a week.

→ Extra-virgin olive oil (½ cup)
→ Red wine vinegar (3 tablespoons)
→ Dijon mustard (½ tablespoon)
→ Minced shallot (½ shallot)
→ Salt and freshly ground black pepper to taste

bitter, but more flavorful than broccoli's. One bunch, cooked, contains 17 grams of plant protein and 12 grams of fiber, plus your daily requirements of vitamins A, C, and K. Boil broccoli rabe in a pot of salted water until it's tender-crisp, about 5 minutes. Drain and sauté it in olive oil, adding garlic and red-pepper flakes. Try it as a simple side with grilled chicken or in a sausage sandwich.

CHARD. Cook up a cup for nearly four times your recommended intake of vitamin K, which can help slow arterial calcification. Vitamin K is fat soluble, so sauté your chard in olive oil for the best absorption.

Root Vegetables

These tubers can help you protect your gourd. In a study published in the *British Journal of Nutrition*, people who ate the fewest root vegetables had three times the cognitive decline of those who ate the most. Many root vegetables—including the most famous, carrots—are rich in beta-carotene, which may be responsible for the brain-boosting benefits, the researchers say.

PURPLE SWEET POTATOES. Skip white potatoes and opt for sweet potatoes instead. Even better? The purple sweet potato derives its rich color from anthocyanins, which boost antioxidant content. Coat the potato lightly in oil, wrap it in foil, and bake at 325°F until soft, about 90 minutes. Top with a pat of butter before serving.

CELERY ROOT. Also known as celeriac, this root might be the weird stepchild of the vegetable world, but flavor-wise it's like the love child of parsley and celery. It infuses wraps and salads with a bright, grassy, crunchy complexity, and it's a great source of bone-building phosphorus.

KOHLRABI. Consider shredding kohlrabi into slaws. Its crisp flesh is rich in high-powered disease-fighting vitamin C and contains cancer-fighting sulforaphane.

JICAMA. You might notice that your grocery store is stocking more and more exotic vegetables, and this tuber is one worth trying. Jicama contains inulin, a prebiotic that may reduce the risk of colon cancer. Dip thick-cut jicama, instead of chips, in guacamole.

RADISH. No hot-sauce-infused potato chip can match the potent punch of a fresh radish root. Eat sliced radishes raw with a good hit of flaky sea salt. Plain radishes have 1 measly calorie apiece. Oh, and save the radishes' green tops. They have a similar spiciness and add bite to a mixed-greens salad.

BEETS. This root may help your endurance so you can redline your 5K time. In a 2012 Saint Louis University study, runners who ate 1¼ cups of baked beets 75 minutes before racing were 5 percent faster toward the end

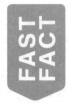

Whole Grains vs. Refined Grains

A whole grain, such as wheat, consists of three components: bran (hard outer layer), endosperm (soft inner layer), and germ (the embryo in the middle). When a whole grain is refined–to make white flour, rice, or pasta–the bran and germ are stripped away. Why? Because the bran creates texture issues, and the germ turns whole-grain products brown. Problem is, all the good stuff (fiber, protein, omega-3s, vitamins) is in the bran and germ. In fact, the endosperm is made up almost entirely of carbohydrates. Bad for your belly–and your blood work.

of the run than placebo eaters. Slice beets $\frac{1}{8}$-inch thick and toss with oil, salt, and black pepper. Bake at 375°F until chip-like, 15 to 20 minutes. Sauté the tops: They provide vitamin A for vision and vitamin K for healthy blood clotting.

Alliums

These little guys do more than boost the flavor of your foods. This class of vegetables, which includes onions and garlic, may help fight stomach cancer, a Chinese study found.

LEEKS. These long, thin bundles have a milder flavor than most onions. They're also a good source of vitamins A, C, and K. Try this: Thinly slice the tender white and light-green parts and swirl them in a bowl of water to wash. Drain and dry. Try them sautéed in butter and added to scrambled eggs or mashed potatoes.

ONIONS. They might leave you with bad breath, but the stink will be worth it in the end. Compounds in onions may have cancer-fighting benefits, blood-thinning properties, and even antibacterial effects, according to a study review published in *Critical Reviews in Food Science and Nutrition*.

GARLIC. Surprise—garlic breath is healthy, too. Specifically, it's good for your lungs. Chinese scientists recently discovered that garlic might protect against lung cancer. Nonsmokers who ate a diet rich in raw garlic were 33 percent less likely to develop lung cancer than those who ate none. Consuming raw garlic releases sulfuric compounds that may prevent cell mutations and tumor growth, according to the study. Even people who ate as little as three cloves a week saw a reduction in risk. Try tossing freshly cooked spaghetti with raw minced garlic, olive oil, and parsley, and season with salt and black pepper. And don't throw away garlic with tails: Garlic cloves that have sprouted contain more cancer- and heart-disease-fighting flavonoids than fresh ones do. Those cloves can be more bitter than fresh ones, so throw them into the sauté pan; avoid raw preparations like homemade salsa.

The Best of the Rest

SWEET PEAS. Peas are packed with vitamin A, and they're unique among vegetables for their protein content. One cup contains 8 grams! Stock up when you're in the frozen food section. Freezing peas actually boosts their antioxidant activity, reports a study in the *Journal of Food Science*. All these need is a little butter and sea salt to taste great.

BUTTERNUT SQUASH. The orange flesh tips you off to its payload of carotenoids, a potent class of antioxidants linked to lower incidences of cancer and heart disease. Look for smaller specimens, which are usually more tender.

JAPANESE EGGPLANT. It's more slender than your average eggplant but has the same flavor and texture. Choose ones that are 6 to 8 inches long and glossy; dull ones are often bitter. Slice them into 1/4-inch-thick planks and grill over direct, high heat until tender, basting with a two-to-one mixture of melted butter and miso paste. Serve sprinkled with black sesame seeds.

BEEFSTEAK TOMATO. This monster can weigh as much as 2 pounds, and it has a massive flavor payload to match. A beefsteak's circumference makes it the go-to pick for a BLT or caprese stack, or as a lycopene-loaded snack. Sprinkle them with salt and olive oil. (The fat in the oil can help your body absorb nutrients.) Sprinkle, drizzle, take a bite, and repeat. The best specimens are glossy, blemish-free, and crimson. Buy organic tomatoes when you can. Tomatoes grown using organic fertilization and organic pest-control techniques contained 55 percent more vitamin C than conventionally grown tomatoes, a Brazilian study found. Plus, the organically grown tomatoes housed 139 percent more disease-fighting antioxidant phenols. Organic

SMART ADVICE

FROM *MEN'S HEALTH* NUTRITION ADVISOR **MICHAEL ROUSSELL, PH.D.,** FOUNDER OF NAKED NUTRITION, LLC

"A lot of people avoid nutrition because they think it's going to be this miserable experience where they're not eating all the foods they enjoy. Over the long haul, nutrition shouldn't be about restriction. It's about the small adjustments you can make to your life to make your diet work better for you. I look at a client's diet and see: What are things they're already doing pretty well, and how can we change them to make them a little bit better? So maybe they're eating breakfast, but they're not eating enough protein at breakfast.

Maybe when they go out and have drinks, they're not drinking drinks that are full of sugar-laden mixers, but they're having too many. We can make small changes, such as adding more protein at breakfast or setting a limit of four drinks a week if they're trying to lose weight, maybe six if they're active. If you start with small, easy changes, you'll gain momentum and see some results. Then we can start tackling bigger changes."

farming can subject crops to more stressful growing conditions, which may boost their natural defenses and antioxidant stockpiles, the researchers say.

Fleshy Fruits

PLUMS. These flavor bombs contain only 30 calories and 8 grams of carbohydrates each. They're 85 percent water by weight, so they can even help hydrate you. Or, ditch the water and try the dried variety—prunes. A study from UC Davis suggests that prunes may help reduce blood levels of LDL (bad) cholesterol.

MANGOES. To squash your triglyceride level, eat more mangoes. In a Mexican study, people who ate about a cup of mango every day for 30 days lowered their levels of these harmful fats by 38 percent. The fruit's polyphenols help reduce oxidation.

GUAVAS. This tropical fruit has sweet white, yellow, pink, or red flesh inside its yellow-green rind. It delivers fiber and vitamin C. What's more, guava's antioxidants are more active than those in apples, bananas, mangoes, or papayas, a study from India reveals. Bite into it like an apple, or slice it in half and scoop out the pulp. You can also blend some of the flesh into a yogurt smoothie for a hint of tropical sweetness.

BANANAS. They're most famous for their blood pressure–reducing potassium content, which is a big benefit: A recent study in the *American Journal of Clinical Nutrition* found that a whopping 95 percent of men don't hit their daily mark for potassium. But they're not a one-trick fruit: Bananas are also rich in manganese and vitamin B_6.

Crisp Fruits

ASIAN PEARS. One large Asian pear has 10 grams of fiber—nearly double what a large apple provides. The best way to pick a ripe one: Ask your produce manager or market vendor for a taste. It should be crisp, not mealy. For a simple slaw, cut a pear into matchsticks and toss them in a bowl with sliced cabbage and shallots, minced chives, and a splash of cider vinegar. Season with salt, black pepper, and sugar. Add mayo or Greek yogurt for a creamy variation.

RED DELICIOUS APPLES. There are 7,500 varieties of apples in the world, and they're all smart choices. They're high in fiber, low in calories, and filled to the core with phytonutrients. However, the Red Delicious is king for a few reasons. One is its thick skin—the peel has five times the antioxidant polyphenols of the flesh. The other is its signature hue, which comes from anthocyanins, a class of heart-disease-fighting polyphenols that are also found in red wine. One study showed that Red Delicious had the highest concentration of polyphenols out of eight common North American varieties, followed by Northern Spy and Ida Red.

Berries

They may be sweet, but berries are actually good for your blood sugar. In a study published last year in the *American Journal of Clinical Nutrition*, the men who ate the most berries had a 35 percent lower risk of type 2 diabetes than those who ate the least. All berries are packed with nutrients. Try these types.

BLUEBERRIES. Blueberries are blue because of anthocyanins—potent antioxidants that may prevent heart disease and cancer, according to a study by Romanian researchers. Can't get 'em fresh? Buy them in the freezer aisle. According to research in the journal *Neurology*, eating these berries regularly may help shield you from Parkinson's disease. In the study, men who ate the most strawberries and blueberries (two or more weekly servings) were 23 percent less likely to develop Parkinson's later in life than those who ate the least. The berries' anthocyanins may trigger the production of protective brain enzymes, the researchers say.

STRAWBERRIES. In addition to the brain benefits noted above, strawberries are powerful in their own right. In a study published in the journal *Food Chemistry*, participants ate about 3 cups of strawberries a day for 16 days. Their conclusion: Eating strawberries can help your red blood cells fight disease-causing oxidative stress. You may see a similar benefit eating fewer strawberries over a longer period of time, the researchers say.

RASPBERRIES. One of the most fiber-rich berries, they boast 8 grams per cup. Plus, recent research published in the journal *Food Chemistry* shows that raspberries have more lutein—an eye-protecting antioxidant—than previously believed.

CRANBERRIES. Don't relegate cranberries to the holidays. They contain A-type proanthocyanidins, an uncommon antioxidant that may explain the berries' inflammation-fighting effects, according to new research in

Do You Eat Too Much?

Simple tricks to cut your consumption without starving.

1. PRELOAD. Going out for dinner? A half-hour before you leave, eat a 200-calorie snack that contains at least 15 grams of protein. With a gut full of satiating protein and fewer hunger hormones circulating, you'll consume fewer calories at the restaurant. Two good snack choices: a whey protein shake, or an apple with string cheese (contains satiating fiber and fat, too).

2. STOP BEFORE YOUR TANK IS FULL. Picture a gas gauge in your belly. "E" means you're ravenous and "F" represents a full tank. Aim to stay between half and three-quarters of a tank by eating before you feel famished and stopping when you're satisfied, not stuffed, says Matt Lawson, M.A., a weight-loss coach for iBehaviorCoach.

3. CHEW ON IT. You've heard this one before: Chew each bite 40 times. Well, there's science behind it. In one study, men who chomped that many times per bite ate 12 percent less than those who chewed 12 times. Researchers believe chewing longer before swallowing speeds the release of gut hormones linked to feeling satisfied.

4. EAT LIKE A RESTAURANT CRITIC. Take time to note the texture, flavor, and smell of your food. Think about where it came from, the source. Saying to yourself, "Wow, this grass-fed rib eye from Wyoming is juicy" can create a vivid meal memory that keeps you feeling fuller longer, a U.K. study found. (Note: That line works best when you're actually eating a grass-fed rib eye from Wyoming.) And eating mindfully automatically will slow you down if you typically Hoover your food into your mouth.

5. PLAN YOUR GROCERY TRIPS. Hungry shoppers really do load their carts with more high-calorie options, a study in *JAMA Internal Medicine* reports. The best time to shop is after breakfast on a weekend, says Anita Mirchandani, R.D., a New York City dietitian. If that's not a good time for you, preload before you go. Also, studies show that going to the grocery store with a list will reduce the likelihood that you will purchase high-calorie foods that catch your eye.

6. BUY NEW DINNERWARE. The average U.S. plate has been enlarged by 23 percent in the last century. No wonder our waistlines have ballooned! The fix: Eat from plates with wide or colored rims. They make small portions seem larger because the plate looks more filled, according to research in the *International Journal of Obesity*.

7. BEWARE OF MEGAPORTIONS. Restaurants often plate oversize portions. Check out the chart below for an eye-opening look at how much extra you're eating when you eat out.

	RECOMMENDED SIZE (FDA)	AVERAGE WEIGHT IN RESTAURANTS	% BIGGER
Hamburger	2.5 ounces	5.3 ounces	110
Bagel	2 ounces	4.4 ounces	120
Muffin	1.5 ounces	6.5 ounces	330
French fries	2.5 ounces	6.7 ounces	170
Pizza slice	5 ounces	7 ounces	40
Beer	12 fluid ounces	15.4 fluid ounces	30
Steak	2.5 ounces	8.1 ounces	220
Soda	12 fluid ounces	23 fluid ounces	90
Pasta	0.5 cup	2.9 cups	480

Advances in Nutrition. Aim for a serving or two of cranberry cocktail or dried berries a day. Just be careful of the intense sugar content of prepared juices and sauce.

Legumes

Beans should be known as heart-savers, not wind-breakers. People who ate a cup of fiber-rich lentils, beans, or chickpeas a day reduced their systolic blood pressure by 4 millimeters of mercury after 3 months, according to a study in *Archives of Internal Medicine.* The potassium and magnesium found in legumes may play a role in regulating blood pressure. Add these legumes to salads, curries, and chili:

NAVY BEANS. They boast the best combo of magnesium and potassium—two nutrients men often fall short in—and vitamin C. Plus, every cup of boiled navy beans contains 19 grams of fiber—more than any other cooked food.

LENTILS. When cooked, they're tender and a bit chewy, with a subtle nutty flavor. A half cup of cooked lentils has about 8 grams of fiber and only 115 calories. Lentils are also a rich source of minerals such as iron, phosphorus, and manganese. Cook according to package directions, season with salt and herbs, and add lemon juice or vinegar to finish. Serve as a side dish with grilled fish, lamb, or sausage.

Nuts

If you ever doubted the nutritional power of nuts, here's your proof: A study published in the *New England Journal of Medicine* showed that there were 20 percent fewer deaths over 30 years among people who ate at least 7 ounces of nuts a week compared to those who ate none. Try the *Men's Health* mix from Planter's or stock up on these:

MACADAMIA NUTS. With a serving yielding 17 grams of monounsaturated fat (the heart-healthiest kind), these steamroll almonds and walnuts in good-fat content. Pair them with dark chocolate for a super snack.

WALNUTS. They're the alpha nuts in terms of alpha-linolenic acid, a polyunsaturated fat that fights inflammation. Yale researchers report that eating about a half cup of walnut halves a day can improve blood vessel function.

Seeds

Don't let their small size fool you: Some seeds are nutritional powerhouses.

CHIA. Beyond their role in growing a 'fro on your desktop pet, tiny black

TRY THIS!

Flip Your Snack Switch

Popcorn contains 15 times the disease-fighting polyphenols of whole-grain tortilla chips, according to a recent study conducted at the University of Scranton in Pennsylvania. The reason: Unlike corn tortilla chips, popcorn includes the nutrient-packed hull of the corn kernel.

chia seeds are a good source of calcium and an excellent source of fiber and manganese. Add chia seeds to a bowl of oatmeal or sprinkle them over sliced fruit.

PUMPKIN. These seeds deliver the immune boosters magnesium and zinc. The roasted, hulled variety adds nuttiness to granola.

HEMP. Just an ounce of hemp seeds delivers 11 grams of complete protein—that's protein with all the essential amino acids, the same ones found in meat, eggs, or dairy. Shake some into a stir-fry or blend them into a postworkout smoothie.

SUNFLOWER. Roasted sunflower seeds are an excellent source of the antioxidants manganese, selenium, and vitamin E, as well as bone-building phosphorus. Sprinkle them into a salad or atop a pureed vegetable soup.

Eggs

Start scrambling. Eggs contain choline, a brain-boosting vitamin. What's more, if you've heard that they're bad for your heart, you heard wrong. In fact, Brazilian research suggests a link between egg consumption and clearer coronary arteries. One guess is that the yolk's payload of vitamins E, B_{12}, and folate may be the key. Just stop at four eggs a day to limit the calories.

Fish and Shellfish

Foods from the sea aren't just protein-rich—they're also packed with omega-3 fatty acids, which have been linked to heart health and brainpower. Consider these:

BLACK COD. Also known as sablefish, this meaty whitefish has more omega-3s per gram than sardines—with far less funk. Plus, they're a sustainable species.

MACKEREL. One 6-ounce fillet contains 2 grams of omega-3s—more than four times the amount in canned light tuna. Too fishy? Douse cooked mackerel with freshly squeezed lemon juice for balance.

SOCKEYE SALMON. Wild salmon might be more expensive, but a 5.5-ounce serving, which is about half a fillet, boasts 175 milligrams of brain-boosting choline, 39 grams of protein, and 2,178 milligrams of omega-3 fatty acids.

MUSSELS. Affordable, sustainable, and protein-rich at about 20 grams per serving, mussels are muscle chow. They also deliver vitamins B_{12} and C, iron, and magnesium, all of which can help you recover from exercise.

SEA SCALLOPS. A 4-ounce serving of cooked sea scallops provides 23 grams of protein for 126 calories. Buy jumbo dry-packed sea scallops (the "wet" variety are treated with an additive), pat them dry and lightly coat with oil, and sear them for just 2 minutes per side in a hot pan. Finish with a squeeze of citrus and a sprinkling of sea salt.

CLAMS. Twenty small cooked clams have only about 280 calories, but they pack a protein punch—almost 50 grams. Clams also contain high levels of vitamin B_{12} and iron. Put scrubbed clams in a pot with white wine, garlic cloves, parsley, and freshly ground black pepper. Cover and steam until they open. Hit them with lemon juice.

Poultry

These cuts will give you plenty of protein with generally less fat than other types of meats. One downside: Poultry is a top cause of death from foodborne illness in the United States, the Centers for Disease Control and Prevention (CDC) reports. Don't become a statistic: Wash your hands before and after handling raw chicken, thaw frozen chicken in the fridge, and cook poultry until a meat thermometer stuck into the thickest parts of the thigh and breast reads 165°F, the USDA recommends.

BONELESS, SKINLESS CHICKEN BREASTS. Roast a batch for salads all week long. A 4-ounce breast contains 36 grams of protein.

TURKEY. It's not just for Thanksgiving. Five ounces of roast turkey contains 108 milligrams of brain-boosting choline.

Beef, Pork, and Game

These meats can give you a hit of protein and vitamins. Just beware of processed versions, like deli meats, bacon, and sausage. A study from Poland published in 2014 showed that men who ate about 2.6 ounces of processed red meat per day were 28 percent more likely to develop heart failure and more than twice as likely to die from it compared to men who ate less than an ounce per day. One theory: The sodium in processed meats increases your blood pressure, which may increase heart failure risk, the researchers say. Plus, the phosphate additives in these meats might impair your body's ability to balance calcium and phosphate, which can harm your heart. Finally, smoked meats are a source of toxic polycyclic aromatic hydrocarbons, which have been linked to heart disease. Buy fresh cuts of meat and cook them yourself.

GRASS-FED RIB EYE STEAK. Research shows that eating grass-fed red meat may improve your inflammation-fighting omega-3 fatty acid profiles. The meat itself may contain triple the immune-boosting vitamin E and seven times the antioxidant carotenoids that grain-finished beef has.

PORK TENDERLOIN. This cut contains the best combination of zinc and iron without being too high in calories.

BISON. Beef's leaner cousin has less than half the total fat while still packing essential nutrients, like zinc, selenium, and B vitamins, needed for optimal testosterone production, immune function, and energy.

Whey Protein

It's one of the rare healthy processed foods. With its protein payoff, whey can help you get big, and it may have even more benefits. In a Washington State University study, people who drank a daily shake with whey protein for 6 weeks dropped their blood pressure by about 8 points. Whey may improve the function of blood vessel linings so they regulate blood pressure better, the researchers say. Take a cue from the study and add 28 grams (1 scoop) to

SMART ADVICE

FROM *MEN'S HEALTH* WEIGHT-LOSS ADVISOR **JEFF VOLEK, PH.D., R.D.,** AN EXERCISE AND NUTRITION RESEARCHER AT THE UNIVERSITY OF CONNECTICUT

"Whey protein is a very effective–if not ideal–source of protein for men. It is an effective supplement that they can use around workouts to enhance the adaptations to training.

"A lot of research shows that in addition to the post-exercise time period, the pre-exercise time period may be beneficial as well to get some protein in. It doesn't need to be a lot–as little as 10 grams of protein split between the pre- and post-workout time periods is enough to trigger an increase in muscle protein synthesis, which over time could translate into greater gains in muscle mass. That's because whey has about 10 percent of the amino acid leucine, the key amino acid responsible for turning on protein synthesis machinery in muscles."

your next postworkout shake. Make it at home in the blender; the premade bottled varieties can be low in protein and packed with sugar you don't need. Scoop in your powder along with ½ cup of plain yogurt and ½ cup of milk. Then add 1½ cups of fresh or frozen fruits, such as bananas, berries, or pears, and ½ cup of vegetables, such as kale, spinach, or carrots. A tablespoon or two of nut butter, nuts, rolled oats, or avocado can also give your smoothie thickness and a boost of fiber. Add ¼ to ½ cup of ice or water, blend until smooth, and if you'd like, top with ¼ teaspoon to 1 tablespoon of ground cinnamon, grated fresh ginger, vanilla extract, honey, or maple syrup.

Grains

SPROUTED GRAINS. These grains have begun but not finished germinating. They can have triple the soluble fiber, a key to blood sugar control. Our favorite is sprouted rice: Find it at health food stores or vitacost.com.

OATS. They pack a powerful combo of fiber, folate, and magnesium. Plus, they have proven cholesterol-lowering properties.

QUINOA. These protein-loaded pearls carry 8 grams of the nutrient per cup. Try tossing cooked quinoa with a little olive oil, diced tomatoes, diced cucumber, lots of chopped parsley, salt, and freshly ground black pepper for a simple tabbouleh salad.

KAMUT. This heart-healthy, nutty-tasting whole grain yields almost double the nutrients of other varieties of wheat, with 10 grams of protein and 7 grams of fiber in each cup. It's rich in potassium, zinc, and antioxidants.

Dairy

Milk isn't just for kids: Men who consumed the most dairy were less likely to become obese, Swedish researchers found in a 2013 study. The reason: Certain natural trans fatty acids in dairy may help reduce risk of insulin resistance.

ORGANIC 1% MILK. Buy milk from cows fed an all-grass, hormone-free diet. It delivers more omega-3 fatty acids than the conventional stuff. Opt for 1% for the ideal amount of protein and calcium without a big calorie load.

KEFIR. This fermented milk packs a two-to-three ratio of protein to carbohydrates. Once in your digestive tract, it acts as a fertilizer, dumping billions of bacteria that benefit your heart, digestion, and immune system.

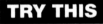
TRY THIS

Add Oatmeal to Subtract Weight

"I don't follow any particular diet, but I do make sure my weight doesn't fluctuate. If I notice I'm up a few pounds, I eat more oatmeal. Obviously, it's great for breakfast, but I also eat it as a snack because it's absorbed slowly, keeping my blood sugar steady and satisfying hunger."

–John Elefteriades, M.D., heart surgeon and director of the Center for Thoracic Aortic Disease at Yale School of Medicine

YOGURT. Eating yogurt can cut your diabetes risk by up to 24 percent, a study from the University of Cambridge suggests. People who ate at least four and a half 4-ounce servings a week were least likely to develop the disease. The researchers say the probiotic and vitamin K in yogurt may play a role. One drawback: Yogurt cups often carry hidden sugar shocks. Added sugars in yogurts go by many names: "fructose," "evaporated cane juice," "cane sugar," or forms of "juice concentrate." Stick with plain Greek yogurt—which has more protein than its plain counterpart does—and have some fruit on the side.

FETA CHEESE. It's a medium-firm, white Greek cheese with a light but tangy flavor. An ounce has 75 calories—less than Cheddar, Swiss, and full-fat mozzarella. In addition, it's a good source of protein. Crumble some feta into a spinach salad, toss it with sautéed shrimp and lemon, or use it as a pizza cheese.

Drinks

GREEN TEA. Research suggests that this grassy variety, which hasn't yet been fermented like other teas, may improve your cholesterol levels, lower blood pressure, fight cancer, promote satiety, and even prevent tooth decay and gum disease. Don't like the bitter taste of green tea? Let the boiled water cool a bit before you brew. The ideal temperature for brewing green tea is between 170° and 185°F.

BLACK TEA. Like the green variety, black tea is good for BP. Plus, this drink might protect your prostate. A study published recently in the *American Journal of Epidemiology* showed that every cup of black tea a man drank per day was linked to a 5 percent decrease in his risk of prostate cancer. The researchers say that might be because black tea contains flavonoids,

COUNTER-INTELLIGENCE
Don't Go for the Fake Cream

If it's cream-filled and sold in a convenience store, skip it—but not just because of the sugar and trans fats that you're probably thinking of. The phosphorus compounds used as additives in junk foods like Twinkies may raise your risks of cardiac and kidney diseases, according to a study in the *Journal of the American Society of Nephrology*. Scan ingredient lists: The additives go by monikers such as "disodium phosphate," "monocalcium phosphate," and "sodium acid pyrophosphate."

which can fight cancer cells—and hamper the growth of new blood vessels that tumors need in order to expand.

COFFEE. A cup of joe does more than perk you up. Coffee is the number one source of antioxidants in the U.S. diet, according to a study from the University of Scranton in Pennsylvania. What's more, a growing body of research suggests that quaffing a few cups a day can reduce your risk of type 2 diabetes, Alzheimer's disease, and even prostate cancer. How do you take your coffee? The answer should be black, without sugar. A touch of half-and-half may not add many calories, but new research from Croatia suggests that milk can reduce the antioxidant levels. Of course, if you doctor your drink with sugar or artificial sweeteners, you're just stirring in calories or chemicals. A better way to handle bitter: Add some ground cinnamon to taste. Finally, remember that, like many other things, coffee is best in moderation. In a study published in *Mayo Clinic Proceedings*, men who drank more than 4 cups a day were 21 percent more likely to die in a 17-year period.

RED WINE. In moderation, red wine is part of a healthy diet. Ten ounces (about two glasses) of red wine after a fatty meal may shield your heart from the meal's adverse effects, say Italian scientists. Red wine reduces the post-meal rise in cholesterol oxidation products in the blood, which are linked to heart disease. Less wine may still provide the benefit. Just don't top two drinks a day, or you're going into heavy-drinking territory—which is obviously bad for your health.

Cooking Essentials

EXTRA-VIRGIN OLIVE OIL. Make this your go-to for salads. Its combo of high monounsaturated fatty acids and good ratio of omega-3 to omega-6 fatty acids make it a healthy choice. Studies have linked olive oil consumption to better heart health and a lower risk of strokes and cancer. Store your

Win the War in Your Gut

Bacteria deep inside your gut play a role in determining whether your belly jiggles. We all have about 5,600 strains of bacteria that break down food as it passes through the 30 feet of our gastrointestinal tract. Research suggests that the makeup of these microbes determines how much energy you harvest from food. That in turn regulates your appetite, satiety, and insulin resistance. In general, the greater the variety of bugs you have, the better. Build up your arsenal with the following strategies:

POUND PREBIOTIC FIBER

All fiber is good at fighting fat, but a special class called prebiotic fiber is great at it. Prebiotics promote the proliferation of good bacteria in your digestive tract. Because you can't digest prebiotic fibers, they pass intact through your small intestine. But when they enter your colon, bacteria feast on them and break them down into gases and short-chain fatty acids—a setup that allows helpful bacteria to flourish. Plus, studies suggest, this process spurs the production of satiety hormones, which help you feel fuller faster. If you're aiming to lose weight, shoot for 15 to 21 grams per day. Good sources of fructan, a natural prebiotic fiber, include sunchokes (15 grams per half cup), leeks (6 grams per half cup), artichokes (6 grams per artichoke), asparagus (3 grams per six spears), and onions (2 grams per 2 teaspoons). Rye bread also contains about 1.1 grams of fructan per slice. In a study from Denmark, men who ate whole-grain rye bran at dinner consumed 11 percent less at lunch the next day than guys who had munched white bread. Their guts' counts of bifidobacteria, a good bacterium, increased, while counts of bacteroides, a less-helpful bug, decreased. You can also find prebiotics in some fiber-supplemented products—many contain inulin, a natural prebiotic fiber extracted from chicory root. Check for this ingredient.

EAT MORE BUGS

Think of your gut as a fragile ecosystem: If you start to lose species, the habitat suffers. Several species of bacteria can carry out similar chemical reactions to process your food. If fewer of them are available to complete these reactions, metabolic changes—and weight gain—result. The solution: Eat more good bacteria every day from fermented foods such as yogurt, kimchi, and sauerkraut. Or pop a probiotic supplement, such as Align.

PROTECT YOUR MICROBES

The antioxidants in produce do more than fight cancer and protect your heart—they also boost good gut bacteria. Plants produce many phytochemicals as antibiotic agents to protect them from infection, and they have antibacterial effects in your gut too. Against the bad bacteria, that is. "Gut bacteria metabolize the phytochemicals, and those metabolites are absorbed and bioactive," says *Men's Health* nutrition advisor Jeffrey Blumberg, Ph.D., director of the Antioxidants Research Laboratory at the Human Nutrition Research Center on Aging at Tufts University in Boston. "It's like a two-for-one." If you nosh on the CDC's recommended 6 cups of fruits and vegetables per day, you're on the right track. You can also drink your phytochemicals: In a Japanese study, people who sipped a cup of green tea daily for 10 days experienced a boom in flab-fighting flora. Prefer stronger stuff? A study in the *American Journal of Clinical Nutrition* found that men who drank 9 ounces (about two glasses) of Spanish red wine a day for 20 days showed improved concentrations of belly-off bacteria.

bottle in a cool, dry cupboard—otherwise, heat and light can break down its healthful compounds.

CANOLA OIL. Neutral flavor and a high smoke point (the temperature at which a fat starts to break down and becomes useless) make this oil great for stir-frying. What's more, its combination of monounsaturated and polyunsaturated fats may help your heart. In a study published in the *Journal of Internal Medicine*, people who added canola to their diets and subtracted other fats reduced their LDL cholesterol by 17 percent and their triglycerides by 20 percent.

CINNAMON. It may look like dirt, but it acts like a drug. Two teaspoons of cinnamon, consumed with food, can tamp down postmeal blood sugar surges, according to a study published in the *Journal of the Academy of Nutrition and Dietetics*. In fact, another study showed that as little as a quarter teaspoon a day can lower blood sugar, triglycerides, and bad LDL cholesterol in people with type 2 diabetes. Researchers believe the methylhydroxychalcone polymers in the spice increase cells' ability to metabolize sugar by up to 20 times. Sprinkle it on coffee and oatmeal.

CURRY. If you've ever been a Marlboro man, you may be able to undo some of the damage: Consuming curry can help former smokers breathe easier. In a study from Singapore, ex-smokers who ate curry monthly scored 10 percent higher on a lung function test than those who didn't eat the spice blend. Even folks who had never lit up took deeper breaths after downing curry-rich food. Credit the antioxidants in the spice turmeric. Not a curry fan? Make yellow mustard your go-to condiment; it's high in turmeric.

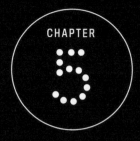
Fortify
Your Fitness
Build Your Better Body

Some guys are built like Joe Manganiello, and others like Winnie-the-Pooh. Most of us are somewhere in between. But no matter which genetic cards you were dealt, you can become a better, fitter man. Fitter is always better—it's the ultimate DIY project. That's why we encourage it and offer useful advice about how to do it right in every issue of *Men's Health*.

■ **Better** INSTANTLY
↓
Standing at your desk for 2½ hours a day helps you burn up to 350 extra calories.

When I joined the magazine, I was in my early 30s. My wife and I had just had our first daughter, which meant I didn't have as much time for the things I loved, whether it was weekly basketball games or weekend ski trips. One morning, not long after I arrived, I looked in the mirror and wasn't impressed with the guy staring back at me. I resolved right then to get back in shape. Our fitness director, Adam Campbell, gave me a 30-minute workout I could do at home 3 days a week, after the baby was in bed. That was more than 12 years ago. My workouts have evolved since then, but my commitment to them has never wavered.

Exercising is critically important to good health these days. No matter how you dice the data, one thing is clear: We're way less active than the generations that have come before us. If you have any doubt that you are moving less than your great-grandfather did, have a look at the chart below, which illustrates the massive reduction in the number of calories humans are burning daily. It comes from a Dutch study that compared the activity levels of modern office workers with those of actors mimicking the daily lives of 19th-century Australian settlers. The actors' activity levels were 1.6 times higher—that's the equivalent of walking up to 8 more miles a day than we office workers do today. The scientists reported their findings in the *International Journal of Sports Medicine*; they show how technological advances like the washing machine and the

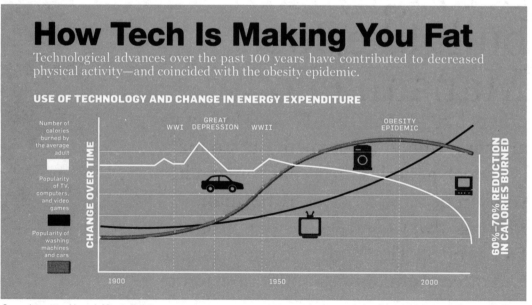

How Tech Is Making You Fat

Technological advances over the past 100 years have contributed to decreased physical activity—and coincided with the obesity epidemic.

USE OF TECHNOLOGY AND CHANGE IN ENERGY EXPENDITURE

Source: International Journal of Sports Medicine

automobile over the past 100 years have contributed to decreased physical activity—and coincided with the obesity epidemic.

Keep looking at that chart. Don't stop until it makes you want to lace up your running shoes. Being fit, after all, offers tremendous health benefits, according to George L. Blackburn, M.D., Ph.D., director of the Center for the Study of Nutrition Medicine at Beth Israel Deaconess Medical Center in Boston. His study, published recently in the medical journal *Obesity Reviews*, describes the many benefits of exercise beyond the effect it has on weight:

→   Improved insulin sensitivity and other hormonal responses to food
→   Stress reduction
→   An overall sense of competence and accomplishment
→   Motivation to improve other behaviors

Those last two benefits suggest how regular exercise that you enjoy can help you stick to a workout program. But other perks to being fit are more nuanced:

→   When you're fit, it's almost impossible to look like a fool on the basketball court, even if you suck at basketball. Same applies to all sports, except maybe golf.
→   When you're fit, you move with the power and ease of a younger man. And that feels great!
→   When you're fit, you look better in clothes, because you fill them out right—muscularly, not lumpily.
→   When you're fit, you're ready for anything—a marathon day at work, chasing a purse-snatcher, climbing a tree to avoid the gnashing teeth of an angry dog, playing soccer with your kids, carrying her over your shoulder and up the stairs to bed (with her permission, of course).
→   When you're fit, everything in life seems to come easier: sleep, healthy eating, women, sex, job opportunities, happiness, and exercise. You exude a confidence that leads to more of everything, from phone numbers at the bar to zeros in your paycheck.

Staying in shape is a lot easier than getting in shape. Once your workouts become regular and you reach a certain level of fitness, you'll find that you'll regret missing a workout. I do. My goal is to exercise at least every other day. If I miss for a couple of days, I start to feel crappy and get cranky. That's because I know how great I feel afterward—tired and yet energized, optimistic and thankful for my health. That's the real reward of fitness: how good you feel about your body, yourself, and your life.

So start a fitness routine. If you already have, great! Never stop. Life is so much better when you're strong and fit enough to climb a tree.

The Fast Five for Fitness

Simple stuff you can do right now.

1 **Never stop moving—ever!**
Take the stairs, park your car in the spot farthest from the door, walk for 30 minutes a day. To lose pounds, to move from couch spud to moderately fit—which is where the biggest jump in health benefits comes from—you need to increase your physical activity. (See "Weight Loss Made Simple" on page 93.) You've heard this before? So, why aren't you doing it? Walking is the easiest, safest way to get back in shape if you are overweight and haven't exercised in a long time. A meta-analysis of studies from seven countries involving nearly 500,000 participants found that walking reduced the risk of cardiovascular events (heart attacks, strokes, and so on) by 31 percent. What's more, other studies show that walking provides protection against dementia, obesity, colon cancer, peripheral artery disease, erectile dysfunction, and depression. Walk this way: Swing your arms and put a little bounce in your step. Canadian researchers found that changing your style of walking to a more energetic, purposeful gait can actually make you happier. Walking more—and sitting less—is a superb strategy for improving your health.

2 **Never sit down on the job.**
I mean that literally. I've been using a stand-up desk at work for a few years now, ever since a study found that the more hours you sit each day, the higher your likelihood of dying an early death. Yes, standing burns more calories than sitting. Equally important, it'll reverse the hunched-over Neanderthal posture that desk jockeys develop over time. Another good option, if you don't mind looking silly, is a Swiss ball, one of those big blown-up beach-ball-looking gadgets you see at the gym. Sit on the ball instead of your chair for a few minutes every day and you'll strengthen your core, which will help you reduce your risk of lower-back problems, says Nicholas A. DiNubile, M.D., a clinical assistant professor of orthopedic surgery at the Hospital of the University of Pennsylvania in Philadelphia.

3 Stretch and strengthen your hammies and glutes.

If you try nothing else in this chapter, do these two exercises to stay limber and prevent pain: the standing hamstring stretch and the hip raise. Keeping your hamstrings flexible and your glutes strong is critical to avoiding lower-back pain. Plus, since your glutes are the largest muscle group in your body, building them up will help you burn more calories (and provide pelvic stability to improve your posture). See the instructions for each of these moves below. Do them twice a day—in the morning, at work, or while watching television. Hold the hammie stretch for 15 to 30 seconds and be sure to stretch both legs.

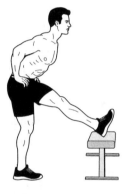

Standing Hamstring Stretch

Rest the heel of your left foot on a bench or chair so your elevated leg is completely straight. Keep your right leg slightly bent. Without rounding your lower back, bend at the hips and lower your chest toward your elevated leg until you feel a comfortable stretch. Hold this stretch for 15 to 30 seconds. Switch legs and repeat. Do 3 sets.

Hip Raise

Lie on your back with your knees bent at 90-degree angles and your feet flat on the floor and hip-width apart. Rest your arms out to your sides, palms up. Tilt your pelvis back so your lower back is flat against the floor, and crunch your abs slightly (a). That's the starting position. Now, push through your heels to raise your hips until your body forms a straight line from your shoulders to your knees. Squeeze your glutes as you raise your hips (b). Pause for 3 to 5 seconds at the top, and then lower your hips to the starting position and repeat. Do 3 sets of 10 reps. To make it harder, do the hip raise with your feet elevated on a bench or Swiss Ball.

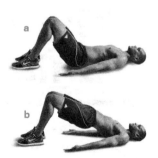

4 **Lift something heavy.**

Each year after around age 30, your muscles start to shrink—if you don't do something about it. The atrophy happens so slowly that you don't notice it at first. Then one day you look down and see your belly where you once saw your feet. This happens because, even if you're just sitting around, your muscles are burning calories. When they atrophy, you burn fewer calories overall. Even if your eating and exercise habits don't change, you're suddenly packing on fat around the middle. Fat burns calories too—but only a third of what muscles burn. Soon you look like the Pillsbury Doughboy. The fix: Strength training 3 days a week can stall the muscle atrophy that comes with aging. And if you want to improve your scores on many of the fitness checks in Chapter 2, weightlifting is your best bet. See the suggestions later on in this chapter and in the DIY Strength projects in Chapter 12.

5 **Be the CEO of your body.**

Treat your fitness like a business by creating clear, measurable goals and implementing a plan to achieve them. Slack off? Then fire your ass! We often, sometimes to a fault, derive our identities from our careers and work. If that's the case, well, then make it work for your fitness. The more closely you associate exercise with your personal identity, the more likely you are to make sweating part of your daily routine, according to a team of U.S. and Canadian scientists. You'll also be less likely to let workouts slide. Would you skip an important meeting? No. Would you not bring work home on the weekend if you had a deadline? No. Would you skip a run because something less important is vying for your time?

The World's Most-Efficient Workout

Trainers like to say the best gym is the one you pass by every day. Even better: the gym you live in. You can pack on some serious muscle and build real strength at home using very little equipment in a small space. All you need is an hour or so per week.

Muscles respond to just about any training, as long as it's hard and isn't the same routine you've been doing since 1987. When it comes to building strength, how often you work a muscle is just as important as how hard you work it, according to research in the *Journal of Strength and Conditioning Research.* You need about 10 to 15 sets per muscle group per week to see results. In other words, you should aim for three total-body workouts a week, and during each one, complete 3 to 5 sets per muscle group.

That's why I love the 4-week get-back-in-shape "density" program developed by trainer and longtime *Men's Health* contributor David Jack. With density training, you condense the amount of work you do into a fixed amount of time instead of, say, counting reps and sets. That way you can keep workouts short—20 to 30 minutes. And as you progress, you'll naturally increase your sets and reps, be able to use more weight, and perform more challenging exercises. In other words, it's impossible to plateau.

Jack's workout on the following pages is efficient and effective—perfect for the busy guy with a spare tire to lose. All four moves—pushup, reverse lunge and press, inverted row, and squat—hit nearly every muscle in your body. When you perform a row, for example, you engage the latissimus dorsi (or lats), the largest muscles of your back. But because your lats also attach to your thoracolumbar fascia—a large, diamond-shaped sheet that connects muscles to the spine and pelvis—you also engage other connected muscles, including your gluteus maximus.

The Plan: You'll need only a pair of dumbbells and a bar for inverted rows. Do three density workouts a week for 1 month (12 workouts) with at least 1 day off in between for recovery. Start with the first workout, and every other day move on to the next option. There are three levels of exercise difficulty: basic, advanced, and expert. Perform each workout as a circuit, completing one exercise after another without any rest (unless otherwise indicated).

TRY THIS!

The Single-Best Exercise Secret Ever!

Readers ask me all the time: How can I stay motivated to work out? Simple. Don't do exercises you hate. Pushing your body is hard enough when you enjoy what you're doing. So, if you hate stationary cycling, get off the bike and play tennis. If you can't stand running, join a fitness boot camp class. If you hate bench pressing, do feet-elevated pushups. Another stay-with-it tip: Recruit friends. Research has shown that you're more likely to stick with a workout if you exercise in a group. Sure, it's more fun, but pride and vanity are factors too. British researchers found that people progress quicker because they push themselves harder when working out with others. And, naturally, it's harder to skip the gym at 6 a.m. when you know a buddy is waiting. If your friends are lazy asses, tap social media. In a study in the *Journal of American College Health,* researchers found that logging fitness activity online for others to see inspired as much motivation as regularly working out with a group.

The 4-Week Workout Schedule

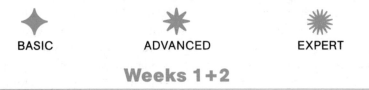

BASIC   ADVANCED   EXPERT

Weeks 1+2

The basic, advanced, and expert exercises start on page 82. Do 5 reps of each exercise, going from move to move without rest. For dumbbell exercises, select a weight that you can lift 10 times. Repeat circuits until the workout time is up.

Workout 1	**Workout 3**	**Workout 5**
Do circuits for 10 minutes.	Do circuits for 10 minutes.	Do circuits for 10 minutes.
Workout 2	**Workout 4**	**Workout 6**
Do circuits for 15 minutes.	Do circuits for 15 minutes.	Do circuits for 15 minutes.

Week 3

Do each exercise for 20 seconds and rest for 10 seconds (that's 1 set).

| **Workout 7** | **Workout 8** | **Workout 9** |
| Do 2 sets. Rest for 1 minute. That's one circuit. Complete two more circuits. | Do 2 sets. Rest for 1 minute. That's one circuit. Complete two more circuits. | Do 2 sets. Rest for 1 minute. That's one circuit. Complete two more circuits. |

Week 4

Do the first exercise for 20 seconds and then rest for 10 seconds. That's 1 set. Complete 4 sets, rest 1 to 2 minutes, then move on to the next exercise. Do that move for 20 seconds, then rest for 10 seconds; do 4 sets, and so on. Don't advance to the more difficult options until you can complete at least 8 reps of each exercise in 20 seconds.

| **Workout 10** | **Workout 11** | **Workout 12** |
| | | Do this final workout using all expert-level exercises. |

The Perfect Total-Body Warmup

Most men (me included) hate stretching before exercise. It's boring. It seems like a waste of time when we're eager to get to the action. And as it turns out, static stretching doesn't improve performance or prevent injury prior to activity, according to Eric Cressey, C.S.C.S., a Massachusetts-based trainer who works with pros and Olympic athletes. "A better approach is dynamic stretching, or what I call mobilization. The key is that you're moving, just like you are during an activity."

Cressey recommends the combo of the four connected movements below to warm up your entire body in just a few seconds. Do 6 reps on each side before every workout. "It increases core temperature, lengthens and loosens tight muscles, and targets the three areas that tend to be most restricted in men—ankles, hips, and the midspine," he says.

STEP 1: Walking High-Knee Hug (stretches your glutes and requires more than 90 degrees of hip flexion, a range of motion that challenges most desk jockeys). Stand with your feet shoulder-width apart, lift your left leg off the floor, and hug your left knee to your chest.

STEP 2: Offset Lunge (stretches your groin and legs). Release your knee, take a long step forward, and lunge deeply until your back leg is close to horizontal, placing the fingertips of both hands on the floor inside your left foot.

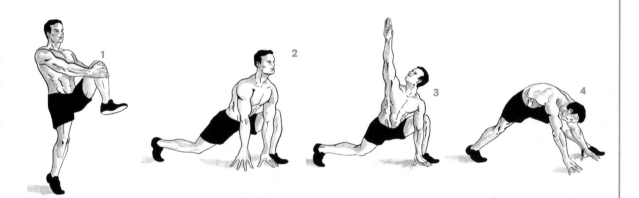

STEP 3: Overhead Reach (targets the middle of your back, stretches your chest, and activates your core). Keep your left fingertips planted as you rotate and reach up with your right hand. Both arms should form a straight line. Bring your right hand back down to the floor so that you're in the Offset Lunge position again.

STEP 4: Hip Lift (stretches your hamstrings). Keeping your hands on the floor, rock your hips back and straighten both legs. Focus on your right leg; straighten it as much as you can to feel your right hamstring stretch. Step forward with your right leg and stand up straight.

Now repeat this four-stretch sequence using the opposite leg and arm for each move. Do a total of 6 reps per side.

The Exercises

Pushup

Pushup

Assume a pushup position with your hands slightly beyond shoulder-width apart, your feet together, and your body in a straight line from head to ankles. Lower your chest until it's an inch above the floor, then push up. That's 1 rep.

Explosive Pushup (shown)

Do a basic pushup, but after lowering your body, push back up with enough force that your hands leave the floor.

Isometric Explosive Pushup

On each rep, hold your body in the down position for 3 seconds before pushing yourself up explosively.

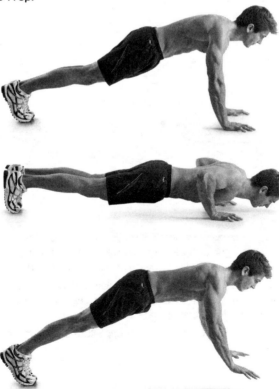

Better INSTANTLY

↓

Postworkout, your body craves a blend of carbs and protein. Chocolate milk is the perfect combination.

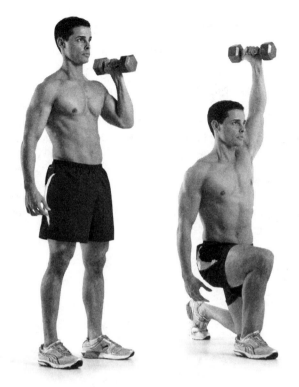

Reverse Lunge and Press

Reverse Lunge and Press (shown)

Stand holding a dumbbell next to your left shoulder. Step back with your left leg. Then press the dumbbell straight above your shoulder. Lower it, and stand back up. Now, with the dumbell in your right hand, repeat with your right leg back and press the dumbbell up. That's 1 rep.

Reverse Lunge with Simultaneous Single-Arm Press

Do a reverse lunge with your left leg while simultaneously pressing the dumbbell in your left hand straight above your shoulder. Stand and then lower the weight. Next, repeat the move with your right leg and arm. That's 1 rep.

Isometric Reverse Lunge and Press

For this exercise, hold a dumbbell in each hand. Do a reverse lunge, but after you lower your body, pause for 3 seconds. Then press both dumbbells above your shoulders. Lower the weights and return to the standing position. Repeat with your other leg. That's 1 rep.

Inverted Row

BASIC	ADVANCED	EXPERT
Inverted Row	**Elevated-Feet Inverted Row (shown)**	**Isometric Elevated-Feet Inverted Row**
Lie underneath a secured bar. Grab the bar with an overhand, shoulder-width grip, your arms and body straight, and your heels on the floor. Pull your body up and then return to the starting position.	Do an inverted row, but first place your heels on a box or bench.	Do an elevated-feet inverted row. But after you pull your chest to the bar, pause for 3 seconds at the highest point. Lower your body and repeat.

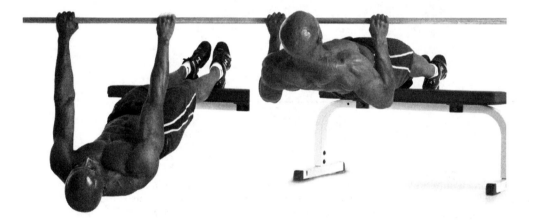

Squat

Prisoner Squat

Place your fingers on the back of your head, pull your elbows and shoulders back, and stand with your feet shoulder-width apart. Lower your body as far as you can. Pause and return to the starting position.

Goblet Squat (shown)

Hold a dumbbell vertically in front of your chest, cupping one end of the dumbbell with both hands. Keep your elbows pointed down toward the floor and do a squat. Then push back up.

Isometric Goblet Squat

Do a goblet squat, but pause for 3 seconds at the lowest point of your squat. Then push back up to the starting position and repeat the move.

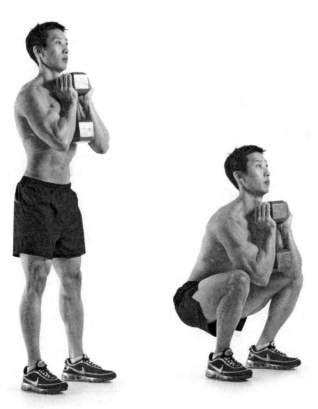

Better INSTANTLY

↓

While watching TV, do something physical during commercials—pushups, squats, even high-knee marching in place. You'll add more than 10 minutes of muscle burn to your day per hour (even more during sporting events).

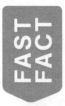
4 Muscle Mistakes to Avoid

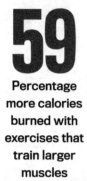
That simple at-home density workout on page 80 will quickly get you back in shape. Gaining muscle and strength is actually quite easy when you start training. "Your muscles go through a learning process, so almost anything you do triggers growth," says Mike Boyle, A.T.C., of Mike Boyle Strength and Conditioning in Woburn, Massachusetts. "But eventually your muscles adapt, and you have to train smarter to see results."

You've no doubt experienced this wall—often called a plateau—where no matter what you do, the progress isn't coming. If you want to keep progressing, you need to challenge your muscles in new and innovative ways. Start by purging your fitness plan of these common pitfalls.

Mistake #1 You don't train your legs

Most guys' workouts are top-heavy. "They focus too much on the mirror muscles—the chest and arms," Boyle says. A sign of true fitness is a muscular backside. "Your largest muscles are in your lower body, and training them releases hormones that build size and strength everywhere else."

TRY THIS: The elevated-back-foot split squat. Hold a bar across your upper back using an overhand grip. Assume a staggered stance, with your left foot forward and your right foot back and on a 6-inch step or box. Lower your body as far as you can and then push back up to the starting position. Do 10 reps, switch legs, and repeat. That's 1 set; do 3.

Mistake #2 You run too much

Logging miles isn't a total waste of time, "but it's close," Boyle says. This is because your body adapts quickly to repetitive movement, and that's running in a nutshell. "Plus, running doesn't activate your fast-twitch muscle fibers," he says, which are great fat burners and body builders.

TRY THIS: Intervals—short bursts of intense activity followed by active rest. Set a treadmill to an 8 percent incline and run for 30 seconds. Then rest for 1 minute. Do this 10 times. This type of training leads to gains in aerobic and anaerobic performance that are significantly greater than with steady-state cardio, according to a recent study in the *Journal of Strength and Conditioning Research.*

Mistake #3 You lift too slowly

Explosive lifting leads to fast gains. Why? "It activates more fast-twitch muscle fibers, which have the greatest growth potential," Boyle says. "So lift like you mean it." You'll also crank up your heart rate, increasing your calorie burn.

TRY THIS: Do the lifting phase of each exercise as fast as possible. The actual speed of the lift doesn't matter. "As long as the movement is explosive," says Boyle, "your body will recruit fast-twitch fibers." Then take at least 2 seconds to lower the weight.

Mistake #4 You stay in your comfort zone

Professional athletes don't sharpen their games by working on their strengths; they also eliminate weaknesses. So should you. "Doing only the moves you're familiar with is a cop-out," Boyle says.

TRY THIS: Do compound exercises (that is, moves that target multiple muscles), like deadlifts, chinups, and dips. "They're some of the toughest ones you can do, and you can't make serious gains without them," Boyle says. Try the deadlift and you'll see what Boyle means. But make it even more effective by using a few simple tweaks. Stand on two 25-pound plates and use a grip that's twice shoulder width. Both variations will increase the range of motion of the exercise, forcing you to perform more total work.

TRY THIS!

Mold Your Results in Foam

A foam roller can help increase your range of motion, which can bolster your form and reduce your risk of injury, say researchers in Canada. When men spent 2 minutes foam-rolling their quads, the scientists found that the men's knees bent nearly 13 percent more afterward. The researchers think foam-rolling warms the connective tissue around the muscle, making it more conducive to stretching. Try rolling your quads, hamstrings, calves, glutes, back, and hips for 2 minutes apiece before your workout, using the moves shown here.

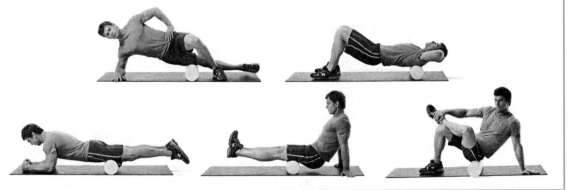

0

**Percentage
increase in your
endurance
capacity after
you consume a
16-ounce
energy drink**
Source: Journal of the
International Society of
Sports Nutrition

Better Workout Results, from Head to Toe

Now that you have a solid strength workout under your belt—and before we get to the goal-specific workouts in the DIY section in Chapter 12—here's a muscle-by-muscle rundown of how to get the best results for every body part. These represent a selection of the best tips and strategies from the top trainers, exercise physiologists, and athletes that we've ever interviewed. Looking to customize your workout for specific results? Start here.

SCULPT BOLDER SHOULDERS. Strong, stable shoulders will help you lift more weight in nearly every upper-body exercise. So start each upper-body workout with the band pull-apart. It trains your rotator cuff and scapular stabilizers, the network of muscles that help create a strong shoulder joint. Keeping your arms straight, use both hands (palms up) to hold a stretch band out in front of your chest. Now squeeze your shoulder blades together and stretch the band out to your sides, without bending or lowering your arms, until it touches your sternum. Reverse the move and repeat. Do 2 or 3 sets of 10 to 15 reps, resting 60 seconds between sets.

BEEF UP YOUR BACK. Most of the fibers in your upper-back muscles are horizontal, which is why rowing exercises work them so well. But the ones in your lats are closer to vertical. The J pull-in hits your lats from start to finish. Attach a rope handle to a high pulley of a cable station. Grab an end with each hand and kneel facing the machine. Keeping your arms straight and your torso upright, pull the rope down toward your groin. (The rope's path of travel should look like a J.) Try 3 sets of 10 reps, resting for 60 seconds between sets.

PUMP UP YOUR PECS. If you're unhappy with your chest development, you may have one of two problems. One possibility: You don't work your chest enough. Sometimes you just need to do more work. Try the $1\frac{1}{2}$-rep bench press, which effectively doubles the workload for your pectoral muscles. On a flat bench, lower the weight to your chest, and then press it halfway up. Lower it again, and then press it up until your arms are straight. Use 70 to 80 percent of your 1-rep max, and perform 3 or 4 sets of 8 reps. Another possibility? Your shoulders are beat-up. Years of dips and bench presses will do that to you. To build your chest and triceps while sparing your shoulders, try the close-grip board press. Duct-tape a pair of foot-long two-by-fours together, creating a square block. Lie on your back at the bench press station, resting the block in the middle of your chest. Grab the bar using an overhand grip, with your thumbs 12 to 15 inches apart. Lift the bar, lower it to the block, come to a dead pause, and then push back to the starting position. You can go heavy: 3 or 4 sets of 6 to 8 reps. The block will prevent the bar from moving too low and hurting your shoulders.

BUILD STAMINA. Remember the squat, curl, push press combo we asked you to do on page 26? To improve your muscular stamina, keep practicing. Perform 2 sets of the drill twice a week, resting 90 seconds between sets. If you can't do at least 16 reps on your first set, lighten the load. Each time, add an extra rep to your first set. Once you reach 20 reps with the lighter weight, grab slightly heavier dumbbells and work your way up to 20 reps again. Continue the slow increase until you can do 20. Here's one way to instantly improve your squat: Press outward against the floor with your feet (but don't actually move them) as you squat. You'll feel your glutes activate, which will boost your power.

ADD TO YOUR ADDUCTORS. You wouldn't be caught dead on the inner-thigh machine. But you also don't want to ignore your adductor muscles, an area of untapped growth potential. Target them by doing pullups while holding a light weight plate between your feet. You'll force your abs and adductors to engage as you work your back, shoulders, and arms.

MAKE YOUR HIPS AGE-LESS. Slip both feet through the center of an elastic exercise band (available at PerformBetter.com). You may need to tighten the band so that, when you slip it around your thighs just above your knees, there's tension when you spread your legs a few inches apart. Now, strike an athletic stand with a slight bend to your knees and your feet hip-width apart. Step to the right with your right foot, stretching the band. Bring your left foot to meet your right. Continue this way for 10 or 20 yards and then come back by stepping to the left. That's 1 rep. Do 6. You'll feel it in your abductors, the muscles on the sides of your hips.

BLAST YOUR BICEPS. To hit all the muscle fibers in your biceps, you need to either lift max weight or lift at max speed. Hint: You're probably doing neither. The next time you do curls, use a weight you think you can lift just 6 or 7 times. Bang your reps out as fast as you can while maintaining good form. That means lifting the weight quickly, lowering it at a normal speed, and immediately starting the next rep. Stop the set when 1 rep is clearly slower than the others. You may pull off 4 or 5 reps on your first set,

TRY THIS!

The Strength Vitamin

A workout in a pill? Maybe. Lack of vitamin D in your system can lead to impaired athletic performance, according to a recent review published in the journal *Nutrients*. Other research shows that men with higher levels of vitamin D tend to have stronger muscles than those with low levels. Odds are that you fall into the latter group; in fact, no less than 77 percent of people in the United States are deficient in vitamin D, according to a National Health and Nutrition Examination Survey. Your goal: 600 IU a day. Fortified milk is a good source. So is the sun.

and fewer on later sets. Rest for 45 seconds between sets, and shoot for 25 reps total.

TRICK OUT YOUR TRICEPS. Try the jackknife pushup. Get in a pushup position, but place your toes on a bench; keep your hands on the floor, thumbs 6 to 12 inches apart, and your body straight. (If you feel the blood rush to your face, you're in the correct position.) Do pushups as fast as you can without rearranging any of your favorite facial features. (That is, don't hit the floor.) Do 5 sets of 10 reps, resting 1 minute between sets.

POWER UP YOUR LEGS. Supercharge any lunge variation by extending your range of motion, making your muscles work harder and grow faster. Two that our experts recommend:

1. *Reverse lunge from step*: Stand with both feet on a 6-inch-high box or step. Take a long step back with your right foot and descend until your knee almost touches the floor. Return to the starting position, and then repeat the move with your left foot. That's 1 rep. Do 3 sets of 10 repetitions.
2. *Bulgarian split squat with front foot elevated*: Place your left foot on a 6-inch step in front of you and your right foot on a bench behind you. Drop straight down until your right knee almost touches the floor. Do all your reps, switch sides, and repeat. Perform 3 sets of 12 repetitions for each leg when using body weight only, or 10 reps when you're holding dumbbells at your sides.

SHIFT YOUR BUTT INTO GEAR. Deadlifts and squats are great for your glutes, but only if you're actually engaging those glutes. If your knees cave in

3 Classic Moves, Improved

Everyone wants to lift more on the classic powerlifts, and nothing beats hard work, of course. But you can also produce big improvements by incorporating even the simplest of tricks.

BARBELL SQUAT: During the move, pull the bar down as if you're trying to snap it in two over your shoulders. This will activate your lats, which provide more spinal stability. You'll move more weight with less risk of injury.

BENCH PRESS: Start with your butt. Clench the bench by contracting your glutes, and keep them contracted throughout your set. You'll find that this tweak solidifies your base and allows you to generate more force on the lift (don't forget to unclench when you're done). Another mind trick: When you bench-press, try to bend the ends of the bar away from you as you press it up. You'll fire more muscles in your upper back, creating a more stable platform on the bench.

DEADLIFT: Find a weight that allows you to do 3 sets of 5 reps. That's right, only 5 reps so you keep your form and go heavy. When you can complete 2 extra repetitions in your last set for two consecutive workouts, move up in weight. Retest your 1-rep max every 2 to 3 months. Here's a gear tip: Lose the shoes and lift in your socks. Shoes increase the distance the bar has to travel. They also lift your heels off the floor, which puts more emphasis on your quads and less on your glutes and hamstrings, where it belongs. If your gym frowns on this, invest in shoes with minimal heel lift. Or find a new gym.

AM I NORMAL?

I feel anxious when I miss a workout.

Normal.

This isn't just normal—it's commendable. "Some anxiety and disappointment over missing a workout is healthy because it encourages us to stick with our goals and to see them to fruition," says Scott Griffiths, Ph.D., a psychologist at the University of Sydney. But the key word is "some" anxiety and disappointment. If skipping a sweat session makes you feel like a failure or causes physical symptoms, such as a racing heart or shortness of breath, then a bigger issue may be at play, says Griffiths. Another red flag: You bail on important events to hit the gym. These reactions could signal an anxiety disorder, says Griffiths. See a professional for cognitive behavioral therapy, which challenges disruptive thinking patterns. Find a psychologist at locator.apa.org.

toward each other, you're doing less with your butt and more with your back. The solution: Grab the floor with your feet, as if you're trying to twist through the outsides of your shoes. That helps you keep your knees out and your glutes working.

SEE YOUR ABS (OR AT LEAST FEEL THEM). Forget crunches and sit-ups. Both create motion around your spine—precisely what your core is designed to resist. To build a chiseled, functional six-pack, do anti-rotation exercises. Here are three favorites:

1. *Single-arm wall push*: Assume a pushup position facing a wall with your hands 2 feet from the baseboard. Place your right hand on the wall and push isometrically for a slow 3-count. Repeat with your left hand. Do 10 reps per side. Too easy? Do a pushup between reps.
2. *Abdominal push press*: Lie on your back with your knees bent and feet on the floor. Lift your right knee so your hip is bent 90 degrees, and press your left palm into your right thigh, near your knee. Now try to lift your thigh to your chest while pushing back with your hand. If you're doing the exercise properly, your core should work to produce a stalemate. Hold for 3 to 5 seconds, switch sides, and repeat until you're sick of it.
3. *Abs prayer*: Stand in an athletic position facing a workout partner. Put your palms together (as if praying) in front of your chest, elbows extended 6 to 10 inches from your body. Have your partner push and pull your hands in all directions, forcing you to adjust. Go for 30 seconds, and switch. You should both feel your mid-body muscles working.

BUILD BIGGER CALVES. Instead of working your calves in isolation, try the bench bridge, which works them in conjunction with your hamstrings and glutes. Lie on your back with the balls of your feet on the edge of a bench and your knees slightly bent. Lift your hips. You should feel it from your calves through your glutes. Lower your hips and repeat the move for as long as you can.

RUN SMARTER INSIDE. Spinning your wheels on a treadmill indoors requires about 16 percent less energy than moving at the same pace outside, report researchers in the *Journal of Strength and Conditioning Research*. When you hit the treadmill, set the incline to 3 percent to mimic outdoor running.

RUN SMARTER OUTSIDE. Running on a shifting surface like beach sand can force you to expend 20 percent more energy than running on grass, according to a study in the *Journal of Science and Medicine in Sport*. The result is more calories burned, because your muscles must work harder to stabilize your body.

RUN SMARTER . . . PERIOD. Take your pick: 5 hours of steady-state cardio or 90 minutes of intervals (alternating sprints with active rest) per week. Both produce similar gains in aerobic capacity (your body's ability to deliver oxygen to working muscles), according to a review in the *Journal of Obesity*.

RACE A FITTER FRIEND. Invite a buddy who's fitter and faster than you to a run or ride. Cyclists competing with an opponent who was slightly speedier pushed hard for 9 minutes longer than those who cycled alone, say researchers at Michigan State University.

FINISH STRONGER, EVERY TIME. Many guys think of strength and cardio as separate entities. But interval training can be beneficial at the end of a resistance workout. That's why many athletes finish their workouts with speedwork. When the last lift is done, hop on a treadmill, rower, or Airdyne bike for 5 to 10 intervals. For each interval, sprint all-out for 30 seconds and recover for 30 seconds, but don't dial it back too much during the recovery. If you're at home, here's a great finisher: Do a single kettlebell swing, then 10 goblet squats. Next, do 2 swings and 9 squats. Keep going until you hit 10 swings and 1 squat.

COUNTER-INTELLIGENCE

Make Recovery a Priority

Giving your body a day of rest between intense workouts is a start, but you'll enjoy even greater gains if you treat recovery as an actual goal. Dedicate an hour each week to recovery activities, such as foam-rolling, massage, or yoga, all of which can ease tight muscles and break up scar tissue, accelerating repair and growth. Between sets, do fillers—low-intensity exercises that enhance mobility and reduce injury risk. Focus on problem areas with moves that hit different muscles than the primary exercise. Do body-weight squats between sets of bench presses, for example, or mountain climbers between sets of chinups. You'll fire up sleeping muscles, loosen tight ones, and move more smoothly.

YOUR BODY, DISSECTED

BY T.E. HOLT, M.D.

What really happens when I get a second wind during a run?

Nobody knows. (Isn't that great?) There are theories, however. One has to do with the ways we power our muscles. Ordinarily, fat and glucose fuel your muscles in a process that requires oxygen. If your energy demands outstrip your oxygen supply, your body falls back on a much less efficient anaerobic process. The second wind may happen when your oxygen intake catches up with demand. That shift to aerobic metabolism is like stomping on a gas pedal. Another theory suggests that a release of endorphins is behind your second wind. These opioid compounds are produced by your body to overcome the pain and shortness of breath that might otherwise slow you down. I like the endorphins theory because it accounts for the euphoria, or "runner's high," that accompanies the second wind, as well as the sensation of recovering your "wind." In the long run, though, the cause may not matter: There's no way to increase the effect.

Weight Loss Made Simple

If losing weight is one of your motivations to get fit, you need to know about your BMR, TEF, EAT, and NEAT. These acronyms describe the four different components that make up your metabolism—that is, your body's energy expenditure.

BASAL METABOLIC RATE (BMR): This is the number of calories that fuel your body's involuntary functions, like breathing, heartbeat, cell division, and growth. It accounts for up to 70 percent of the calorie expenditure. Your BMR is related to your body mass.

THERMIC EFFECT OF FOOD (TEF): Your body uses a significant number of calories to digest and process the food you eat. The TEF of protein is about 25 percent, which means that a quarter of the calories that this nutrient provides are burned during digestion. The TEF of carbs and fat is about 10 percent and 5 percent, respectively. So you can see how eating several small, protein-rich meals over the course of the day can elevate your metabolism and help you burn more calories.

EXERCISE-ACTIVITY THERMOGENESIS (EAT): This is the energy you use during planned exercise like lifting weights or going for a run. If you've made it this far in the book, you know that not all exercises are created equal.

Those that work the largest muscle groups, like squats, EAT a ton. Isolation exercises, like biceps curls, barely EAT at all.

NONEXERCISE-ACTIVITY THERMOGENESIS (NEAT): This is the amount of energy burned during any incidental muscular movements, like walking upstairs, tapping your foot to music, holding up this book. Doesn't seem like much, but it can really add up. Here's an example of five simple strategies you can infuse into your daily life to instantly—and almost effort-lessly—burn about 10 percent more calories a day:

+ **DO THIS:** Go for a brisk 20-minute walk.
- **NOT THIS:** Sit for your entire lunch hour.
= 49 extra calories burned

+ **DO THIS:** Stand during three 10-minute phone calls
- **NOT THIS:** Put your feet up on your desk.
= 33 extra calories burned

+ **DO THIS:** Play vigorously with your kids or pet for 15 minutes.
- **NOT THIS:** Watch TV before dinner.
= 82 extra calories burned

+ **DO THIS:** Spend 15 minutes washing the dishes.
- **NOT THIS:** Head straight to the couch.
= 27 extra calories burned

+ **DO THIS:** Take 10 minutes to straighten up one room.
- **NOT THIS:** Check your e-mail one last time.
= 21 extra calories burned

Total extra calories burned: 212
Metabolism boost: about 10 percent

For more fitness tips and goal-specific workouts, visit Chapter 12's DIY projects.

Pounds and the Pavement

If you like running, go ahead and hit the trail—but if that's your main weight-loss activity, it's time for a rethink. You should consider mixing some weight-lifting days into your schedule and incorporating lots of explosive exercises into your routine. Fitness-loving guys tend to overestimate their calorie burn and do too much of the same training. To compound the problem, they'll then reward themselves with excessive recovery meals, says Janet Hamilton, M.A., C.S.C.S., an exercise physiologist at Running Strong in Atlanta. If you're sticking to running, Hamilton says it's a matter of mixing things up: "To build your body so it can tolerate longer and harder bouts of exercise—and burn more calories—mix up your training with hard and easy days." Try Hamilton's prescription: Use this weekly calendar to vary your runs, and throw in some yoga and weights, too.

SUNDAY

Hard—6 to 8 miles at a pace where it's easy to converse in sentences

MONDAY

Easy—Yoga, tai chi, or another training activity that speeds muscle recovery

TUESDAY

Hard—4 miles at a pace where you can still converse in sentences; run hills if you like

WEDNESDAY

Easy—2 miles at a recovery effort

THURSDAY

Hard—4 miles; may include up to 1 mile at a 10K-race effort in the middle

FRIDAY

Easy—general strength training with body-weight resistance

SATURDAY

Rest

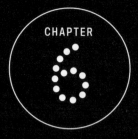

Improve
Your Health
*Take Charge; **Don't Rely on Docs***

Editing *Men's Health* magazine has its perks, besides the endless supply of protein powder. A big one is the healthy, active culture that our corporate parent, Rodale Inc., has created. Rodale also publishes *Runner's World*, *Bicycling*, *Women's Health*, and other wellness-focused magazines. In all, about 800 people work at the company, and the vast majority are health nuts and fitness enthusiasts.

■
Better
INSTANTLY
↓
Quit smoking now and your heart rate and blood pressure will improve within 20 minutes.

You don't have to look very hard to find a good example. In fact, just spend a lunch hour at our headquarters. You'll find the *MH* team at the fitness center or playing basketball at a local gym. The *Runner's World* and *Bicycling* folks never miss their midday run or ride. The cafeteria serves all-organic food. There are more stand-up desks than office fridges.

In other words, my colleagues take full responsibility for their health; they don't rely on a doctor to do it for them. This is probably the most important lesson I've learned at *Men's Health*. Yes, my daily to-do list is always 2 miles long, but no matter how much I have going on, taking care of my health is always near the top. If you rely on your family doc to do it for you, you're going to be disappointed—or dead.

Don't get me wrong: I'm a big fan of doctors. Many have saved my ass over the years. And I have a terrific family doctor. I don't need to have an arrow stuck in my thigh to get an appointment. He actually listens, asks questions, and talks about prevention. But he's also overwhelmed with patients, and even he admits he can't give them all the attention they need.

That means that getting the most from every doctor's visit falls to you. Which is to say: Speak up. Demand more. Today, there are dozens of diagnostic tests that can tip you off to emerging problems long before they need treatment—and early enough for you to reverse them. But many doctors won't recommend these tests unless you have symptoms. They aren't thinking about prevention. They aren't looking for the runaway cement truck (i.e. heart disease or diabetes) that's barreling toward you as you meander through the intersection checking Instagram. They're all about diagnosing and treating, the model they learned in med school.

Here's a real-world example: A few years ago, a colleague of mine who was working on a story about diabetes was curious to know his hemoglobin A_{1c} number. HbA_{1c} is a measure of your blood sugar levels over the previous 3 months. Some doctors believe it's a good indicator of potential longevity because it paints a highly accurate picture of your diabetes risk. Unfortunately, it's rarely used as a routine test in people without obvious risk factors. My colleague insisted on being tested, and it turned out his number was high at 5.9, indicating that he had pre-diabetes and was on the path toward full-blown type 2 diabetes. This fit 52-year-old thought he was doing everything right in exercise and diet. The HbA_{1c} blood test was his wake-up call. Thankfully, and thanks to *Men's Health*, he knew to set the alarm.

Do you know your HbA_{1c} level? I thought not. I don't know mine either, even though diabetes runs through my mom's side of the family. We both should get on that, huh? To improve your health in a meaningful way, you need to become your own best health advocate, and it starts by becoming more knowledgeable about your body and aware of changes in it.

This chapter will help you keep your machine purring all the days of your life.

The Fast Five for Better Health

Simple stuff you can do right now.

1 Check your wallet.

Dig into your pockets and find your last grocery receipt. Was at least half the total for items from the produce department? That's a good indication that you're eating for good health, says Marisa Moore, M.B.A., R.D.N., L.D., a food and nutrition consultant based in Atlanta. What you swallow has the greatest immediate impact on your health, good or bad, outside of smoking or placing the barrel of a gun in your mouth. Keep reminding yourself to eat more plants.

2 Check your gut.

Your waist-to-height ratio is a quick measure of your health. It should be 0.5 or lower. Check it by wrapping a tape measure around your waist halfway between your ribs and your hips. Divide that number by your height in inches. If you are over 0.5, do 3 sets of eight resistance exercises 3 or 4 days a week—see Chapter 5 for some good options.

3 Make a handful of promises to yourself.

→ "I promise to avoid doing stupid things that put me at risk of deadly accidents, one of the biggest killers of men."

→ "I promise to hand the car keys to someone who hasn't been drinking when I've had a few."

→ "I promise to wear my seatbelt and stay off my phone."

→ "I promise to think twice before popping a pill—because a lot of good men (and women) die after inadvertently overdosing on or mixing common medications."

→ "I promise to dive with my arms outstretched when I jump head-first into a pool and to check to make sure the water's deep enough before I do."

4 **Get up, stand up.**
Here's a fitness test that has significant bearing on your health. Sit cross-legged on the floor and then try to stand without using your hands. "Researchers in Brazil found that if you are able to do it, you're six times less likely to die prematurely than if you can't," says *Men's Health* sports medicine advisor Jordan Metzl, M.D., author of *The Exercise Cure.* Why? "Because the better your musculoskeletal fitness, the better your health." Can't do it? Build muscle by starting a regular program of body-weight exercise circuits.

5 **Grab a hammer.**
Find a friend who needs a hand with his deck or putting up drywall or coaching a Little League team. Social involvement is critical for good mental health, says Thomas Joiner, Ph.D., a professor of psychology at Florida State University in Tallahassee who studies causes of depression and suicide. The suicide rate among men ages 35 to 64 rose 27 percent between 1999 and 2010. Joiner says we're experiencing a crisis of connection. "Work and the pursuit of success can be isolating. If you find yourself disengaging socially, take action." Building strong friendships can actually add years to your life. A recent study at Brigham Young University found that the health-protecting effect of having lots of fulfilling relationships is comparable to that of quitting smoking.

Play Doctor

Even if you're a car nut, you wouldn't know if your vehicle's air-fuel mixture was really lean or you had a vacuum leak—until you hooked up your car to a diagnostic code reader. Same goes for your body's fluids, engine, and electrical system. You need to regularly screen for "silent diseases" that often begin small and develop slowly, making them difficult to detect.

Luckily, we live in an era when it's easy to become your own doctor. "Now, for the first time, you can generate your own health-related data," says *Men's Health* cardiology advisor Eric Topol, M.D., the chief academic officer at Scripps Health. There are apps that can measure your blood pressure, heart rate, lung function, brain waves, and eye pressure. Soon you'll be able to do lab tests and have parts of your physical exam administered over your phone,

Their History May Be Your Future

A simple conversation can tell you if a disease may be in your DNA. Find out if any of your immediate relatives had one of the following conditions and then check for your percentage of increased risk.

	FATHER	MOTHER	BROTHER	SISTER	BOTH PARENTS	TESTING TIMETABLE
Heart attack	45%	57%	206%	315%	128%	Have your cholesterol levels checked once a year rather than every 5. Blood pressure checks should be at least every 2 years, or anytime you visit your doctor.
Type 2 diabetes	96%	101%	168%	183%	399%	If you're younger than 45 and have a family history, get tested now, especially if your BMI is 25 or higher. No history? Have your blood sugar tested at age 45.
Stroke	309%	170%	51%	51%	*	The schedule is the same as it is for a heart attack: Have your cholesterol levels tested annually and your blood pressure checked every 2 years.
Colorectal cancer	105%	105%	105%	105%	397%	A family history of colon cancer earns you an early colonoscopy: Go for your first probe at 40 instead of 50. Then it's every 5 years thereafter.
Prostate cancer	78%	–	84%	–	–	If your dad or bro stepped on a gland mine, talk to your doctor about whether you might benefit from a PSA test at age 45.

These numbers represent your increased risk of developing a disease if you have a family history, compared with the risk of the average guy who has no affected relatives.

* Currently no data exist for this scenario, but it's safe to assume that if both parents have had a stroke, you're at a much higher risk.

Sources: BJU International, Circulation, Circulation: Cardiovascular Genetics, Diabetes Care, European Heart Journal, Gastroenterology, Journal of the American College of Cardiology, U.S. Preventive Services Task Force

tablet, or other device. "Pick what you need to manage a condition better and take an active role, or to prevent the condition from happening in your lifetime," says Dr. Topol. "These technologies are inexpensive, portable, and many, if not most, are FDA-approved or -assured that they're accurate and valid."

Becoming Dr. You doesn't mean you have to go it alone. The point is to become your own best health advocate by becoming a partner with your physicians—and by keeping them on point. You accomplish that by doing

SMART ADVICE

FROM *MEN'S HEALTH* CARDIOLOGY ADVISOR **JOHN ELEFTERIADES, M.D.,**
CHIEF OF CARDIOTHORACIC SURGERY AT YALE UNIVERSITY

"I'm a surgeon, so I often see men after a catastrophic event has occurred. It's usually a tear in the aorta that occurs as a result of neglected hypertension. The other thing that happens with long-term neglected hypertension is that the heart muscle enlarges, becoming thick and stiff. That's okay for your biceps, quads, or other muscles that run the body's skeleton, but it's very bad for the heart muscle. It's like this: If a person with normal BP is doing a curl, say with 15 or 20 pounds, then it's like someone with high BP is doing the same thing with 40 or 50 pounds. It puts a great strain on the heart, which becomes thickened, and that makes the heart stiff. It can't accept blood to be pumped forward. To avoid this fate, keep track of your BP. I don't recommend checking your BP 10 times a day. But even for a healthy young man, check it once a month or once every couple of months, especially in the morning after awakening, when it tends to run highest."

your homework, investigating your family history, assessing what might be lurking in your genes, and pressing your doctor to prescribe the right screening tests. On the following pages, we'll look at some of these key tests.

An extra note about being proactive even when you are in perfect health: It's often wise to establish a "baseline" by having these tests so you have solid information you can compare to future results. That's often the only way to identify telling changes in your physiology over time. While it's never fun to be poked, pricked, and scanned (unless you're into that sort of thing), if you skip these tests when you're healthy, you'll need more of them when you're sick.

The Heart Tests

Here are the typical cardiac blood tests and some others that may contribute to a broader assessment of your heart health.

Blood Pressure

You've donned the arm cuff dozens of times, and you should do so every time you see a doctor. Between visits, check your own pressure at a kiosk in a pharmacy or with a home BP monitor. Your blood pressure indicates the force of your circulating blood on the walls of your blood vessels. Systolic, the top number, measures the pressure in the arteries when the heart muscle contracts. (Remember "S" for "sits on top," and it's the pressure when the heart "squeezes.") Diastolic, the bottom number, measures pressure between heartbeats, when the heart muscle is resting. (Think "D" for "down," as in lying down to rest.) Measured in millimeters of mercury, it's read as "118 over 77." A normal BP reading is less than 120 for systolic and less than 80 for diastolic. Prehypertension is anything 120 over 80 to 139 over 89. Untreated, high blood pressure can increase your risk of heart attack, stroke, and other problems. Ask your doctor to measure your BP in both arms. A study from Boston University confirms that having a different blood pressure in each arm is associated with a higher risk of heart problems. Differences of 10 points and up may indicate narrowing arteries.

Cholesterol

You probably know that the total cholesterol blood test—with best results being under 200 milligrams per deciliter (mg/dl)—is a pretty useless way to gauge the health of your heart.

Much more useful are the individual numbers derived from a typical lipid panel. Scientists at Cedars-Sinai Medical Center say you can get the best general estimate of your artery-clogging blood lipids by finding out what's called your non-HDL cholesterol: Subtract your HDL (good) cholesterol number from total cholesterol. Over 130? Nosh like you're Nordic: A European study found that a diet rich in whole grains, berries, and fish reduces non-HDL cholesterol.

In a typical lipid test, you'll also find out your LDL (low-density lipoprotein), the so-called bad cholesterol, and triglycerides, another type of blood fat that puts you at risk for heart disease. Your body turns extra calories and alcohol into these insidious fats and dumps them into your blood. Your triglycerides should be less than 150, and your LDL should be under 100 mg/dl. Even more telling is the size of your LDL particles. The small LDL buggers are most worrisome, because they are more likely to infiltrate the blood vessel walls and trigger the atherosclerosis process. Your HDL, by the way, should be 40 mg/dl or higher. If your HDL is below 35 or your triglycerides are above 250, there's a significant likelihood that your blood contains these small, dense LDL particles. Ask your doctor about a specific test for small, dense LDL.

Homocysteine

Your body is a temple, not the homocysteine chapel. High levels of this amino acid can damage blood vessel walls and cause hardening of the arteries or even blood clots. It's yet another indicator of your risk for heart disease, Alzheimer's disease, and stroke. The buildup of homocysteine can come from too much coffee or not enough B vitamins. Lower yours by eating more folate and foods rich in vitamin B_{12} like salmon and spinach.

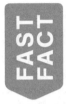

FAST FACT

1 in 9

Number of American men brought to their knees at least once in their life by the pain of kidney stones. Here's your defense: Drink 8 to 12 glasses of water a day, reduce sodium intake, limit animal proteins, and get more calcium to reduce a high oxalate level, which creates the stones.
Source: UCLA study

Know Your Numbers

How much dietary fiber are you swallowing a day? Aim for 14 grams for every 1,000 calories you take in. A study in the *American Journal of Clinical Nutrition* found that for every 10 grams of fiber men ate daily, their risk of death from major diseases like diabetes, heart disease, and cancer dropped by 10 percent over 13 years. To get more, add fiber-rich foods like navy beans (19 grams per cup), lentils (16), and artichokes (14) to your diet.

High-Sensitivity C-Reactive Protein

Your liver produces C-reactive protein in response to silent inflammation. Your goal for this blood test: less than 1 milligram per liter. "When someone scores between 1 and 5, it usually indicates inflammation in their coronaries," says Florence Comite, M.D., author of *Keep It Up*, a book about precision medicine. In that case, your doctor may order a CT scan of your arteries to check for plaque and blockages.

Carotid Duplex Ultrasound

Strokes are the fourth leading cause of death in the United States, and this noninvasive 20-minute test could show if you're at risk. This device isn't much different from a pregnancy ultrasound. The technician puts gel on your neck and then rolls a handheld device over your skin that sends high-frequency sound waves to the carotid arteries. The scan provides two views of the arteries in your neck, which can reveal damage from plaque buildup and show how that damage is affecting bloodflow to your brain. Your doctor probably wouldn't order this test unless you have had a stroke or he or she hears an abnormal sound called a bruit through a stethoscope placed over your neck arteries. Still, if you have a family history of stroke or symptoms of heart disease, you may want to consider this test. Eighty percent of all strokes are due to blood clots caused by plaque, and a quarter of the time your first symptom is your last.

EKG or ECG (Electrocardiogram)

A nurse or technician places sticky patches on your chest, arms, and legs and then attaches electrical leads that are connected to a machine that records the electrical activity of your heart. It then diagrams this activity in line tracings of spikes and dips, called waves. You typically don't need an EKG if you are healthy and have no symptoms of heart disease.

Endothelial Function

A noninvasive test, such as the EndoPAT, analyzes the health of the thin lining of your blood vessels (called the endothelium) and the ability of your blood vessels to dilate. Blood vessels that aren't very pliable may be the first observable manifestation of vascular disease. Check for it while you still have an opportunity to protect the lining of blood vessels with diet, exercise, and certain medications. This test is good for anyone who wants concrete evidence of a greater risk for heart disease and the knowledge that he needs to institute changes in his lifestyle.

Exercise Stress Test

By monitoring your heart rate and blood pressure while you exercise on a treadmill, a doctor may be able to identify the presence of a blockage. You'll have this test if you are experiencing any symptoms of heart disease, such as chest pain, shortness of breath, or light-headedness.

256-Slice CT Scan

A computed tomography scan taken after dye is injected into a vein gives detailed 3D images of the heart and arteries. The pictures are much clearer than x-rays and can spot plaque buildup. Some doctors recommend this test if you have a family history of heart disease or if a stress test is inconclusive.

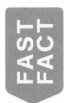

Percentage of American adults with pre-diabetes who aren't aware they have it

Source: Centers for Disease Control and Prevention

The Diabetes Tests

It's estimated that 15.5 million American men have diagnosed or undiagnosed diabetes, a scary statistic because diabetes is a leading cause of all of these horrific problems: blindness, kidney failure, non-traumatic lower-limb amputation, heart disease, and stroke. If you are overweight or have a history of diabetes in your family—or you're simply curious about your blood sugar level—ask your doctor about these tests.

Glucose Tolerance Test

Your fasting glucose tolerance test—a predictor of insulin resistance (pre-diabetes)—should yield a score between 60 and 100 mg/dl. Ask for a baseline and if it's normal, have it checked every couple of years. Improve your number with cardio workouts: A U.K. study demonstrated that 6 weeks of treadmill interval training three or four times a week reduced glucose tolerance in men by 14 mg/dl.

Hemoglobin A$_{1c}$

Whereas the glucose tolerance test measures your body's ability to clear glucose from your blood, this test measures how sugar-coated your blood cells are (never good). Your score should be well below 5.7 percent.

The Cancer Tests

Screening tests can find some types of cancer before they cause symptoms. Generally, when a cancer is caught early, treatment is more effective.

Colonoscopy

This is the gold-standard screening test for colorectal cancer. It can literally save your butt. During the procedure, a doctor checks your colon for suspicious growths using a camera probe that has the ability to clip and remove any precancerous polyps that are found. Don't worry. It's painless, and you're sedated for the probing. The only unpleasant part is the bowel prep beforehand, when you take a laxative to clean your insides so your doctor has a clear view. Those few hours spent running to the bathroom are a small price to pay for a decreased risk of a deadly cancer. A study in the *New England Journal of Medicine* shows that the removal of precancerous polyps during colonoscopy reduces your risk of dying of colon cancer by 53 percent. Everyone should schedule this test by age 50. But if you have a family history of colon cancer, you'll want to have your first a decade before the age when your youngest relative was diagnosed.

Digital Rectal Exam

This test is used to check the health of your prostate. Your doctor inserts a lubed gloved finger in your rectum to feel the size and surface of your prostate, a walnut-size gland that wraps around your urethra. It should feel smooth. Bumps could indicate prostate cancer. An enlarged prostate could be caused by an infection or a common enlargement called benign prostatic hyperplasia. This exam is typically performed yearly during your annual physical exam starting at age 45 for white men and 40 for African American men or any man with a family history of prostate cancer. The test is also used to screen for colorectal cancer using a fecal hidden blood test.

Prostate-Specific Antigen

This blood test used to screen for prostate cancer has become highly controversial. (See "Should You Have the PSA?" on the opposite page.) The test measures your blood level of prostate-specific antigen, a protein made by the prostate, a small sex gland located near the bladder. The test is usually done every 1 or 2 years beginning at age 50. African American men and men with a family history of prostate cancer may wish to begin screening earlier, at age 40. It's normal for the PSA level to rise as a man ages, so knowing your baseline makes it easier to spot trends. A high PSA level can indicate cancer

■
Better
INSTANTLY
↓
Keep your nose running. When your nasal passages become dry, their natural ability to repel viruses becomes less effective. Keep them moist by spritzing your nose four times a day with a saline spray or gel.

Should You Have the PSA?

The prostate-specific antigen blood test is a screening test for prostate cancer, but it is extremely controversial. Some experts believe the PSA isn't useful and can actually do more harm because of false positive results that may lead to painful, unnecessary biopsies and even unnecessary surgeries. But if you skip it, you'll have no way of knowing if there's aggressive cancer in your prostate until it's too late. What should you do? "While many men risk being overdiagnosed and overtreated, PSA testing can undeniably save lives," says *Men's Health* urology advisor Judd Moul, M.D., director of the Duke Prostate Center at Duke University. "I'm in favor of having a baseline PSA. You get a lot of information by getting a baseline value in a younger man. A baseline PSA can be a useful tool for active surveillance (sometimes called watchful waiting), which can be employed to avoid active treatment and involves additional PSA tests over time to see if the numbers increase dramatically. This monitoring concept recognizes that not all prostate cancers need to be treated," says Dr. Moul. Here's how to make the best of a flawed test.

GET A BASELINE. Ask your doctor for a baseline PSA blood test at age 40, so when you are tested again (usually at age 45), you doctor can observe whether your levels have risen, and, if so, how quickly. This is known as your PSA velocity. The greater the velocity over the course of several follow-up PSA tests, the more likely it is that you have not only prostate cancer, but an aggressive cancer.

RULE OUT IMPOSTERS. Only one of four men with an elevated PSA level of 4 to 10 actually has the disease. So if your score falls in that range, be sure your doctor eliminates other possible PSA-boosting culprits, such as benign prostate enlargement, infection, or trauma.

CONSIDER RISK FACTORS. Race, age, and family history of prostate cancer can all play a role in your risk. African Americans' prostate cancer rates are nearly 60 percent higher than those of Caucasians; Asian Americans have among the lowest rates. Between ages 40 and 60, your odds of developing it are 1 in 40; if your father or brother has had a prostate tumor, your risk doubles.

SCHEDULE THAT "OTHER" TEST. While the digital rectal exam (DRE) is a little unpleasant, combining that test with the PSA boosts the accuracy of screening. Consider scheduling a DRE with an experienced urologist if your PSA velocity is high and you've ruled out noncancer causes.

in the gland, but not always. Sometimes, the cause is prostatitis or a natural enlargement of the gland called benign prostatic hyperplasia.

Testicular Self-Exam

Do this one monthly in the shower. Hold one testicle between your thumbs and fingers of both hands, rolling it gently between your fingers. Feel for hard lumps, smooth rounded bumps, or any change in shape. Next, do the other testicle. Note that one testicle is typically larger than the other and hangs lower. If you feel something, don't freak: The epididymis, a small, coiled tube on the upper or middle outer side of the testicle, can feel like a suspicious bump. If you're concerned, see your doctor.

The Bone and Muscle Tests

Osteoporosis doesn't only affect women; men can develop weak, brittle bones, too. Check your bone mineral density and the vitamin that supports it.

DEXA Scan

This noninvasive procedure can do two things: check your bone density to determine your risk for osteoporosis (brittle bones) and compute your body fat percentage and muscle weight (collectively called your body composition). It's not typically given to men until age 70, but you may want to ask your doctor to send you for one (few family docs have a scanning machine) in midlife for an accurate picture of your body fat percentage. Knowing this can be valuable motivation to lose weight and get fit: It's often much higher than most guys realize. Body fat scales, which measure the echoes of electrical impulses, are not particularly accurate. However, they're a useful way to spot trends.

Vitamin D

Known as the sunshine vitamin, vitamin D is produced by the body in response to the skin being exposed to sunlight. We also get it from some foods, including fortified dairy and grain products. Vitamin D is important for strong bones and muscles, and new research suggests it protects you from obesity, dementia, certain cancers, cardiovascular disease, and even erectile dysfunction. Unfortunately, many of us are deficient. A simple blood test can determine your level—normal is between 25 and 80 ng/ml (nanograms per milliliter). If you're low, a vitamin D_3 supplement can help; the Endocrine Society recommends 1,500 to 2,000 IU of vitamin D. But first, try to boost your vitamin D with these foods:

FATTY FISH. You can do better than bland white fish like flounder: Fatty varieties, such as salmon and mackerel, contain up to four times the vitamin D of lean fish. What's more, these oily options also offer higher levels of omega-3 fatty acids—and omega-3s act in concert with vitamin D to promote weight loss and inhibit cancer-cell growth. "Of course you get the added benefit of appetite-suppressing protein, too," says Chris Mohr, Ph.D., R.D., a consulting sports nutritionist for the Cincinnati Bengals. Pick wild rather than farm-raised salmon. A Boston University study found that farmed salmon has just 25 percent of the D of its wild cousins. Wild salmon derive their D from eating nutrient-rich plankton; farmed fish eat feed pellets, which are low in D.

DAIRY. Most milk products boast calcium as well as vitamin D, and you've already read about how calcium helps reduce levels of fat-storage hormones. Dairy is also rich in the amino acid leucine, which helps stimulate muscle growth and fat burning. The D and leucine may be why dairy sources of calcium are twice as effective as calcium supplements at promoting weight loss, says Michael B. Zemel, Ph.D. Choose D-fortified dairy products. All milk is fortified with 100 IU of vitamin D per serving, but yogurt and other dairy foods are hit or miss. Some yogurt brands are fortified with as much as 30 percent of the daily value per 6-ounce serving, while others aren't fortified at all. This is also true of cereal, orange juice, and other fortified foods. Check labels to make the best choices.

EGGS. Like fatty fish, eggs contain omega-3s and protein as well as vitamin D. Small wonder that eating an egg at breakfast while reducing calories can improve weight loss by 65 percent and reduce appetite throughout the day, according to two Saint Louis University studies. Pick omega-enriched eggs, not conventional eggs. Eggland's Best eggs, for example, are higher in omega-3s and also contain double the D.

The Hormone Tests

Made by your endocrine glands, hormones are chemical messengers that influence your muscle growth, metabolism, immune system, and other critical body functions.

Total Testosterone and Free Testosterone

Symptoms of low T include a drop in sex drive, a reduction in erectile function, decreased muscle size, and fatigue. If you have these, talk to your doctor about T testing.

Low T won't just make you fat and limp. Italian scientists say it may boost your risk of an early death. You need 300 to 1,000 nanograms per deciliter (ng/dl) of total testosterone and 9 to 30 ng/dl of free testosterone. If you're low *and* you have symptoms, talk to your doctor about testosterone replacement therapy. Options include gels (applied daily), biweekly injections, or implantable pellets that last 3 to 6 months.

DHEA

This pro-hormone is like a trainer for your T. You need DHEA to make testosterone. If your DHEA falls below 250 micrograms per deciliter (mcg/dl), your M.D. may prescribe supplements.

AGE	NORMAL DHEA RANGE
20s	280–640 mcg/dl
30s	120–520 mcg/dl
40s	95–430 mcg/dl

Thyroid-Stimulating Hormone, Free T3, and Free T4

Next to your gonads, your most important hormone factory is your thyroid, which regulates metabolism. When your thyroid sputters, a range of problems results: low libido, weight gain, fatigue. The problem could be with the thyroid itself—producing too much or too little T3 (triiodothyronine) or T4 (thyroxine)—or with the pituitary gland, which releases the thyroid-stimulating hormone (TSH) that tells the thyroid to get it in gear. These hormonal imbalances could lead to hypothyroidism (a sluggish thyroid) or hyperthyroidism (a Richard Simmons thyroid). Both can be controlled with medication. If you're out of range—2.3 to 4.2 picograms per milliliter for T3, 0.8 to 1.8 ng/dl for T4, and 0.4 to 4.0 milli–international units per liter for TSH—see an endocrinologist to determine why. Inherited defects and auto-immune disorders are common causes.

Stay Young Longer

Diagnostic tests can give you a snapshot of what's happening in your body right now, and genetic tests can tell you what to watch out for in the future. But we don't need either to get a good sense of what the future will likely bring. We know what happens to the human body. Aging slows the heartbeat, erodes the brain, dulls the skin, and steals our muscle. Just look at your parents, uncles and aunts, and their friends. What you see is typical, but it's not necessarily inevitable. You can fight back. You can slow the clock—and live more like a seagull—by understanding what happens as you get older and by using proven strategies to keep critical body parts young.

So, let's take a peek inside your body and examine what happens as you age by comparing typical young parts to typical old parts in some key areas like your arteries, your brain, your face, and your muscles. Remember, this little exercise isn't designed to bum you out, but to empower you to be . . . what? That's right: a better man!

Your Heart and Arteries

Your heart beats more slowly and becomes less efficient with age, both of which will kill your basketball game but probably not you. The real danger is reduced bloodflow in the pipes (coronary arteries) that supply your heart with fuel. "Fatty streaks often start to develop in childhood," says John Elefteriades, M.D., chief of cardiothoracic surgery at Yale University. As you age, the lining of your arteries deteriorates, making them more prone to inflammation and the buildup of plaque, which restricts bloodflow.

KEEP THEM YOUNG: You don't smoke, do you? Good. Smoking wreaks havoc on the lining of your arteries. To avoid deterioration that comes with aging, increase the intensity of your exercise. According to a study in the *Journal of the American College of Cardiology*, high-intensity interval training (HIIT) may prevent declines in the condition of the protective lining of your arteries. What's a good HIIT workout look like? Try this: Do four 4-minute intervals of running, cycling, or rowing at 85 percent of your maximum heart rate, with 3 minutes of gentle-paced exercise in between. Do it three times a week. Another strategy that'll help keep your arteries pliable is stretching your muscles. A study in the *American Journal of Physiology* shows a correlation between a person's ability to touch his toes and the health of his arteries. Try incorporating the total-body stretch on page 81 into your daily routine.

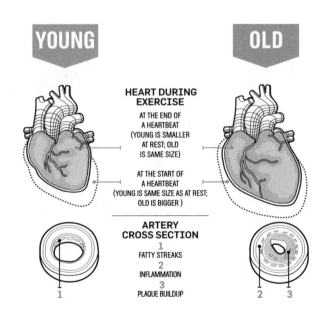

During exercise, the young heart is smaller between beats (at rest); the older heart stays the same size at the end of a heartbeat. As you grow older, arteries progressively deteriorate, as shown above.

Starting in your 40s, the prefrontal cortex begins losing its ability to share messages among neurons. Also, myelin, the stuff that boosts the conductivity of your wiring, starts to deteriorate, says George Bartzokis, M.D., a professor of neurology at UCLA. In addition, the hippocampus—the part of your brain that forms and stores memories—begins to shrink. By the time you reach your 50s, the white matter, the wiring that connects the different parts of the brain, shows signs of eroding. High blood pressure and high cholesterol speed this breakdown.

KEEP IT YOUNG: You can reduce age-related declines in everyday functions by engaging in cognitively demanding tasks twice a week for at least an hour, a National Institute on Aging study found. The exercises have to be challenging, at the level of learning a foreign language. Hey, why not learn a foreign language? You can also strengthen your memory with aerobic exercise. Researchers at the University of Illinois at Urbana-Champaign say getting an hour of sweat-breaking exercise 3 days a week can increase hippocampal volume and improve spatial memory. In addition to staying fit, boost your diet with foods rich in omega-3 fatty acids, such as cold-water fish, and antioxidants.

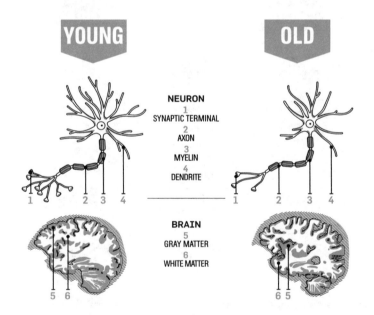

As you age, dendrites retract and myelin deteriorates, slowing speed of transmission of nerve signals. While the effect on gray matter from white matter changes are poorly understood, researchers say a healthy diet and exercise slow the erosion.

Your Face

Look at a snapshot of yourself 5 years ago. Compare it to what you see in the mirror. Your dermis doesn't lie. Even if you just tan and don't burn, the sun's ultraviolet rays have penetrated your skin and begun breaking down its scaffolding of collagen and elastin. This eventually leads to wrinkles, if they aren't there already. What's more, around age 35, your rate of cell renewal naturally slows, making your skin appear dull.

KEEP IT YOUNG: It's all about blocking and tackling. First, block the sun. Use a sunscreen that protects against UVA and UVB rays and contains either a block like titanium dioxide or zinc oxide or the ingredient Mexoryl or avobenzone, says Deborah S. Sarnoff, M.D., clinical professor of dermatology at New York University School of Medicine in New York City. Apply an SPF 15 moisturizer daily, and slather on SPF 30 sunscreen before you go outside. Then tackle the dead skin cells at night. Use a gentle exfoliant to slough off dullness and add a light moisturizer for a cleaner, younger appearance. Oh, one more thing: Stop squinting. Habitually making the same facial expressions eventually imprints fine lines on your face, says Dr. Sarnoff. For instance, chronic squinting overworks the orbicularis oculi muscles around your eyes, causing crow's-feet. That's why sunglasses are critical—they prevent squinting and protect your eyes.

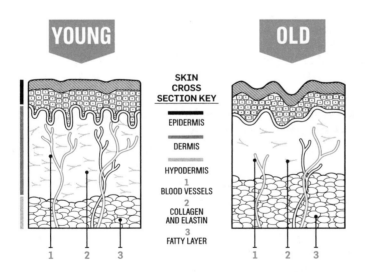

A thicker dermis layer full of collagen and elastin keeps skin smooth and youthful. In the "old" diagram, you can see how the epidermis changes as the fatty hypodermis layer grows and blood vessels shrink.

Scan Your Skin

Be your own dermatologist. If you see a new mole, give yourself the alphabet exam.

→ Is it **A**symmetrical?
→ Is the **B**order irregular?
→ Is there any **C**olor variation?
→ Is it larger than 6 millimeters (¼ inch) in **D**iameter?
→ Is it **E**volving?

One "yes" and you need to see a real dermatologist, stat. However, a "no" on all of them doesn't necessarily mean you're safe, so answer these follow-up questions.

→ Is it inflamed? The skin around the mole may look red and/or feel warm. Your body can develop an immune reaction to abnormal pigment cells. White blood cells flock to the area and release inflammatory chemicals to fight off invaders.
→ Does it itch? This is another side effect of an immune reaction. The scratchy sensation will be local, as it is with a bug bite.
→ Is it oozing? That's a possible sign of later-stage melanoma. Cancers need blood to grow, and if a tumor's growth outstrips its blood supply, the surface of your skin can break down. Puslike liquid, and possibly blood, seeps out and may cause crusting.
→ Are you suspicious? If you're concerned about a mole, symptoms aside, request a biopsy.

Your Muscles

Most men lose 5 to 10 pounds of muscle between ages 30 and 50. "Decreased testosterone and growth hormone precipitate this loss, and inactivity and poor nutrition speed it up," says William Evans, Ph.D., an adjunct professor of geriatrics at Duke University. On the opposite page, you'll see a picture of what muscle looks like in youth and old age.

KEEP THEM YOUNG. There are two key components to building and preserving muscle mass as you age. One is gained in the gym, the other in the kitchen.

GYM: Continuing to do weight-bearing exercise is crucial as you get older. Any of the strength-building workouts in this book will help you to build age-defying muscle.

KITCHEN: After you've stressed and damaged your muscle fibers with exercise, you need to rebuild them to be bigger and stronger. That means eating protein, and a lot of it, for the amino acids needed to repair and rebuild muscle fibers. This process is known as protein synthesis. Here's an easy rule of thumb: Eat 1 gram of protein a day for every pound of your target weight, says Alan Aragon, M.S., a *Men's Health* nutrition advisor. "So if you're a soft 200 pounds but want to be a hard 180, eat 180 grams," he says. Consume about a quarter of that in both your pre- and post-exercise snacks or meals. A chicken breast or 2 scoops of protein powder deliver about 45 grams of protein. Also, be sure that you consume enough potassium as you get older. Well known for its blood-pressure-regulating ability, potassium appears to be a critical nutrient for maintaining muscle mass. Researchers at Tufts University found that people older than 65 who consumed 5,000 milligrams of potassium a day had nearly 4 pounds more muscle than those who took in half that. Go-to sources: spinach, sweet potatoes, and lima beans. Each contains close to 1,000 milligrams per cup.

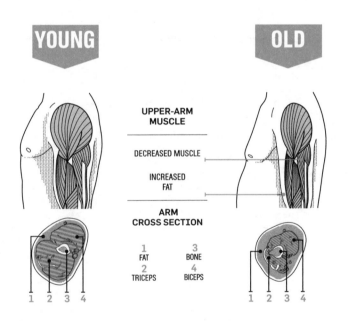

Which body would you rather have? The "old" illustration shows the results of "sarcopenia," the slow muscle loss that begins around age 30. Fortunately, the remedy for sarcopenia is easy: strength training.

Beat the Grin Reaper

To keep your teeth healthy for a lifetime, you need to do more than brush and floss twice a day. You have to do them both correctly, starting with the string. Flossing before you brush will lessen the chance that you'll skip this part and ensure that whatever flotsam is stirred up doesn't stay in your mouth, says David Kim, D.D.S., D.M.Sc., an associate professor at the Harvard School of Dental Medicine. Also, after flossing first, the fluoride from your toothpaste is more likely to reach the areas between your teeth, where it can help fight the bacteria that cause cavities.

FLOSS

1. Use about 18 inches of floss. Wind most of it around the middle finger of one hand and the rest around the same finger of the other hand.
2. Hold the floss taut between your thumbs and forefingers. Guide it between your teeth with a gentle rubbing motion. Don't snap it down quickly.
3. When floss reaches the gumline, curve it against the tooth in a C shape. Gently slide it into the space between the gum and the tooth, moving the floss away from the gum with up-and-down motions.

Repeat on each tooth, including the back of the last tooth. Periodically wind clean floss off one finger and take up dirty floss with the other.

BRUSH

1. Hold a soft-bristled toothbrush at a 45-degree angle against your gums.
2. Brush back and forth gently in short (toothwide) strokes, four or five times per surface.
3. Brush the outer, inner, and chewing surfaces of all teeth.
4. For the inside surfaces of the front teeth, move up and down gently with the tip of the brush.
5. Brush your tongue and gums to scrape away odor-causing bacteria.

Survive the Biggest Man Killers

We spent some quality time on strategies for self-preservation. After all, preventing disease is always preferable to treating it. And prevention will only get easier: Over the next decade, the emerging science of precision medicine will spot health problems earlier than ever, when lifestyle tweaks and minor medical interventions can keep you operating at 100 percent.

STILL, STUFF WILL HAPPEN. ALL HUMANS BREAK. AND WHEN YOU do, you'll need an all-star health care team to put you back together. That's the focus of the next chapter. But before you turn there, let's take a look at two of the biggest killers of men: heart attack and stroke. In many cases the Grim Reaper announces his heavy-footed approach in advance of swinging his scythe. But you need to be aware enough to hear it and know what actions to take quickly in response. That's the goal of this brief report. You may feel that you've heard this stuff a zillion times. But do you know it? Really? Review these signals so you can recognize them in yourself or in others.

Heart Attack Warning Signs

→ Pressure, fullness, or a squeezing pain in the center of your chest that lasts for more than a few minutes
→ Pain extending beyond your chest to your shoulder, arm, back, or even to your teeth and jaw
→ Increasing episodes of chest pain
→ Prolonged pain in the upper abdomen
→ Shortness of breath
→ Sweating
→ Impending sense of doom
→ Fainting or nausea and vomiting

DO THIS
if you think you're having a heart attack

→ Call 911. You'll get faster treatment at most emergency rooms if you arrive by ambulance, and the paramedics can begin treating you en route. If you don't have access to emergency services, get someone to drive you to a hospital. Don't drive yourself unless it's your only option.
→ Chew an aspirin. While you're waiting for the ambulance, chew and swallow a regular aspirin to speed the blood-thinning medicine to your bloodstream.
→ Get comfortable. Loosen your collar and sit in a comfortable position—often with knees bent—to help yourself breath more easily.

Stroke Warning Signs

→ Sudden numbness or weakness of the face, arm, or leg, especially on one side of the body

→ Sudden confusion, trouble speaking or understanding

→ Sudden trouble seeing with one or both eyes

→ Sudden severe headache with no known cause

→ Sudden trouble walking, dizziness, or loss of balance or coordination

→ An easy way to remember stroke symptoms and your action plan is with the acronym FAST.

FACE. LOOK FOR AN UNEVEN SMILE.

ARM. CHECK IF ONE ARM IS WEAK.

SPEECH. LISTEN FOR SLURRED WORDS.

TIME. CALL 911 AT THE FIRST SIGNS.

DO THIS
if you think you're having a stroke

→ Call 911. Do this immediately. Forty-four percent of stroke victims do not arrive at the hospital in time for doctors to administer clot-busting drugs effectively.

→ Check the time. You'll want to know the time when the first symptoms appeared. A clot-busting drug called tissue plasminogen activator (tPA) can reduce long-term disability for the most common type of stroke, but it has to be given within 3 to 4.5 hours of the onset of symptoms (with certain restrictions).

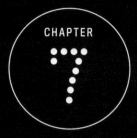
Your All-Star Health Care Team

Draft a Strong Offensive Line

Every Thursday, a bunch of *Men's Health* editors meet at a local gym at lunchtime to play pickup basketball.

Last time I played, one of the guys asked me to make the teams. "Sorry, but I don't need teammates," I told him. "I'll take you all on myself."

Of course that's not what I said, because it'd be stupid to play basketball five-on-one. And yet, that's what most men do with their health—until we have our first holy-shit medical moment. It's time to be more proactive. When it comes to your health and longevity, you're the player–coach. And this chapter will teach you how to draft your fantasy health care team.

Why is this so important? Imagine the following scenario: You blow out your knee. You go to the ER. A bunch of people you've never met work on you and then recommend an orthopedic surgeon to fix you. Sounds par for the course, right? Doesn't make you blink, right?

Would you take your car to a shop without Googling it?

Would you trust your 5-year-old to a preschool without asking around?

Would you dump your aging mother in the first nursing home that put a flyer in her mailbox?

Then why would you trust your health to whomever happens to be on duty in your moment of need?

Maybe you have a terrific primary-care physician; maybe you have no such animal. But the way to protect yourself is to draft a first team of health experts and develop at least rudimentary relationships with these providers—through 3,000-mile oil changes and such—during good times. Then, you'll be familiar with each other when you *really* need them.

Scouting Steps

You don't have to do this all at once, but over the next year or so, recruit your team. Start with a primary-care physician (your utility player for acute medical problems) and a dentist. Then move on to a cardiologist, urologist, ophthalmologist or optometrist, physical therapist, and maybe even massage therapist. Where to begin? Here are four steps to find and evaluate prospects, and what to look for from each specialty health care provider.

CHECK THEIR RECORDS. Visit docfinder.docboard.org/docfinder.html, a website created by the Association of State Medical Board Executive Directors that provides access to records of disciplinary actions and, in some states, malpractice suits brought against physicians (and the settlement amounts, if any). Remember, though, that a malpractice suit doesn't necessarily mean a doctor screwed up. Harvard University researchers recently found that doctors in high-risk specialties—such as urology—are almost guaranteed to face at least one malpractice claim over the course of their career. If your potential provider has shelled out some dough, ask about the amount. A study published in the *New England Journal of Medicine* found that when claims were determined to be the result of medical error, doctors paid out an average of about $522,000, versus only $313,000 for claims that were ruled not to be the physician's fault.

READ ONLINE REVIEWS. For a barometer of a doctor's bedside manner or the amount of time you'll spend in the waiting room, go to RateMDs.com. It has more patient narratives than other sites, and those stories trump numerical ratings for assessing whether a doctor is right for you, says Guodong Gao, Ph.D., associate professor of decision, operations, and information technologies at the University of Maryland in College Park. A doctor's personality and demeanor can be important, since doctors need to communicate well to give good care, Gao says.

LOOK FOR BOARD CERTIFICATION. Check CertificationMatters.org to see if the doctor is board certified. A recent *Archives of Internal Medicine* study showed that certification is a reliable indicator of physician proficiency.

QUIZ A NURSE. "Nurses have a good bead on quality in health care generally, especially in places where they work," says Matthew D. McHugh, Ph.D., R.N., an associate professor of nursing at the University of Pennsylvania in Philadelphia. Ask: Would you go to this provider? Would you want this provider to care for your family?

The First Team

Primary-care physician

WHY: Think of your primary-care physician (PCP) as home base. Establish a regular relationship with someone you trust just like you might with a barber or a car mechanic, suggests *Men's Health* family medicine advisor Ted Epperly, M.D. Anytime you feel sick, your PCP can evaluate your symptoms and refer you to specialists as necessary. In addition, your PCP will screen you for cholesterol problems, hypertension, and other chronic health issues that need attention.

Better INSTANTLY

↓

Stick your arm out your car window. Many local health organizations are offering drive-thru flu shots. Walk-in vaccinations are also available at drugstores. It's quick protection. More than 200,000 Americans are hospitalized each year with complications from the flu, and not all are the elderly.

What to look for

18

Number, in
minutes, of
the average
doctor visit
Source: Medical Care

→ **CONNECTIONS.** Any good PCP is well connected with other health professionals. Make sure your PCP has admitting privileges at one or more good hospitals in your area and strong relationships with specialists. Ideally, your doctors should operate as a tightly knit network, but in reality, PCPs and specialists tend to issue separate orders based on records that aren't shared, says Stephen Schoenbaum, M.D., M.P.H., an advisor at the Josiah Macy Jr. Foundation, a nonprofit that helps train health care professionals. If your doctors are out of sync, your risk of encountering medical error—being prescribed the wrong drug, for example—can be up to two and a half times higher than if your doctors work together, a recent Harvard study found. Seek better-coordinated care from a "certified medical home," suggests Dr. Schoenbaum. (Find one at recognition.ncqa.org.) These facilities emphasize patient-centered care and extended hours. And the extra effort pays off: In a study in the *Annals of Family Medicine*, people who belonged to similar types of practices were significantly less likely to die during a 6-year follow-up period, possibly because of reductions in improper care. No certified medical homes near you? Find a traditional practice that uses electronic medical records, which make it easier to keep all of your doctors on the same page. And don't be shy about insisting that your records be shared.

Cardiologist

WHY: If you wait until you have a heart issue to find a cardiologist, you've waited too long. Men with risk factors for heart disease or a strong family history of heart troubles should establish a relationship now—even if you feel fine and have no symptoms, says *Men's Health* cardiology advisor Prediman Shah, M.D., the Shapell and Webb Family Chair in clinical cardiology at Cedars-Sinai Medical Center in Los Angeles. What do we mean by risk factors? "Men who are smokers, men who are overweight, men who have diabetes, men who use recreational drugs, men who have high cholesterol, and men who have a family history where a brother, a sister, or a parent has had heart disease or an aortic aneurysm," says Dr. Shah. (A study in the *Journal of Clinical Lipidology* shows that people with high LDL cholesterol are more likely to hit their target if they work with a cardiologist than with just a primary-care doc.) At your first visit, your cardiologist will probably run an electrocardiogram to check for heart enlargement or arterial blockages. (It's wise to have a baseline EKG even in your 20s so doctors can spot changes.) He or she may also order other specialized tests, such as a coronary calcium scan, which can detect dangerous deposits on the linings of your arteries.

What to look for

→ **SUBSPECIALTY.** Before you search for a doctor you can trust with all your heart, talk to one you already know: your primary-care physician. Your PCP can tell you the type of cardiologist you need based on your risk factors, explains Stephanie Moore, M.D., F.A.C.C., a cardiologist at the Massachusetts General Hospital Heart Center in Boston. "Some specialize in heart muscle damage while others focus on heart rhythm disturbance," she says. Remember, heart disease isn't one single problem. "Heart disease is a menu [of conditions], and many of those require different approaches to detection," says Dr. Shah. "For example, one form of heart disease is from blockage of the arteries, which may be picked up by a CT scan of the heart. But if you have a problem with a heart valve, you need an echocardiogram. If you have an aneurysm of the aorta, you may need an MRI. If you have a heart muscle disease, you may need an echocardiogram." Once you know the subspecialty, ask your PCP which local doctors have given their past patients the best results, and then confirm that they're certified in their subspecialty by the American Board of Internal Medicine. (Go to CertificationMatters.org.)

→ **CARE COORDINATION.** Zero in on a doctor who takes your insurance (natch) and who is committed to keeping your PCP in the loop. "Care coordination is the most important part of getting the right diagnosis and tests completed when you have multiple doctors," says Dr. Moore.

Urologist

WHY: Urologists handle urinary issues and reproductive issues for men of any age. They're your go-to if you're experiencing erectile dysfunction, premature ejaculation, delayed ejaculation, or penile curvatures, says Larry Lipshultz, M.D., a *Men's Health* urology advisor and professor of urology and chief of male reproductive medicine and surgery at the Baylor College of Medicine in Houston. Or, if you have blood in your urine, you need to see a urologist, stat—this can signal problems from your kidneys down to your penis, and cancer could even be the cause, says Dr. Lipshultz. A urologist can also help you track age-related changes in your prostate, and assess your prostate cancer risk. That's why the American Urological Association recommends that men see a urologist at age 40. "Recently there's been talk about moving it to 50, but as a practitioner, I'm still using 40, especially if you've got risk factors for prostate disease, such as a family history of prostate cancer or if you're African American," says Dr. Lipshultz. "Those are high-risk groups, so those men should definitely start at 40." Finally, consider calling a urologist if you're trying to become a dad but your seed hasn't planted after a year of trying—or maybe even less. "If you're with a woman who's over 35 and her biological clock is winding down or changing, then 6 months is enough time before you start looking into it, because you don't want to miss the opportunity to correct something," says Dr. Lipshultz.

What to look for

→ **EXPERIENCE.** Call the office to find out what your potential doctor specializes in. Some urologists treat mostly urinary issues. Others mostly deal with prostate cancer. Others work with fertility. Others may deal with sexual function or testosterone deficiency. "If you know what your problem is, you want to make sure that the doctor you're going to deals with that particular problem," Dr. Lipshultz says.

Optometrist or ophthalmologist

WHY: First, let's clarify a common source of confusion. Optometrists are not medical doctors. Ophthalmologists are. Find the former if you need glasses or contacts; go to the latter if you're experiencing a change in vision or if you have other worrying symptoms. When either looks into your eyes, they can see your future. Your eyes can be a window to health problems elsewhere in your body, because they give rare direct access to your blood vessels, says Kimberly Cockerham, M.D., F.A.C.S., an adjunct clinical associate professor at Stanford University Medical Center. In fact, an eye exam is an essential (and painless) tool for early disease diagnosis. Diabetes can show up as small areas of bleeding in your retinas, while irregular, narrow blood vessels in your retinas are one of the first signs of high blood pressure, says Dr. Cockerham. In fact, people who had narrow blood vessels in their retinas were 60 percent more likely to develop severe hypertension over the next 10 years than those with wider vessels, according to an Australian study. A gray or white arc around your cornea can also spell trouble. One study in the *American Journal of Ophthalmology* found that people with high LDL (bad) cholesterol were 94 percent more likely to have the telltale arcs around their corneas. Your eye doc will also check your optic nerve. Swelling in your optic nerves can indicate very high blood pressure, a brain tumor, or a brain infection.

What to look for

→ **REFERENCES, RESEARCH.** Ask your primary care physician to recommend several optometrists or ophthalmologists who have specific experience in your particular problem. Then contact your state association of optometrists or ophthalmologists for a list of accredited eye doctors with additional information on specialty and experience. A doctor who participates in medical research and continuing education is likely to be on the cutting edge of diagnosing and treating eye disorders.

Dentist

WHY: You probably spend most of your visit with the dental hygienist, who flosses, brushes, and scrapes plaque off your teeth. But don't discount those precious few minutes you spend with the dentist. He or she is doing more than hunting for cavities. "We look for risks of gum disease, particularly associated with diabetes, and we can see those effects early in many patients," says Mark Wolff, D.D.S., Ph.D. If your tooth doc finds gum disease, he'll probably ask you to come back every 3 months, rather than every 6, so you can clear it up faster. Your dentist will also screen for oral cancer by looking throughout your mouth, including under your tongue, for color changes or lumps. He or she will also feel under your chin and down the front of your neck, searching for lumps and tender spots. Dentists also look at the lips to make sure they're smooth and supple and check minor salivary glands on the inside of the lower lips because low saliva production can be a sign of an autoimmune disease, says Dr. Wolff.

What to look for

→ **DIGITAL X-RAYS.** On the hunt for a new tooth doc? Narrow the field by asking your regular doctor for a recommendation. Who would your GP open wide for? Then call the practice and inquire about the x-ray equipment it uses. Digital x-rays use about half the radiation other systems do.

The Utility Players

Doctors aren't the only people who can guide you down the path to better health. In fact, many doctors are so overworked that they don't have time to get to know you that well. That's why other health care practitioners can be extremely helpful. They can spend more minutes with you, which means they might be able to detect subtle changes over time that a doctor could easily miss. Build a better relationship with these people, and you'll be better off.

Pharmacist

WHY: The person working the Walgreens window does more than just dole out pills—he or she has an expanding arsenal of weapons to help customers diagnose and prevent disease, says Marie Chisholm-Burns, Pharm.D., M.P.H., dean of the college of pharmacy at the University of Tennessee in Memphis. Your doctor prescribed your medication, but your pharmacist knows it best, including whether that weird rash is a side effect or if your headache could be the result of a drug or food interaction. Bottom line: If you ever suspect that something's amiss with a med—be it Rx or OTC—call the expert. Pharmacists have access to drug databases that alert them to interactions and side effects (often discovered after a drug is approved), and they talk to dozens of people who take the same meds you do. To make your pharmacist's job easier, alert him or her to any allergies or sensitivities you have as well as any supplements or nonprescription drugs you take. "I can't tell you how many medication lists I've taken, and people just think about the prescription drugs," Dr. Chisholm-Burns says. Then they'll say, 'Oh yeah, I take this herbal product. I've been taking it for years.' And it turns out it's a problem."

Your pharmacist can also help you figure out how to take your medicines in the smartest way. Say your PCP prescribed you one pill and your urologist prescribed another. Should you take them at the same time, or space them out? What if the drug irritates your stomach? "There are little tricks of the trade," says Dr. Chisholm-Burns. "Take with food. Don't take with food. Those are things that the pharmacist can help with as well." And sometimes medicines say, "use as directed," but your doctor forgot to direct you. Ask your pharmacist. What's more, pharmacists are increasingly playing a role in delivering preventive care. Some pharmacists can check your blood pressure, blood sugar, and testosterone levels (saliva swab), and your prostate function and cholesterol levels (blood tests), according to the American Pharmacists Association. You don't need an appointment, and some screenings are even free, with results given on the spot.

What to look for

→ **SOMEONE WHO TAKES YOUR INSURANCE.** Visit your health insurance company's website to find the pharmacies that are in-network.

→ **PROXIMITY.** Scout out locations close to home and work—you're more likely to make it to a spot close by, says Dr. Chisholm-Burns. A 24-hour pharmacy is ideal for off-hour prescription emergencies.

→ **A TALKER.** Don't be shy—talk to your pharmacist! A good one will take time to answer your questions, no matter how busy things are behind the counter.

■ Better INSTANTLY

↓

For a dry cough, take a remedy containing dextromethorphan, or go natural with a spoonful of honey, which will spur saliva production. For a phlegmy cough take a product that contains an expectorant, which thins mucus.

Massage therapist

WHY: A good rubdown is relaxing, but that's just where the benefits begin. Studies show that massages can relieve neck and back pain, lower your blood pressure, and even boost your immune system. Heck, a deep-tissue massage could even save your hide. "When we have a chance to spend an entire hour touching and observing a person's body, we can see things that aren't right," says Robert Haase, L.M.P., who teaches massage nationwide. Your massage therapist may feel something unusual and refer you to a doctor, and it can turn out to be anything from a sebaceous cyst to a swollen gland to a cancerous tumor, he says. A massage therapist can't replace your dermatologist's mole check, but many are trained to spot problems you can point out to your doctor. "If it's a regular client, we're able to see changes in those moles over time," he says. That's especially beneficial on your back, a spot you may not inspect often enough. The back is the number one area where melanoma pops up on a man's body, according to University of Pennsylvania research.

What to look for

→ **EDUCATION.** Some states have more rigorous licensing requirements than others, so depending on where you live, you might need to do some extra recon, says Haase. "You have to find a therapist who's gone to a good school and knows what they're doing," he says. "All massage therapists are not alike, by any means." If you live in Washington, Florida, or New York, for example, all licensed massage therapists trained in your state should have the training needed to notice larger issues. Otherwise, look for a therapist certified by the National Certification Board for Therapeutic Massage and Bodywork (ncbtmb.org). This guarantees that they have met certain standards of ethics and qualifications, including more hours of education than some states require.

Physical therapist

WHY: Physical therapy may not be on your to-do list, especially if you're fit and healthy, but perhaps it should be. PTs don't just treat people who are injured or recovering from surgery—they also help otherwise healthy folks who just need to increase their fitness level or improve their posture. For those problems, they prescribe exercises and stretches you can do at home. But that's not all PTs do. They can also help you recover from other health problems linked to muscle dysfunction, such as temporomandibular joint dysfunction, a common cause of jaw pain, or pelvic floor weakness, a common cause of urinary problems, says David Kietrys, Ph.D., P.T., O.C.S., an

35

Age when men are most likely to be diagnosed with testicular cancer. Remember to check your stones monthly.

associate professor in the department of rehabilitation and movement sciences at Rutgers University in Newark.

Over the course of your treatment, your PT will spend more time with you than your doctor probably does, and closely scrutinize your body and its movements. That gives him or her the chance to spot not only musculoskeletal problems, but others as well. "Physical therapists are trained to screen patients for medical diseases that might require referral to another health care practitioner, such as a physician," says Kietrys. "Sometimes we pick up things that are kind of coincidental that might require a medical intervention, such as a lesion on the skin or hypertension that needs to be managed. Sometimes there's a scenario where someone comes to the physical therapist thinking that they have mechanical back pain, leg cramps, or some muscle spasm or swelling in their leg that just needs some physical therapy, but the PT realizes they might actually have a more serious disease." For instance, if you have leg pain, your PT may check for signs of deep vein thrombosis, a potentially deadly blood clot.

What to look for

→ **SPECIALIZATION.** Check the American Board of Physical Therapy Specialties (abpts.org) to find PTs in your area with special advanced training. Physical therapists can specialize in fields such as cardiovascular and pulmonary therapy, clinical electrophysiology, orthopedics, and sports. It's a good place to start, although there are plenty of good PTs out there who don't have this advanced training, says Kietrys.

→ **EXPERIENCE.** Call the practice and ask a few key questions. Has a PT on staff treated patients with the problem you're experiencing? (The answer should be yes.) Will you see the same PT for every session so that they can monitor your progress? (The answer should be yes.) How much one-on-one time will you get with your PT during the initial consultation? (The answer should be at least 30 minutes, says Kietrys.) Finally, ask them to explain how they keep up with current practices and the literature in their field. You don't want someone who isn't paying attention to the latest scientific studies and innovations, says Kietrys.

Get Your Money's Worth from Your Next Checkup

COME PREPARED. Anytime you visit a doctor, walk in with a list of all medications and supplements you take, major illnesses or surgeries you've had, and the family health history we mentioned back on page 101. This info will arm any health professional to recommend the best tests, treatments, and interventions for you. Before you go in, search your symptoms on reputable sites, such as cdc.gov (as opposed to randomly typing symptoms into Google), to put your b.s. meter on high alert.

START THE CONVERSATION. According to a study published in *JAMA*, you have a mere 23 seconds to speak before your doctor redirects the conversation. That's a problem, because your doc might miss something important. So start by saying: "I have three things I'd like to discuss with you today," suggests Howard B. Beckman, M.D., coauthor of the *JAMA* study. Start by describing the most important or bothersome question or symptom first. The reason? Doctors are trained to start dissecting the first symptom you bring up.

ASK QUESTIONS. Don't just accept whatever your doctor says—ask for an explanation of your options before you accept a treatment plan. Some doctors may dole out pills too quickly. Prescription numbers have jumped 39 percent from 1999 to 2009, the Kaiser Family Foundation reports. For example, over a 15-year period, the amount of sleeping pill scripts rose 21 times faster than sleeplessness complaints did. "Many doctors just assume you want a prescription," says Leana Wen, M.D., coauthor of *When Doctors Don't Listen*. So explain that you would rather understand your diagnosis first so you can address the underlying cause. Another thing to ask—is there a cheaper version of this drug? If the doctor likes a costly brand-name drug, ask why. Then go to projects.propublica.org/docdollars to see if he or she has taken money from pharmaceutical companies. If he insists on a drug that he has a financial stake in, get a second opinion.

BE TRANSPARENT AND ASK FOR THE REAL DEAL. More than half of doctors say they sugarcoat health predictions, a *Health Affairs* study reveals. What's more, 11 percent admit to lying to patients in the past year. Tell your doc to give you the real lowdown. It also helps if you're honest about your end of the bargain. More than half of Americans don't always take their medications as instructed—even though 87 percent consider them critical to their health, according to the National Council on Patient Information and Education. If you're part of the noncompliant majority, fess up and explain: The pills are too big, you're experiencing unwanted side effects—whatever. Your doctor can switch your medication or tweak your dosage to address any concerns.

COPY HIS NOTES. Reading your doctor's notes can help you stay healthy. Harvard researchers found that people who accessed their doctor's notes after appointments took better care of themselves and were more likely to take meds as prescribed. Physician visits tend to put people on edge, so it's easy to forget key details. At the start of your visit, tell your doctor you'd like a copy of his notes. Hopefully he'll pay attention to his handwriting but don't count on it.

DITCH A RUDE DOC. If your doctor is rude and doesn't want to work with you, book your next appointment elsewhere. If the disrespect was severe, file a report with your state's medical board.

Survive the Hospital

A hospital is supposed to be a place filled with highly educated experts who are there to help you get better, but that's not always the reality. Studies suggest that between 98,000 and as many as 400,000 Americans die every year as a result of medical mistakes, and I'm not talking about a slip of the scalpel. In an emergency, you may have no choice but to go to the closest ER. But for anything else, here's what to do.

PAUSE BEFORE YOU POP THAT PILL. It might be the wrong dose—or the wrong drug. Medication errors can and do kill people. The scariest part: Hospitals hide these mistakes from patients 98 percent of the time, according to a study from Johns Hopkins University. Make sure you have bedside scanning. With this protocol, nurses match bar codes on your ID bracelet to labels on medication bottles. The computer then verifies that the scanned drug is the correct one and that it hasn't expired, which cuts back on mistakes.

CARD YOUR DOCTOR. Doctors in training look the same as doctors in charge. There's no universal way to distinguish med students and residents from staff physicians. In some hospitals, trainees wear shorter white coats than senior docs; other facilities use color-coding to signal rank. This lack of standardization means a resident can easily be mistaken for a staff doctor. So card 'em. Hospitals often list the employee's title on the ID badge, so a quick glance may help establish rank. If you feel uncomfortable being seen by a student or the caregiver's badge displays no clues, it's okay to say: "I've never met you. What's your role on the team taking care of me?" Jot down the name of the attending doctor and consult him or her if you have any concerns. The one time to always request the head honcho: before scheduling surgery. Residents may not be able to clearly outline risks and benefits.

LEARN THE HOSPITAL'S RHYTHMS. The call button isn't a surefire SOS. You see the call light as an emergency flare, but your nurse may see just another blip on an already crowded radar. Heck, you may have time to watch another half-episode of *Judge Judy* before help arrives: A University of Michigan at Flint study of four hospitals found that patients waited for up to 18 minutes for a nurse or another staffer on the floor to respond to a call light. As soon as you arrive, find out when nursing shifts change (some hospitals have 8-hour shifts; others rotate nurses every 12 hours) and when mealtimes begin. Both are peak times for calls, a study in the *Journal of Nursing Care Quality* reports. Then time your nonurgent requests, like bed adjustments, to avoid those periods. You should also ask how to summon the hospital's rapid response team. This crew, which can include a doctor, nurse, respiratory therapist, and pharmacist, is supposed to arrive at your bedside quickly. Rule of thumb: You (or a family member) shouldn't hesitate to call for them if your symptoms or vital signs have changed or you feel that something just isn't right. Still concerned? Seek out a hospital with a wireless call system, where nurses are equipped with devices that immediately notify them of patients' needs.

PICK A FACILITY NURSES FAVOR. You're sharing your nurse with 12 other patients. Nurses are the front line of hospital care. As a result, they usually account for the largest slice of a hospital's labor costs—so when budgets are cut, one nurse may end up caring for more than a handful of patients. The consequences go beyond a long wait for pain meds: Patients on understaffed floors are 2 percent more likely to die when their nurses are overworked, a study in the *New England Journal of Medicine* found. Choose one of 395 "Magnet hospitals"—these are hospitals where nurses rank highly in such categories as quality of care, leadership and education, and a positive working environment. (Find one at nursecredentialing.org/magnet/finda-magnetfacility.) That translates to better care for you: Surgical patients in Magnet hospitals are 14 percent less likely to die, according to a study in *Medical Care.*

CHOOSE YOUR DOCTOR IN ADVANCE. In a true medical emergency, the best ER is the closest ER. Report critical symptoms—trouble breathing, uncontrollable vomiting, a seizure—first so your care isn't inappropriately delayed. For less-urgent attention, such as a gash or broken bone, have a nearby ER already picked out. It should be staffed with board-certified emergency medicine doctors, as well as specialists for any preexisting problems, like heart disease or diabetes. Need a tiebreaker? Choose a facility where you've been treated before so the staff has fast access to your medical records.

ASK YOUR DOCTOR ABOUT HIS HANDS. Your doctor's hands may be filthy. No one expects a hospital to make them sick. Yet 1 in 20 patients develops an infection that can be blamed on lax hospital hygiene, the CDC reports. One major factor: Hospital staff fail to follow hand-washing guidelines 60 percent of the time, a study review in *Infection Control and Hospital Epidemiology* found. Sink visits tended to occur after rather than before patient contact, and physicians were less likely than nurses to lather up. Unless you actually see your doctor scrub up, request that he or she hit the sink or at least apply hand sanitizer. If you're really uncomfortable, try a funny approach: Say, "I know you'll want to wash your hands after touching me—would you mind doing it beforehand too?" And after your doctor obliges, be sure to express your thanks.

If you're having surgery . . .

Remember science class in high school, when the teacher handed you a scalpel and you learned anatomy by dissecting a frog? Don't be the frog. Instead, find out:

→ **HOW MANY OPERATIONS HAS THE DOCTOR PERFORMED?** Studies of gallbladder-removal surgeries have found that physicians don't hit their stride until about the 50th procedure. Studies show that 50 is also the magic number for coronary angioplasties. For knee replacements, it's 65. Coronary angiography? Eighty-two. Anterior cruciate ligament repair? A hundred and twenty. Robotic prostatectomy? Three hundred. Minimally invasive laparoscopic radical prostatectomy? Seven hundred and fifty.

→ **IS YOUR DOCTOR BOARD CERTIFIED?** To be certified by the American Board of Surgery (ABS), a surgeon must complete 5 years of surgical residency training after medical school and pass written and oral ABS exams. Also, as of 2009, the ABS requires completion of a program called Fundamentals of Laparoscopic Surgery (FLS). To check a surgeon's current status, go to home.absurgery.org and click on "Check a Surgeon's Certification." If the certification was granted prior to 2009, find out if the doctor completed the FLS program.

→ **CAN EVERYONE TELL THEIR RIGHT FROM THEIR LEFT?** It's not that easy when a patient is draped for surgery. So take a Sharpie and write "cut here" or "this knee" on the body part to be operated on. Operations on the wrong side have happened. From the time you're admitted to the time you're wheeled into the OR, ask everyone you meet, "What operation am I here for?"

→ **DO YOU HAVE A PAIN PLAN?** Before the surgery, discuss with your nurse or doctor how to manage any pain you may have afterward. Although loading up on narcotics might be tempting, some drugs may slow your brain so much that they knock you out.

If you're hooked up to an IV . . .

It's one of the most common hospital procedures: You're intravenously given medication, fluid, or blood through either a peripheral line in your arm or a central venous catheter below your neck. While infections and complications can occur with both methods, the latter is the riskier one. Roughly 20,000 people die from central-line infections each year, according to the CDC. So ask:

→ **WHAT'S THE HOSPITAL'S INFECTION RATE?** If you're scheduled for a procedure that will require a central line, ask your doctor for the hospital's "rate of central-line infection." Less than 1 in 1,000 is ideal. If it's above three, consider going elsewhere.

→ **WILL ULTRASOUND IMAGING BE USED?** Ultrasound isn't just for seeing infants in utero—it's increasingly being used as an aid for inserting central lines. Instead of having to rely on feel and experience, a doctor can now see the catheter entering the vein, which greatly increases accuracy and safety.

→ **HOW'S THE HYGIENE LEVEL?** Before starting an IV, doctors and nurses should wash their hands and put on gloves (plus a mask in the case of a central line). If they don't have the necessary instruments handy and end up touching other things in the room, they should put on new gloves before touching you. And after disinfecting the injection site, they should not touch it again. This is a common error and a prime reason for infection. Finally, watch for bracelets, watches, and long-sleeved lab coats, all of which can harbor bacteria. Don't hesitate to request that sleeves be rolled up and bling removed.

→ **IS IT IN?** Certain intravenous drugs, as well as some of the contrast agents given for CT scans, can be extremely toxic to soft tissue. Run through two checks: After the IV is in, make sure you see blood in the syringe when the nurse draws back the plunger. And before you receive the medication, fluid, or blood, ask the nurse to run some saline as a test. Now look at the skin around the injection site. Does it appear to be bulging with fluid? If it does, the IV is not in correctly.

→ **IS IT STILL NECESSARY?** Your risk of infection rises with each day you have a central-line catheter in place. So ask every day if the benefits are still outweighing the risk.

If you're in the ER . . .

The emergency department is a bustling place. Make sure you know what's happening for you. Find out:

→ **IS THIS AN ACCREDITED TRAUMA CENTER?** The American College of Surgeons classifies trauma centers from Level I to Level IV. According to the CDC, receiving care at a Level I center lowers your risk of death by 25 percent over facilities that aren't equipped for trauma care. Find (and remember the name of) the best trauma center near you at cdc.gov/traumacare.

→ **IS YOUR WRISTBAND ACCURATE?** Because the pace is so fast in an ER, watch that they don't confuse you with someone else. Check the name and birth date on your wristband. If the hospital also uses other wristbands (to identify allergies or diabetes, for example), be sure they're accurate, too.

→ **ARE ALL THESE TESTS NECESSARY?** Most ER docs take a shotgun approach to diagnostics, and they do a lot of excess imaging with CT scanners. Those machines put out a lot more radiation than traditional x-rays do, and there's increasing concern about that. So always ask why a test has been ordered and if it's absolutely necessary.

→ **IS THIS MEDICATION CORRECT?** One of the most common errors in a busy ER is giving the wrong medicine. Before taking anything, ask: What is this medication? Who is it for? Why am I getting it? They'll probably double-check.

Sleep Better, Wake Up Healthier

Overhaul Your Downtime

I hope this chapter puts you to sleep.

If you are among the 50 million to 70 million Americans who are shuffling around like extras in *The Walking Dead*, you may need to go to bed earlier. Getting high-quality, restorative sleep is critical to good health and longevity. Although scientists still aren't sure exactly why we and millions of other animals sleep, they know what happens when people chronically don't get enough. They get sick.

■
Better
INSTANTLY
↓
Try no caffeine after 3 p.m. and see how you feel at 6 a.m.

Sleep deprivation is detrimental to the immune system. (Isn't it curious that you often catch a cold after taking a red-eye on a business trip or pulling a few all-nighters?) Habitual bad sleep ages your arteries and puts you at increased risk for heart disease. Not enough sleep makes you more likely to nod off behind the wheel just as that cement truck in front of you decides to stop. (See "Accidents" on page 35.)

Seven to eight hours of solid sleep is the gold standard for men. I know: Yawn (see, it's working!), you've heard this all before. Sleep isn't like exercise, where even a little does a body good. You need to be out for an hour before you get into the phase where the good things start to happen. What "good things"? A good night's sleep reboots your life. Deep sleep coincides with the release of growth hormone, which is essential for muscle building. It triggers the body's cells to increase production and proteins to help restore and repair tissue (more muscle building). Solid sleep correlates to positive changes in the structure and organization of the brain, a phenomenon known as brain plasticity, which enhances learning and task performance. A bad night's sleep, in contrast, can leave you foggy and mud-footed. Some guys wear sleep deprivation like a badge of honor. That's a sign of deep-seated stupidity. Over time, it will destroy you. Consider this your wake-up call: Men in a Penn State University study who logged 6 hours a night or less were four times more likely to die of any cause over 14 years than those who slept longer. Lack of sleep can disrupt your metabolism and cognitive function, and also increase your risks of hypertension, obesity, and diabetes.

Even if it doesn't kill you, a lack of sleep can fatten you. Research from Japan shows that night-to-night sleep consistency is crucial for weight control. In the 3-year study, people with the most variation in sleep duration put on weight, while those with more consistent sleep patterns actually lost pounds. Erratic sleep patterns may interfere with appetite-regulating hormones, such as leptin. One study at the University of Colorado showed that people consumed more carbohydrates and 6 percent more calories if they didn't get enough sleep. You never knew watching the Giants on *Monday Night Football* could be even more painful than it already is, did you? TiVo the game and hit the hay. Start with this handful of strategies to improve the quality of your sleep; you'll be a better man in the morning.

The Fast Five for Better Sleep

Simple stuff you can do tonight.

1 Go to bed at the same time every night.

Every. Single. Night. Your sleep clock is like a mechanical timepiece: Without your attention and some discipline, it won't keep accurate time. If you don't sleep soundly, go to bed 15 minutes later the next night, says *Men's Health* sleep medicine advisor W. Christopher Winter, M.D. If you sleep great but feel groggy in the a.m., go to bed 15 minutes earlier. Repeat to find your ideal amount—and then stick to your schedule, even on the weekends. Since you don't have the threat of being late for work, set up a reward for rolling out of bed on time—breakfast at your favorite diner, say. Eventually you'll start waking up earlier on your own. Don't try to catch up on sleep on weekends. You can't. Snoozing late on a Saturday won't erase a lousy week of sleep, according to a Penn State College of Medicine study. Even when sleep-deprived men "caught up" by logging two 10-hour nights of shut-eye, they still struggled on a test of attention and reaction time. So while you may feel more rested after sleeping in, your brain remains bleary.

2 Use your bed for only two things—sleep and sex.

If you need to do work at home, sit at a desk. If you want to watch TV, stand or sit on a chair or a couch. Sleep experts say that you need to program your mind to associate your bed with sleeping. If you think of your bed as a home office and entertainment center, you may have more trouble nodding off at night.

TRY THIS!

Eliminate Dark Under-Eye Circles

Rough night last night? Keep your paws off your peepers. Every time you rub under your eyes, you open up little packets of soft pigment that are deposited into your skin to give it a darker appearance. Plus, rubbing increases pressure in the blood vessels under your eyes, making them more visible. Instead, apply a facial moisturizer with sunscreen to protect the delicate skin under your eyes. If this is a common problem, apply a cream with vitamin C or caffeine instead.

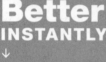
3 Turn out the lights—all of them.

If you fall asleep with the lights on, you won't sleep as soundly. That's because light suppresses your production of melatonin, the hormone that tells your body to snooze. But don't stop there: Block outside light with room-darkening curtains. And switch off your smartphone, tablet, and other light-emitting gadgets 2 hours before bedtime. The shortwave blue light they emit is like kryptonite for melatonin. What's more, e-mailing and checking sports scores will keep you from winding down mentally. Finally, get smart about nightlights. If you need them in your room—say, to guide your way to the toilet—switch to red bulbs. Red light is least likely to suppress sleep-initiating melatonin, an *International Journal of Endocrinology* study found.

4 Don't think too hard.

When your head hits the pillow, resist the urge to run through tomorrow's to-do list. Pick a diversion to ponder—but don't select something that can add stress (thinking about your incorrigible boss, for example). Instead, think of something distracting and fun. Start a train of thought that's open-ended—like mapping out your fantasy itinerary for a 3-week vacation with supermodels.

5 Stay cool.

The ideal room temperature for shut-eye is about 72°F, sleep scientists say. That's because your body clock regulates your core temperature, and its fluctuations tell you when to sleep and when to wake up. If you're too warm, your internal alarm assumes it's time to rise, and sleep becomes fitful. If your bedroom veers from oven to icebox, coat the walls with radiant barrier paint. It's similar to the stuff used in spaceships to insulate and help keep temperatures constant. Or, use a mattress pad that can heat and cool your bed. If you sweat at night, opt for bamboo viscose sheets—they're more absorbent than cotton, say Turkish scientists. They're also the softest sheets in the world.

Silence Your Sleep Saboteurs

A hundred things could mess with a good night's sleep. The following tips will help you stake out your bedroom as sacred ground.

CHECK THE AIR. Fifty percent humidity equals maximum melatonin release, say scientists in Japan. Each day at the same time and in the same spot, gauge the humidity in your bedroom with a hygrometer. Too dry? Use a humidifier that shuts off when the humidity hits a set level. Too damp? Buy a dehumidifier with auto shutoff to avoid overflow.

FIND YOUR IDEAL SLEEP SURFACE. Sealy, Serta, Sleep Number? The truth is that there's no universally perfect mattress. Test different models by lying in your normal sleep position for 15 minutes, ideally with your bedmate. Pick one firm enough to support you but without any pressure points. If you're a side sleeper, narrow the field to soft mattresses, which can help ease pressure on your hips, shoulders, and knees. A back or stomach sleeper needs a medium-firm model for spine support. Next, lie down and check for gaps between your body and the mattress. (There shouldn't be any.) Finally, make sure the store accepts exchanges if sleeping on your new bed turns out to be a nightmare.

THINK PINK. One intruder a security system can't keep out: noise. Squealing brakes or a blaring horn will wake up your brain, so drown out clatter with rhythmic "pink noise," which is thought to synchronize brain waves.

SMART ADVICE

FROM *MEN'S HEALTH* SLEEP ADVISOR **W. CHRISTOPHER WINTER, M.D.,** DIRECTOR OF SLEEP MEDICINE AT MARTHA JEFFERSON HOSPITAL IN CHARLOTTESVILLE, VIRGINIA, AND CONSULTANT TO THE SAN FRANCISCO GIANTS

"Our brains respond to bright light by inhibiting the production of melatonin, a chemical that makes us sleepy. When I'm traveling, I request a hotel room that faces away from the morning sun and is located in the quietest part of the building. I always pack earplugs and a sleeping mask, and I bring duct tape to block out light under doors and around curtains so that the room is pitch black."

You've no doubt heard of "white noise," which is the sound produced when different frequencies are combined. Pink noise is sound in which every octave carries the same perfect consistent frequency. Think of a tree's leaves blowing in the wind or a steady rain on pavement. It's called pink noise because light with the same power spectrum would appear pink. In a Chinese study, 75 percent of participants reported more restful sleep when exposed to pink noise. Check out SimplyNoise.com's free color noise generator.

MOVE THE MUTT. She kicks, snores, and drools—not your honey, but your hound. People sleep worse when their dog is on board, an Austrian study found. To convince Fifi to park it on the floor, flail your limbs and yell when she jumps on the bed. Then give her a treat when she curls up in her own bed.

LAY ON LATEX. It's time to toss that subpar pillow. People in an Australian study who snoozed on feather pillows reported the worst sleep quality. Where did the sound sleepers lay their heads? On latex pillows. If you're staying in a hotel, bring your own pillow to create a sense of home for multiple senses—touch, smell, and sight.

MAKE THE DAYS BRIGHTER. Turn up the lights in your office. In a Harvard study, researchers exposed people to either low or normal light during the day, followed by a few hours of bright light at night. Those exposed to low daytime light were more susceptible to the melatonin-suppressing effects of bright nighttime light. In fact, a Swiss study found that the better illuminated your waking hours are, the more soundly you'll sleep at night. So when

YOUR BODY DISSECTED

BY T.E. HOLT, M.D.

Why do I drool when I sleep?

When you salivate and don't swallow, you drool. Rabid dogs drool. Sleeping people shouldn't, because salivation slows during sleep and reflexive swallowing continues all night long at a rate of about three swallows an hour. (It's triggered by saliva accumulation over special nerves in the back of your mouth.) All of this should keep us from sleep-slobbering, but clearly the system has flaws. Turning your head to the side during the night, for instance, keeps saliva off those nerves, letting it puddle on your pillow instead. Also, people with obstructive sleep apnea (and those who simply snore) have impaired nighttime swallowing reflexes. Finally, smells of food, even if you're only dreaming them, can make you salivate in your sleep. So if you wake up next to a puddle, odds are that (1) you're lying on your side, (2) you're a serious snorer, or (3) somebody's frying bacon in your dreams.

you arrive at work, raise your blinds and replace your bulbs with the "cool white" type (look for 4100K on the label); these bulbs emit light from the blue part of the spectrum, which delays your melatonin production. This advice is even more important if you slog away in a cubicle. Working in a windowless environment can stunt your nighttime sleep, a Northwestern University study found. People who toiled in an office that lacked sunlight slept 47 fewer minutes a night, on average, than those with office windows. Again, researchers believe the lack of light is bad for melatonin production. Spend about a half hour outdoors on your lunch break to take in some natural light.

STAY COOL WHEN NECESSARY. To fall asleep faster on hot nights, rest your head on something cool. Pop your pillowcase into a plastic bag and put it in the freezer 2 hours before you plan to hit the sack. Bonus: Freezing may kill some odor- and acne-causing bacteria lurking on the fabric.

QUASH HEARTBURN. If daytime heartburn is a pain, a midnight attack is a nightmare. Symptoms of gastroesophageal reflux disease, or GERD, occur when the valve between your stomach and esophagus malfunctions, allowing acid to seep past. Some patients wake up choking or coughing, while others don't consciously rouse but still feel drained in the morning. You can also wake up with a bitter taste in your mouth or a sore throat. Beyond avoiding oversize meals and spicy food before bed, try a sleeping wedge to elevate your head a few inches above the rest of your body. When you lie flat, it's easier for acid to creep from your stomach to your esophagus. If you like to sleep on your side, curl up on your left. On your right side, the sphincter between your stomach and esophagus may stay open longer, letting acid flow freely, a study review in the *Archives of Internal Medicine* found.

SEQUESTER YOUR BEDMATE. A limb-flinging, snoring, blanket-stealing partner will undeniably disrupt your sleep, but your bedmate may also be guilty of subtler offenses. Your partner's teeth grinding, frequent bathroom trips, or even body heat can also spoil your slumber. If she tosses and turns, top your mattress with memory foam, which won't shift with her body. If that's too warm, choose a mattress with pocket coils; these aren't tied together, so movement won't create a chain reaction. If she's a kicker, ask her to sleep on her back or stomach. Or consider "sleep vacations," where you sleep apart a few nights a week. If you set the dates in advance, you won't have to feel awkward or guilty (and she may be happy about it).

TRY THE RIGHT MIDNIGHT SNACK. If you're having trouble nodding off at night, maybe you are hungry. A few hours before bedtime, try having a snack containing melatonin or ingredients that trigger the release of the natural sleep-inducing hormone in your brain. Turn the page for some healthy melatonin-rich combos to ignite your sleep cycle and ease your appetite.

■

Better
INSTANTLY
↓

For more satisfying sleep, listen to music in the 60 to 80 beats-per-minute range, which is a close match to your resting heartbeat, say researchers at Case Western Reserve University. Suggestions? Mozart, Jane Monheit, or the Beatles' "I'm So Tired."

→ **TART CHERRIES.** Swirl them into plain Greek yogurt. Tart cherries are one of the best natural sources of melatonin. The yogurt is packed with protein and tryptophan, an amino acid that will lull your nervous system to sleep. Not much for cherry? Try kiwifruit instead. Research from Taiwan reported that eating two kiwis an hour before bed helped people conk out 35 percent faster. Kiwis contain serotonin, a chemical that regulates your sleep cycle.

→ **CHERRY JUICE.** Juices made with cherry concentrate have 10 times more melatonin content than a handful of tart cherries.

→ **A HANDFUL OF ALMONDS, HAZELNUTS, OR WALNUTS.** They're rich in healthy fats and tryptophan, which will trigger sleep-inducing serotonin and melatonin.

QUELL STRESS. Do you wake up in the middle of the night worrying? Warning: This is going to sound like psychotherapy, but it beats most guys' go-to solution (tequila). You need to establish a 15-minute "worry window" during the day. Schedule this block of time for the afternoon or early evening. Whenever a worry pops up throughout the day, promise yourself that you'll deal with it, but only during this pre-assigned time. As you examine the worries, ask yourself: How likely is it that this fill-in-the-blank catastrophe will happen? (Use facts, not your feelings, as evidence.) What would you do if it did happen? By applying a dose of objective reality to both the perceived danger and the possible consequences, you'll find the calm and perspective you need for a good night's rest. If you do wake up during the night, jot down your worries on a piece of paper so you won't forget what you need to address the next day.

COUNTER-INTELLIGENCE

Too Much of a Good Thing?

Sleep is good, but in a study in the journal *Sleep*, men who logged 9 or more hours a night were 43 percent more likely to have heart disease than 7-hour sleepers—regardless of their age, BMI, physical activity, alcohol use, and preexisting diseases. Now, it's possible that you're in the minority of people who naturally need a lot of sleep—and that's fine, as long as you feel refreshed when you wake up. If not, you might have a disorder like sleep apnea or restless legs syndrome, which can fragment sleep and make you snooze longer. If that's the case, see your doctor. Otherwise, use an alarm clock with a light. A timed dose of light can boost a.m. alertness, according to a study in the *Journal of Sleep Research*. When sleepers were exposed to gradually intensifying light in the half hour before waking, they felt more alert than those who were blasted with light when their alarms went off. Gradual light exposure may rev your sympathetic nervous system to help you wake up.

Sign of Trouble
Morning Pit Stains

Snoring is one of the most common symptoms of obstructive sleep apnea, but what if you snooze solo and no one's there to hear you sawing wood? Wake up and check your pits: Nighttime sweating can be a sign of sleep apnea, according to new research from Iceland. People with the sleep disorder were three times as likely as healthy people to report heavy perspiration three or more nights a week. One theory: When your airway is obstructed, you work up a sweat just trying to breathe. Steaming up your pajamas? Seek out a sleep lab that's accredited by the American Academy of Sleep Medicine (sleepeducation.com/find-a-center).

GIVE YOURSELF SOME GOOD AIR. Love those pretty red sunsets in your town? Often they're caused by air pollution, which can seep into your home and keep you awake long after the sun dips below the horizon. According to a study from Harvard, poor air quality can increase your risk of disordered sleep breathing—repeated lapses in respiration during the night. Air pollution increases inflammation, which can make your throat more likely to close, reducing your oxygen levels during sleep, the researchers say. HEPA filters can help, but only if you choose the right one. Standard HEPA filters offer a "minimum efficiency reporting value" (MERV) of 1 to 4. Upgrade to a higher-efficiency MERV 13 filter that also traps tinier particles (which can travel deeper into your lungs). If you have allergies or asthma, consider a GAPA filter, a more powerful type that uses electrostatic energy to attract fine particles.

SAY NO TO NSAIDS. Workout soreness can keep you awake, but so can the painkillers you might pop to relieve it. There's evidence that taking a nighttime dose of a nonsteroidal anti-inflammatory drug (NSAID), such as aspirin or ibuprofen, may suppress the part of your nervous system that releases melatonin. Fight evening aches with acetaminophen (Tylenol), which may have less of an effect on melatonin. Remember: Never take acetaminophen when drinking; it can harm your liver. Next, check your prescription bottles: If taken in the evening, beta-blockers can turn down melatonin production. Some antidepressants such as fluoxetine (Prozac) may also have this effect. If you're often tired during the day, ask your doctor if you can take your meds earlier.

HIT SNOOZE, AND LOSE. A warning for morning zombies: If you need an alarm to wake up in the a.m., you may be at risk for weight gain. In a study from Germany, 69 percent of people reported "social jet lag," a situation in which your daily schedule is at least an hour off your internal body clock. Socially jet-lagged folks were three times as likely to be overweight. Sleep times that don't regularly sync up with your body clock may alter

Wake Up Healthier—And Better Looking, Too!

→ **SHELVE WORK WORRIES.** Turn off your computer and smartphone on schedule. People who stop reading e-mails and checking their phone at a set time each evening sleep better than those who don't put limits in place, according to a Northern Illinois University study. A deadline helps you detach from work psychologically, the researchers say.

→ **DON'T BE ON THE LOSING SIDE.** Try a new position in bed: An Australian review concluded that sleeping on your stomach can increase eye fluid pressure, which can raise glaucoma risk and worsen nearsightedness. Snooze on your back–unless you have sleep apnea. In that case, sleep on your right side, Turkish researchers say.

→ **IRON OUT WRINKLES.** Before you hit the hay, save your face. Apply prescription Retin-A and a vitamin C serum, such as SkinMedica Vitamin C+E Complex, on alternating nights, recommends Ted Lain, M.D., a dermatologist based in Austin, Texas. Why at night? Because sunlight can break down the active ingredients in these skin-improving products.

→ **SKIP THE RINSE CYCLE.** Saliva washes away germs and bathes your teeth in restorative minerals. But as you sleep, you produce less spit, says Marilynn Rothen, M.S., R.D.H., a dentistry researcher at the University of Washington in Seattle. Before bed, brush with fluoride toothpaste. Then spit but don't rinse. You'll leave a protective layer of fluoride.

metabolism, the researchers say. Our advice: Go to bed an hour early tonight and see if you wake up before the alarm sounds.

DON'T IGNORE A SNORE. Sawing logs is no laughing matter. Johns Hopkins University research reveals that snorers are nearly three times as likely as nonsnorers to develop obstructive sleep apnea, in which you stop breathing for brief bouts periodically through the night. Snoring is the vibration of something at the back of your upper airway—your tongue, tonsils, or soft palate—that makes breathing difficult.

Even in the absence of sleep apnea, snoring may raise your risks of heart disease and stroke, say researchers at Henry Ford Hospital in Detroit. Snorers without obstructive sleep apnea were more likely than silent snoozers to have thickened, narrowed carotid arteries, a precursor to atherosclerosis and blood clots. One theory: Your palate vibrates when you snore, inflaming the nearby carotid arteries. If you're a snorer, ask your doctor to refer you for a sleep study.

Obstructive sleep apnea is when your airway isn't just narrowed—it's blocked. This reduces the amount of oxygen you take in overnight. Research shows this can have short-term effects—like making sleep less refreshing so you still feel crappy after seemingly adequate hours of slumber. Plus, as you might imagine, starving your body of oxygen every night can have serious long-term effects. In one study, researchers from the U.K. and Australia who analyzed the MRIs of 60 people with severe sleep apnea found that they had lost about 8 percent of their gray matter in two brain areas, including one critical for motor function. Nighttime oxygen deprivation could be the cause. The good news: In an Italian study, people who used continuous positive airway pressure for 3 months regained lost brain cells. Have a checkup with an otolaryngologist or sleep specialist, who can detect the cause of your snoring and figure out if you have sleep apnea.

In the meantime, practice your "Don't Stop Believin'." Research from Britain suggests that

The Art of the Perfect Nap

A midday doze doesn't make you old. It makes you smart. One City University of New York study found that people who nap have sharper memories. But not just any nap will do: Use our guide to find your sweet spot.

→ **10 MINUTES**
A QUICK FIX: Napping for 10 minutes immediately wards off fatigue and boosts brainpower for at least 2½ hours, an Australian study found. A 5-minute nap? No help.

→ **20 MINUTES**
DELAYED BENEFITS: Doubling down will improve your reaction time and performance on alphanumeric tasks. But not right away—it takes at least 35 minutes to shake off the postnap mental fog from "taking 20."

→ **30 MINUTES**
A HEALTHY BOOST: You'll feel drowsy for about 5 minutes afterward, but then more alert and mentally fit for 90 minutes. Still, a 10-minute nap is better; you avoid the hangover effect of a deeper sleep.

→ **45 TO LESS THAN 90 MINUTES**
NO HELP: During a 45- to less than 90-minute nap, you drift into deep sleep without completing a full sleep cycle. You might feel worse when you wake up than you did before.

→ **90 TO 110 MINUTES**
SIGNS OF TROUBLE: The average person's sleep cycle lasts 90 minutes, the ideal duration for a longer snooze. But habitual long napping may be a sign of a sleep disorder.

And remember this: A nap is most effective when your circadian cycle dips—typically between 2 p.m. and 4 p.m. Napping earlier or later may disrupt your nighttime slumber. It's also more effective if you set the mood. Your brain links certain spaces with certain tasks. So skip the TV-centric couch and hit the bed. Keep the room dark, quiet, and cool, and add a fan to drown out noises. Napping at work? Prepare a postnap to-do list first. That will help you clear your mind and fall asleep more quickly. One more thing: Set an alarm, and when you wake up, hands off that snooze button! Do whatever it takes to get yourself moving: Try some quick exercises, splash some water on your face, or sip a caffeinated drink to wake up. Or, listen to music: A Japanese study found that people who listened to music after a nap were less sleepy than those who didn't tune in. If you're routinely sleepy after your 30-minute naps, you probably need to sleep more at night.

Think Twice about Sleeping Pills

You might think that the solution to sleep problems is easy. Just ask your doctor for a script, right? Wrong. Don't rely on Ambien to put you to bed. In a study from the Scripps Clinic in La Jolla, California, people who took hypnotic sleep aids, such as Ambien and Restoril, were nearly five times as likely to die over the next 2½ years as those who didn't take them. In addition to the potential for overdose and dangerous sleepwalking and sleep driving, these meds may increase your risk of respiratory infections and even cancer, the researchers say. The over-the-counter options, such as diphenhydramine (Benadryl), may not be innocuous either. A new study from Arizona State University linked use of these pills to an increased stroke risk.

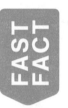

Percentage increase in shooting accuracy in basketball players who slept nearly 2 hours more each night for 5 to 7 weeks
Source: Stanford University

20 minutes of daily vocal exercises can curb snoring by strengthening the muscles in your throat. It also reduces sleep apnea. Sing along with the radio on the way to work, sound off in the shower, or hit the karaoke stage more often.

GEAR UP. Even if you sleep naked, you should consider wearing a few things to bed: an eye mask and earplugs. A little moonlight or a distant car alarm might wake you enough to disrupt your shut-eye but not enough for you to remember, and these tools can keep them out. Researchers in France found that when patients in a busy recovery room were masked and plugged, they scored about 30 percent higher on sleep quality. If you just can't bear the thought of sleeping with your eyes covered, install room-darkening shades to keep light out.

SWEAT FOR SLEEP. A good workout can elevate your performance in bed. The more calories you burn while awake, the sounder you may sleep. In a Dutch study, people who torched 2,500 calories a day spent more time in bed sleeping (not just lying awake) than those who burned 1,500. If you sap your energy stores during the day, you need to replenish them during rest, which is associated with better sleep efficiency, the researchers say. Try evening exercise: The spike in body temperature may help initiate sleep.

SCREW JET LAG. We surveyed 860 pilots about their secrets for staying energized during travel. A few pilots wrote in to tell us that sex helped them adapt to new time zones. Ejaculation releases prolactin, a sedating hormone that can override your circadian clock and help you conk out easier. And yes, you can fly yourself to your destination.

RUN TO THE DOCTOR IF YOU WALK TOO MUCH. Sleepwalking is often linked to stress or sleep deprivation, and it can be induced by anything that messes with your sleep cycle. It's usually not a problem; however, frequent nocturnal wandering is associated with depression, alcoholism, and insomnia, a Stanford study found. See a doctor if it's a common occurrence.

Should You Try Melatonin?

Melatonin is a hormone produced by the pineal gland in the brain that helps regulate the internal clock that controls your sleep and wake-up cycles. You can get more natural melatonin in your system from eating certain foods and also by taking a dietary supplement available in pharmacies, grocery stores, and health food stores.

First experiment with eating foods that either contain melatonin or induce its secretion, such as tart cherries and nuts. If they don't do the trick, consider a melatonin supplement. Melatonin supplements have been used effectively to treat jet lag and some types of insomnia, and they may help some people struggling with restless legs syndrome. Research from the Mayo Clinic found melatonin to be useful for treating a REM-sleep behavior disorder that causes people to act out their dreams violently—often by yelling, screaming, or jumping out of bed. Melatonin may be your solution when you have trouble falling asleep, but before you pop, take these tips.

→ **TIME IT RIGHT.** Melatonin supplements aren't "sleeping pills." They won't knock you out a few minutes after ingesting them. They work by initiating a sleep cycle, which begins several hours before you're actually in bed, so you'll need to take your supplement a few hours before darkness falls—or about 2 hours before you plan on hitting the sheets. As the melatonin enters your bloodstream, your body will think dusk has arrived early, so you'll fall asleep easier once your head hits the pillow.

→ **FOLLOW INSTRUCTIONS.** Some guys think, "If one pill works, five will work better." Not true. Research shows that big doses of melatonin can diminish the response you're aiming for, and regularly taking a megadose may actually cause you to stop responding to melatonin supplements entirely. Studies by Richard Wurtman, M.D., the MIT neuropharmacology professor who discovered melatonin's role in sleep, show that the effective dose for sleep is 0.3 milligram. Problem is, you won't find a dose that small in drugstores, he says. So pick up a pill cutter and quarter or halve a 1-milligram pill, as long as it isn't a time-release formulation (which can't be divided).

→ **KEEP IT AWAY FROM KIDS.** Although melatonin is not toxic, and the worst side effect users report is oversleeping, U.S. poison centers receive more calls about melatonin than any other supplement because the sleep aid looks like candy. "Most are unintentional ingestions—say, a child who raids the medicine cabinet," says Alvin Bronstein, M.D., of the American Association of Poison Control Centers. If Junior takes the supplement when you're not looking, most poison control pros will tell you to let him sleep it off, says Dr. Wurtman. If there's vomiting, make sure he drinks plenty of clear liquids to avoid dehydration while riding it out.

YOUR BODY DISSECTED

BY T.E. HOLT, M.D.

Why is yawning contagious?

We don't know for sure, but recent neuroscience research suggests that it involves specialized neurons ("mirror neurons") in the brain that play a role in cementing social relationships. (That may be why chimpanzees, in addition to grooming one another, also yawn contagiously.) Some researchers speculate that such behaviors are the foundation of empathy. So next time you yawn in response to your girlfriend's yawn, you can tell her you're not bored—it just shows what a sensitive guy you are.

Keep Your Brain Healthy

Stifle Stress, Strengthen Synapses, Wise Up about Your Mental Health

I know a guy in the health and fitness industry

who, over the past decade or so, has become pretty well known in the field. Ask him anything about fixing or improving the human body, and he'll rattle off a half-dozen great tips. He runs a brand you've heard of and has dedicated his life to inspiring others to live happier, healthier lives.

■
Better
INSTANTLY
↓
Mess with your mind and try something different today—a new route to work, a new sport, and a new food. Brains need to be challenged like muscles.

Until recently, however, he was a walking ball of stress. He had a bad habit of staying connected to his work 24-7, getting mired in small details instead of focusing on the big picture. That had consequences at home, naturally. Eventually, something would wake him up—a fight with his wife, missing one of his kids' activities—and he'd yank himself back toward a better balance. But it never lasted.

Then, one day in 2013, he had a revelation: He could chase his to-do list all he wanted—like he had been for the past decade—but his work would never be done. There would always be e-mails to answer, ideas to vet, and competitors to sweat. Worrying about it all, day after day, was no way to live. Fact was, he couldn't be physically healthy if he wasn't mentally healthy too.

That day, he left work at 5:15 p.m. It felt good. He didn't check his work e-mail that night. That felt even better. Since then, he's been leaving the office by 6 or 6:30 p.m., no matter how much work is on his desk. His kids' activities go directly to the top of his to-do list, even if they're in the middle of the workday. He's in bed every night—always with his wife, often with a book, never with his iPhone—before 10 p.m.

I don't want to overstate his transformation. He's not perfect, and his stress level at his job ebbs and flows. So, yes, he still falls into some of the same traps, as any hard-charging executive might. But his quality of life has undoubtedly improved—so much so that he decided to write the definitive book on men's health.

You're holding it.

So take it from me: It's easy to forget your brain. You want to lose weight, shred your body, get those abs and biceps showing. But are you paying attention to your brain? Your emotional health? I wasn't.

Your mind is like the electrical wiring that runs through your car. Seriously—it runs through a system of electrical signals that control virtually everything else in your body. One fault can make the whole thing run poorly. An unhealthy brain or a stressed mind can set off a chain reaction throughout the rest of your body. Don't believe me? In an Oregon State University study, researchers found that chronically stressed middle-aged men were almost 50 percent more likely to die during an 18-year period than those who experienced fewer stressful events.

But stress isn't the only killer. In a Johns Hopkins study, people who'd experienced a bout of depression had a 69 percent greater risk of cancer than their sunnier counterparts. Over time, depression may interrupt the stress hormones involved in cell growth and cell cycle regulation, potentially leading to cancer, the researchers say. Other studies have linked depression to heart disease.

What about worrying? That's dangerous, too. A British study found that

BRAIN TRAINER

Try to sign your name perfectly—with your eyes closed. Can't do it? Keep practicing until you can. Closing your eyes while you write awakens dormant neural circuits, which can slow age-related cognitive decline. Once you master this challenge, close your eyes and try it with your non-dominant hand.

anxiety can raise your risk of dementia. That's because chronic mental tension spikes your levels of glucocorticoids—and an excess of these hormones may wipe out brain cells and shrivel your memory center, the scientists say.

Over time, these troubles can team up with other health problems—like high blood pressure—to reduce your mental function and usher in diseases like dementia and Alzheimer's. Age-related brain plaques, which may play a role in Alzheimer's disease, can start forming *in your 40s*.

Start with these five steps, and you'll be on the way to a better brain.

The Fast Five for Brain Fitness

Simple stuff you can do right now.

1 Embrace hobbies old and new.

It sounds like a cliché, but it helps relieve stress. Play that guitar you haven't picked up in a while. Perfect your pizza crust recipe. Activities that give you a sense of mastery can also activate the mesocorticolimbic system, deploying a rush of dopamine. Moreover, as you practice a skill, you enter a healthy psychological state known as flow. Trying something new has additional benefits. Cognitive performance in almost every category declines after your mid-20s. However, you may be able to make your brain more resilient if you're constantly learning new, mentally complex things. Our favorite experts suggest taking dance classes, doing yoga, juggling, playing chess—whatever makes you think. In a study from Germany, people who spent more time on brain-stimulating activities cut their risks of Alzheimer's and mild cognitive impairment by 62 percent, compared with people who spent less time on these activities.

2 Work out your stress.

Do at least half an hour of moderate-intensity cardio three times a week. Exercise can have a soothing effect similar to that of anti-anxiety meds, a Southern Methodist University study review concluded. The effects can even be immediate: Research from the University of Maryland shows that 30 minutes of cardio can immediately reduce stress and help shield you from stressors afterward. Physical activity boosts bloodflow to your brain and promotes the release of feel-good chemicals called endorphins. To keep the good vibes coming, try something new: Sign up for a martial arts class, check out an indoor rock-climbing center, or go mountain biking. The benefits will keep piling up. For example:

→ Forty minutes of aerobic training three times a week for a year can increase the size of an older adult's hippocampus by 2 percent, which is important because the increase may lead to improved memory. Experts suggest moderate-intensity cycling, running, rowing, or swimming.

→ Strength training for 60 minutes three times a week for 6 months can help improve short- and long-term memory performance and attention as you age, according to a Brazilian study published in *Medicine and Science in Sports and Exercise.* The need to focus on technique when doing different lifts provides a cognitive challenge you may not get while doing a repetitive exercise like running.

→ Doing high-intensity intervals or resistance training—with your heart rate at 80 to 85 percent of its max—spikes your levels of brain-healthy hormones. In fact, another study in *Medicine and Science in Sports and Exercise* found that the level of BDNF— brain-derived neurotrophic factor, a protein that boosts the function and growth of neurons—increased 13 percent after 30 minutes of high-intensity exercise, but showed no significant increase after low-intensity exercise. Aim for two 30-minute sessions a week. Team sports that demand interval-like intensity—say, hoops or soccer—add a social aspect and are even better for your brain.

3 Lean on your friends.

You may have 2,000 Facebook friends, but if you don't feel connected, you'll know it in your heart. In a recent University of Chicago study, lonely people saw their blood pressure rise faster over 4 years than socially satisfied people did. What makes that so scary: The isolated folks' increase in BP was significant enough to raise their risk of a heart attack. "The health effects of loneliness are a lot bigger than people understand," says *Men's Health* mental health advisor Thomas Joiner, Ph.D., a distinguished professor of psychology at Florida State University. "Researchers are starting to understand that the effects on health of loneliness are bigger than

Better INSTANTLY

↓

Quick refocus: Close your eyes and take three deep, long breaths. Open your eyes. Whatever you're doing just got easier.

the effects of something like smoking or obesity—it's just a huge, huge effect." Loneliness is bad for all people, but it often hurts men most. Why? "Men tend to be lonelier with age because they don't replenish or nurture their relationships, their family relationships, their friendships, whereas women tend to do that a little bit more," Joiner says. Volunteering is one way to socialize with other people. Or just hang out with buddies. If they're pals from work, don't spend the time bitching about your boss. Venting can actually be counterproductive; with men, it often turns into a stress-inducing "who has it worse" showdown.

4 Meditate.

If you say "om" once in a while, you'll feel less stress the rest of the time. For 5 minutes, sit with your spine straight and eyes closed, and concentrate on observing your breath (without changing the flow of your natural breathing pattern) until the alarm sounds. Teaching yourself how to breathe deeply can help boost your performance. It seems simple, but most people don't breathe properly. To do it right, expand your belly and ribs fully as you inhale through your nose for a four-count, hold for a two-count, and then exhale for a six-count. Try to make the pattern second nature.

5 Beware of false coping mechanisms.

Sometimes when you're sad, worried, or stressed, your brain craves instant gratification, often in the form of a quick fix such as high-carbohydrate foods, alcohol, or risky behavior. The trouble is, chomping a doughnut, swilling a bourbon straight up, or hitting the slot machine will just mask your problems, not help them. In all likelihood, it will make things worse. For instance, in a University of Chicago study, stressed-out men injected with alcohol felt anxious longer than guys in a placebo group. Booze may disrupt your body's calming process, prolonging the mental misery. Do the things I just suggested instead!

BRAIN TRAINER

These matchsticks are arranged in incorrect mathematical equations. Your job is to correct the equations by moving only one stick in each equation. This puzzle was created by psychologist Carlo Reverberi, Ph.D., and has been shown to spark creativity. (See the solution on page 169.)

$$IV = III - I$$
$$IV = III + III$$
$$VI = IV - II$$
$$III = III + III$$

Raise Your Mental Health IQ

We all experience stress, anger, and other negative mental states. It's unavoidable. However, some guys handle it better than others. The following section will show you a plethora of ways to combat each one. Don't be afraid to try them. Good mental health sometimes requires an open mind. For starters, check out these six suggestions from top psychologists and other mental fitness experts for simple ways to think more clearly, build mental muscle, be happier, and become more successful.

1. **REVIVE YOUR SPIRIT.**

   "I keep a smiling baby Buddha on my desk. It reminds me that the real source of happiness is inner peace. Any object that holds deep emotional resonance can help you find clarity and stay centered during the day."—P. Murali Doraiswamy, M.D., professor of psychiatry, Duke University

2. **HIT REBOOT.**

   "Make a list of things that are important in your life and check how you feel about each one. Shuffle your commitments based on your answers. Note the things that bring you happiness, and don't just criticize."—William Pollack, Ph.D., associate clinical professor of psychiatry, Harvard Medical School

3. **SLEEP ON THE JOB.**

   "There's no doubt that daily 15- to 30-minute naps can boost productivity. To zonk out faster, sleep deeper, and wake up fresher, spray lavender oil on your pillow or sleep mask. I use this with my NBA patients."—W. Christopher Winter, M.D., director of sleep medicine, Martha Jefferson Hospital in Charlottesville, Virginia

4. **THINK MORE CLEARLY.**

   "Before an important task, use mindfulness-based breathing to help focus. Sit with your eyes closed and breathe normally. Focus on each breath. If your mind wanders, return the focus to your breath. After 60 seconds, blink your eyes open."—James N. Dillard, M.D., D.C., author of *The Chronic Pain Solution*

■ Better INSTANTLY

↓

Eat a small handful of walnuts every day. People who did that in a Spanish study improved their working memory by 19 percent. Polyphenols in walnuts are thought to improve communication between neurons.

5. **MAKE MORE FRIENDS.**

"Loneliness may be as dangerous for your health as smoking is. Join a book club or rec sports team to meet like-minded guys. Nurture your network daily."—Thomas Joiner, Ph.D., professor and psychology clinic director, Florida State University in Tallahassee.

6. **LIE ABOUT YOUR AGE.**

"Don't accept the premise that growing older equals feeling worse. Chronological aging is inevitable; physical and psychological aging, less so. To stay younger longer, pick an age when you felt the most vigorous and keep this as the focal point for the way you live your life."—Larry Lipshultz, M.D., professor of urology, Baylor College of Medicine in Houston

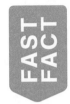

Percentage decrease in the stroke risk of men who had the highest blood levels of the antioxidant lycopene (found in tomatoes) compared with those who had the lowest
Source: Neurology

Ease These Brain Bruisers

Stress

SHOW YOUR PEARLY WHITES. Smiling when you're stressed can calm your heart rate, say scientists from the University of Kansas. Luckily, you don't have to grin like an idiot: Even a half smile—an expression similar to holding a pencil between your teeth—can help.

TURN ON SOME TUNES. Call it music therapy: A study in *Nature Neuroscience* found that listening to favorite tunes or anticipating a certain point in a song can cause a pleasurable flood of dopamine. Listen to a few songs in a row several times a day to reduce stress and boost your mood.

SQUEEZE A STRESS BALL. Yes, it can work when used correctly. Squeeze it for 15 seconds, then relax for 30 seconds. Do this for a few minutes at least five times a day.

TAKE A WALK IN THE PARK. Frequent exposure to nature may help you recover from stress and mental fatigue, especially if you live in an urban area. Dutch researchers found that city dwellers living near parks and gardens were 25 percent less likely to be diagnosed with depression than those with nary a patch of grass in sight. Another option: Bring the outdoors in.

Research from Japan shows that after touching a houseplant for 2 minutes, men felt calmer and had reduced bloodflow to brain regions activated during stress. We're wired to constantly assess whether our surroundings are pleasant (calming) or unpleasant (stressful), with nature falling into the "pleasant" column. Any plant with smooth, soft leaves, like a philodendron or peace lily, should work.

OUTSMART ANXIETY. Pumping yourself up—rather than trying to remain calm—may be the best way to combat performance anxiety, according to research from Harvard. Instead of stressing out about the prospect of a big presentation, date, or meeting, think positively and embrace your nerves as "energy."

Anger

TAKE A DEEP BREATH. It reverses your body's response to anger and slows your racing heart. Breathe in to a count of 10, and breathe out for 10. Do this for 10 to 20 breaths. Then roll your shoulders to ease tension. If your fists are clenched, shake them out. Release your tight muscles, and everything else will relax.

TAME YOUR GROWLING STOMACH. Being hungry won't do you any favors. In an Ohio State University study of married couples, researchers found a link between low blood sugar, aggressive impulses, and aggressive behaviors. Moreover, when researchers at the University of Kentucky let people blast others with various intensities of white noise, those who downed a sugary beverage showed the most mercy. The researchers believe a spike in blood sugar provides more energy to regulate anger. If you're planning to have a difficult talk with your spouse or partner, eat a handful of raisins first. You'll increase your blood sugar without crashing later, thanks to the fiber.

PUT OUT THE FIRE OF RAGE. What do you do when you're angry? Is your reaction physical? Do you spew a few choice words? Whatever your MO, use it as a cue to step back and pretend you're a referee. This self-distancing can reduce angry thoughts and aggression, an Ohio State study found. That's important because anger has long-term consequences—beyond making others think you're a hothead. Nope, anger doesn't just hurt others. It hurts you. In one study in the journal *Pain*, researchers found that anger can intensify back pain. That may be because anger activates neural pathways that transfer mental tension to the muscles surrounding your spine.

Anger may also raise your diabetes risk, reports a study in the *Journal of Behavioral Medicine*. People who often lost their cool were more prone to develop insulin resistance than those who kept calm, because anger spikes hormones that hinder blood sugar control. Say this mantra that reversed rage in a Romanian study: "I wish this weren't happening, but I can tolerate it." Or reassess your feelings: Australian researchers found that angry people reported being able to chill out when they positively reappraised the event that set them off instead of dwelling on the negative aspects.

Depression

GO A LITTLE EASIER ON YOURSELF. Overconfident people have an elevated risk of depression, a University of Pennsylvania study reveals. That's because self-inflation may set you up for disappointment and blind you to ways you can improve. A healthier approach? Accept failure as a possibility—but one you can influence. Once you acknowledge your weaknesses, you can then find ways around them, say British researchers.

PLAY WITH A PUP. Dogs can help you get out of the dumps. No matter how bad you feel, most pooches will be glad to see you. Even if you don't have a pet, ask a friend if you can play with his dog. A simple game of fetch can help you relax and focus on positives.

FRESHEN YOUR BREATH—AND YOUR OUTLOOK. Chewing gum may function like a happy pill. In a study from Japan, people who chomped on gum twice a day for 2 weeks lowered their scores on tests of depression and mental fatigue by as much as 47 percent—while those who sucked on a mint instead saw almost no change. The act of chewing may keep you happy—and alert—by increasing bloodflow to your brain and reducing your levels of stress hormones, the researchers say. Chew for at least 5 minutes. (Choose sugar-free gum to protect your teeth.)

DIAL BACK ON THE XXX. Regular porn users are more likely to report depression and poor physical health than nonusers are, a CDC study found. For some guys, porn may become a substitute for healthy face-to-face interactions, social or sexual. Save most of your viewing for when you're with your partner: Watching porn together can boost satisfaction, research shows.

BRAIN TRAINER

Wrap your head around this puzzle from Scott Kim, coauthor of The Playful Brain. Use a sheet of 8½- by 11-inch paper to build something capable of supporting a full glass of wine at least 4 inches above the surface of a table. This kind of puzzle activates your brain's right hemisphere, which is associated with creativity. (Find the answer on page 169.)

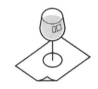

AM I NORMAL?

I can't do real work unless my office is completely in order.

Normal.

Do you mean you need 5 minutes to tidy up every morning? Fine. You're just a conscientious guy—especially if your effort is efficiency related, such as filing documents. But if the sight of an out-of-place paper can keep you from completing tasks at hand, you may have a problem, says Michael Chmielewski, Ph.D., an assistant professor of psychology at Southern Methodist University in Dallas. Think about your home life:

Do you feel anxious if the floor isn't freshly vacuumed? Do you spend hours cleaning each day? If you're nodding yes, then you may want to talk with a psychologist (find one at locator.apa.org). But if your fixation is limited to office cleanliness, then it may just be an excuse to put off work. Establish a time for tidying up, like the first 10 minutes after lunch, and limit yourself to that window.

SPEND LESS TIME AT THE SCREEN. If you have an iPhone in one hand and an iPad in the other, you may be setting yourself up for trouble. Multitasking with digital devices may be linked to depression, say researchers at Michigan State University. People who multitasked most with several media devices, like tablets and smartphones, reported a 70 percent greater number of depressive symptoms, on average, than those who multitasked least. While some people with the blues may be overusing the devices to artificially boost mood, the scientists warn that even emotionally fine folks can be so distracted that they stop properly coping with setbacks. If this sounds like you, use one device at a time.

DO SOMEONE ELSE A FAVOR. And you'll benefit, too: Performing five acts of kindness every week could boost your happiness by 40 percent, research from the University of California at Riverside reveals. You don't even have to spend cash! Let a car merge ahead of you in traffic. Pick up litter. Give advice to a colleague.

SEEK HELP WHEN YOU NEED IT. Women are diagnosed with major depression more frequently than men, but researchers don't think females are actually more likely to be depressed. They're just about three times as likely as men to seek professional help (75 percent vs. 26 percent), according to a study in *Depression and Anxiety*. Psychologists have a few theories about this. One is that men don't talk about their emotional problems because we've been socialized to avoid showing weakness. Or, we might just fail to recognize that behaviors like anger and irritability can signal underlying depression. If you think you're depressed—check "4 Sneaky Signs of Depression" on page 165 for some signals—see a doctor. There's no shame in talking out your problem.

SAY "THANK YOU." A few years ago, Martin Seligman, Ph.D., director of the Positive Psychology Center at the University of Pennsylvania in Philadelphia, came up with the idea of writing a gratitude letter. He recruited 411 people who'd visited the website of his 2002 bestseller, *Authentic Happiness*, and asked them to perform one of five tasks purported to foster well-being. The gratitude task was this: Write a letter expressing thanks to someone who has been especially kind to you but who never received proper thanks. Deliver that letter, in person, and watch the person read it. This wasn't an easy assignment, but the payoff proved to be huge. Of all the positive interventions, this task provided the biggest boost to happiness and the biggest decrease in depressive symptoms—and the 80 respondents who were assigned the task were still feeling the afterglow at 1-week and 1-month follow-ups.

Low Self-Esteem

CONDUCT A REALITY CHECK. A lot of men—check that—most men base their self-worth on their careers and tangible accomplishments like money, power, and possessions. They equate their worth as a human being with what they are or are not accomplishing in the world, and if they can't measure up to their own high standards, they view themselves as failures. Sound familiar? Just as a bad coach belittles you, you may be belittling yourself for no reason. Recognizing this in yourself is a step in the right direction. You're becoming more in tune with reality, which is essential when it comes to blocking negative self-talk. Ask yourself honestly, "Am I really a loser? Where's the evidence?" By challenging negative thoughts, you may find that there's little evidence to support them. Let's say you feel you've made a fool of yourself at a company meeting. "Challenge your knee-jerk beliefs," says Mario Alonso, Ph.D., a psychologist and consultant specializing in family businesses. Did everyone start whispering to one another that you are an idiot and should be fired? Of course not. "When the ANTS invade—that is, the automatic negative thoughts—choose to be kind to yourself by questioning the validity—the reality—of those thoughts." I remember once when I thought I said something stupid while being interviewed on live morning TV. I beat myself up over it, thinking that millions of people had made a judgment about me when in reality they were probably drinking coffee or rushing off to work and didn't give me a second thought. In the end, I realized that none of those viewers thought I was too important to be above making a mistake, so why should I think that way?

FAST FACT

2050

Year by which Alzheimer's disease diagnoses are expected to triple

Source: Neurology

Are You Truly Blue?

Doctors overdiagnose depression in men. Here's why.

It is estimated that 4.4 percent of men suffer from depression, yet 6.7 percent are taking antidepressant medication. Why are more men taking happy drugs than have clinical depression? Part of the disparity is due to the fact that SSRIs (the most commonly prescribed antidepressants) help treat other problems, including premature ejaculation and migraines. But that still doesn't account for all the scrips being written. "There's a lack of knowledge about what these drugs are appropriate for—and many illnesses have symptoms that mimic depression, including thyroid disorders and celiac disease," says Michael Addis, Ph.D., director of the Men's Coping Project at Clark University in Worcester, Massachusetts. Compounding the problem is the fact that a third of primary-care doctors say they won't ask about mental health at all and half say assessing psychological issues causes them to lose time and money, reports a new study by University of Cincinnati researchers. That disinterest may prompt a lot of knee-jerk prescription writing. Don't let your primary-care doctor jump to a quick diagnosis. If he or she does, consider a second opinion from a psychiatrist.

BECOME YOUR OWN VINCE LOMBARDI. The antidote for negative self-talk is positive self-talk. One of the greatest football coaches of all time, Vince Lombardi, famously said, "The greatest accomplishment is not in never falling, but in rising again after you fall." Wow. Powerful stuff. Give yourself such a halftime pep talk regularly. Write down and rattle off what you're particularly good at. High-five yourself when you've done good. Studies of high-achieving men with high self-esteem show that they regularly give themselves internal pep talks, reminding themselves of their positive traits and accomplishments.

LIFT YOUR CONFIDENCE. Low self-esteem is not just a worthless *feeling*; it actually manifests itself in inaction. When you feel pessimistic and inadequate, you tend to avoid trying anything worthwhile that may result in failure. Combat that inaction with something men are good at: action. Try fitness and sports activities. Lift weights, start a running or cycling program, join a tennis league. Being physically active raises your self-esteem because you are accomplishing something tangible. Also, physical activity improves your mood by releasing brain chemicals during a workout. And by improving your strength and endurance and losing some weight, you may find your feelings of self-worth strengthened as well.

VISUALIZE (AND PRACTICE) SUCCESS. Men, it seems, are genetically wired to wing it. But we are often at our best when we practice to be our best. Look at any successful athlete. He practices until he becomes so confident in his ability that there is no fear or self-doubt. And another thing that almost every champion athlete does: He visualizes a successful performance. Con-

4 Sneaky Signs of Depression
Is it normal or a warning signal?

WAKING UP EARLY

NORMAL You're excited or anxious about a big meeting. Or you're going fishing.

WARNING SIGN It's 4 a.m. and the alarm is set for 6. And this early-morning awakening has become routine. This is a classic sign of depression; a bad case of the blues can disrupt sleep-regulating hormones, including cortisol and melatonin. If you experience this warning sign or the others below, see a mental health professional who specializes in treating men; find one at locator.apa.org.

DRINKING

NORMAL You grab a beer or two with a buddy after a stressful day at work.

WARNING SIGN You drink every day, sometimes alone.

AGGRESSION

NORMAL You can barely resist telling someone off.

WARNING SIGN You can barely resist clocking someone.

OVERWORKING

NORMAL A big project has you logging major hours in the office.

WARNING SIGN Regardless of your workload, you practically live at your desk—hey, it beats having to deal with your life.

sider Seattle Seahawks quarterback Russell Wilson, one of the smallest (at 5'11") in a sport where the average NFL QB is about 6'2". The third-round draft pick silenced the naysayers by winning the starting role after just two preseason games and leading his team to the first Super Bowl championship in franchise history. His secret: Unsurpassed preparation and a huge imagination. "I'm a big visualization person," Wilson says. "I'll sometimes go out on the field late at night. I call the plays in my head and walk 'em out." You can do the same whenever you feel challenged. Imagine yourself in the stressful situation, then playact—that is, mentally adopt the confident attitude you hope to feel and physically create the tone of voice, posture, and actions you want to display. Practicing the response you wish to achieve over and over helps establish pathways in the brain that become self-fulfilling.

FIND YOUR PURPOSE. Many men experience bouts of self-doubt in mid-career or midlife. It's often triggered by the death of a parent, divorce, illness, or being denied a promotion at work. The life event causes him to realize his limitations and even his own mortality. This is so freaking common there should be a college course warning young men that this is on the horizon. How you deal with it when it occurs may set the tone for the second half of your life. Psychologists say middle life is a time to redefine success. Is it money, a VP title, and a beach house, or is it a good marriage, well-adjusted, happy kids, your health, and your own happiness? Which counts for more at the buzzer depends on your perspective. And your perspective can change. Take some time to reflect on what makes you happy and fulfilled. If you've been doing the same work for 15 or 20 years, consider trying something new that will energize you and provide a profound sense of satisfaction. Carl G. Jung, the famed Swiss psychiatrist, called age 40 "the noon of life." He believed it was the beginning of a process when a person becomes more uniquely individual, and it offered a man an opportunity to toss off societal trappings of success and pursue his own true desires and lead a more balanced life.

Age-Related Brain Changes and Strokes

DIG UP THOSE FLASH CARDS FROM HIGH SCHOOL. A study in *Neurology* reports that speaking more than one language may stave off dementia by $4\frac{1}{2}$ years. The researchers speculate that being bilingual boosts cognitive reserve, your brain's resistance to age-related decline and dementia.

PROTECT YOUR EARS. Hearing loss, which can start in your 20s, may

TRY THIS!

Improve Your Memory Now

NAMES

Try to focus as soon as you shake hands with someone new. Attention at the time of learning is the most critical thing. Second is rehearsal; third is relating the name to something. So repeat the name ("Nice to meet you, Frank"), and then create a mental image linking it to an object (e.g., Frank eating a frank).

PASSWORDS

Too many PINs? Turn them into words that correspond with the ATM keypad (like 2274 for CASH). For your website log-ins, create a smartphone album of visual triggers; for example, if a photo of friends represents Facebook, you could use "Buds4Life." Image-based codes are difficult to crack and highly memorable.

FACTS

All that cramming in college was about as smart as the rounds of vodka shots. If you study for 5 consecutive hours, you won't remember nearly as well as if you study for an hour five times a week. Learn a fact in the a.m.? Review it before bed: Shut-eye helps bolster memories.

play a role in cognitive decline as you age—the extra effort needed to process speech may detract from other brain functions. So don't use earbuds with the volume past 50 percent for extended stretches. And try an app like Hearing Check; if you test poorly, see an audiologist ASAP.

WEAR ROSE-COLORED GLASSES. Looking on the bright side is a bright idea: Pessimists have a higher risk of stroke than people who are more positive do, a Finnish study found. Perpetual negativity may damage your blood vessels and disrupt the part of your nervous system that controls your heart rate, making you more likely to have a stroke, the researchers believe. So build your optimism muscles: Each week, pick one part of your life—career, dating—and envision the next decade if all goes well. This exercise can improve your whole-life outlook, say scientists from the University of California at Riverside.

TART TO FEEL BETTER. Squeeze this into your diet: Citrus fruits may lower your stroke risk, a Harvard study reports. Women whose daily diet included high levels of flavones (one or two oranges' or grapefruits' worth) had a 19 percent lower risk of ischemic stroke than those who ate little of the compound. And yes, men would benefit too, the scientists say. Flavones may strengthen blood vessels and decrease inflammation.

TRY THIS!

Close Eyes, See Clearly

The next time you find yourself struggling to remember something, close your eyes. Research from England's University of York reveals that doing this can significantly enhance your recall because it reduces your cognitive load. The result: Your brain can focus on retrieving the information you're seeking.

AM I NORMAL?

When I watch a movie, I end up rooting for the villain.

Normal.

Good news: Unlike the bad guys on the big screen, you actually have a heart. "It's a pretty natural reaction to feel bad as you watch someone's downfall," says Glenn R. Fox, Ph.D., who studies affective neuroscience at the University of Southern California's Brain and Creativity Institute in Los Angeles. And the more you know about the scoundrel, he says, "the more sympathy you're likely to have. When you have a good amount of background information on someone, you understand his behavior a little more. That's what's going to elicit the empathic response." But feeling pity is one thing. "The line might be where you actually approve of the character's bad behavior," says Fox. Plus, not caring about the good guy's troubles while cheering on the crook could be a sign of a personality disorder. If this sounds like you, think about seeing a mental health professional who focuses on addressing problematic behaviors. To find one, go to locator.apa.org.

Mind Over Bladder
Overcome stage fright in a crowded restroom

Difficulty urinating in the presence of other people happens when the external sphincter muscle tightens and restricts you from relieving yourself. You might know it as "shy dick" or "bashful bladder," but there's a medical name for it—paruresis. Almost everyone experiences it at some time or other. When it happens to you, try these ways to loosen up:

→   Visualize a waterfall or something else that relaxes you. Try to envision yourself turning on a faucet.

→   If you feel like you are standing at the urinal for an eternity, try timing yourself at home when you're not under pressure. What seems like a long time may not be.

→   Hit the stall. Minus the phone numbers and creatively positioned stick figurines on the walls, nothing beats a stall as a reminder of home privacy. If that doesn't work, try sitting down.

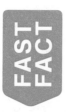

59

Percentage
increase in
stroke risk of
people with the
highest levels of
chronic stress
Source: Stroke

LET YOUR MIND WANDER. Go ahead, daydream. Brain scans show that daydreaming actually exercises more of your brain than doing crossword puzzles. That's because it activates the same neural circuits you use to form memories. Aim for a couple of 5-minute sessions a day.

CHECK YOUR BP. We already suggested this on page 102, but it's important for keeping your brain ticking too. The higher your systolic blood pressure is when you're younger, the more likely you are to lose gray matter in key areas as you age, say scientists at UC Davis. Chronically high BP (above 120/80 mm Hg) deprives your brain of blood and nutrients.

WATCH YOUR SUGAR. Forget that can of soda now, or you may have no choice later. High "normal" blood sugar could raise your Alzheimer's risk, say scientists in Australia. In a 4-year study, healthy people with the highest levels in the "normal" range (92 to 110 mg/dl) had the most shrinkage in brain regions critical for memory. Even if you don't have pre-diabetes or diabetes, excess sugar in your bloodstream promotes clotting, which can deprive your brain of blood and oxygen, the researchers say. In addition to cutting back on highly processed carbohydrates in general, ditch the soft drinks completely—corn syrup speeds into your bloodstream even faster.

BE LIKE POPEYE. Learn to love olive oil. In a study from Spain, men who ate about 4 tablespoons of extra-virgin olive oil a day showed better language comprehension, attention, and abstract thinking than those on a low-fat diet. Its antioxidants (Italian olive oil has the most) may reduce brain inflammation.

IMPROVE YOUR D. Research from France reveals that consuming more vitamin D may reduce your risk of developing Alzheimer's disease. In the 7-year observational study, people whose diets contained the highest levels of vitamin D were less likely to develop dementia than were those who consumed the least. The difference in D intake between the two groups? Just 400 IU a week. That's the amount in about four glasses of 2 percent milk.

EAT SMART. Your brain is a fuel-guzzling engine, and to keep it from misfiring, you need to eat the same foods that keep your heart healthy. These include lean protein, good fats, whole grains, and plenty of antioxidant-rich and inflammation-fighting vegetables and fruits. Here's an example of a day's worth of brain food:

→ **BREAKFAST:** Eggs and steel-cut oats
Eggs contain choline, an essential nutrient that helps brain function; steel-cut oats are high in fiber, which helps regulate blood sugar.

→ **SNACK:** A handful of blueberries and eight almonds
Blueberries are high in epicatechin, which has been shown to promote bloodflow, improve mood, and hone focus. The almonds provide protein and fiber.

→ **LUNCH:** 6 ounces wild Alaskan salmon with three-bean salad
Salmon is laden with omega-3 fatty acids, which appear to promote brain health. Beans are loaded with the fiber you need to keep your blood sugar off the roller coaster.

→ **SNACK:** 2 ounces dark chocolate
Dark chocolate (at least 65 percent cocoa) is rich in flavanols, antioxidants that may improve cognitive function, and it contains a little caffeine, which may help concentration.

→ **DINNER:** Five-vegetable curry stir-fry with brown rice
Toss eggplant, onions, broccoli, and yellow and red bell peppers into a wok to unlock the maximum variety of antioxidants. Sprinkle on turmeric for anti-inflammatory protection.

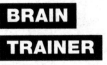

BRAIN TRAINER

To strengthen your working memory, play the 2-Back card game, says Richard Restak, M.D., coauthor of The Playful Brain: The Surprising Science of How Puzzles Improve Your Mind.

1. Shuffle a deck of cards and place it facedown. This is your draw pile.

2. Name two cards— for example, aces and kings—as trigger cards.

3. Turn the cards over one at a time and place them on a discard pile. When you draw a trigger card, try to name the card you turned over two cards previously. Check to see if you're correct, and if you are, hold on to it. Keep going until you're through the deck. A perfect score is eight cards

BRAIN TRAINER ANSWERS:
Page 157. IV−III = I; VI = III + III; VI−IV = II; III = III = III

Page 161. Fold the paper accordian-style and stand it on its edge so it forms a standing tube with star-like points. Rest glass on top.

CHAPTER

10

A Better Man
in Bed

*A Guide to a Lifetime of
Happy, Healthy, and Hot Sex!*

My favorite day of the month here at *Men's Health:* the afternoon when we gather at the couches outside my office with a printout of the cover (the image only, no words) taped to a flip chart and brainstorm cover lines for the new issue.

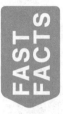

If you're a regular *Men's Health* reader, you've probably noticed how different our cover lines are from those on most men's magazines. Ours don't describe the story; they describe the benefit you'll get if you read the story. A sampling: "Get Back in Shape!" "Score a Raise!" "Eat Pasta, Lose Pounds!" "Boost Your Brainpower!" You get the idea.

But then there are the sex cover lines. That's where we take some creative license—to entertain ourselves and our readers. One of my all-time favorites: *"Sex So Hot the Fire Trucks Will Come!"*

It made us all howl when we came up with it, not just because it was hilarious, but also because we all knew we'd just crystallized the tone that good sex coverage should take in our magazine. All guys, straight or gay, want to get laid. Often. How can any average guy get better at the one thing he wants constantly? How can he approach women (or men) he believes are out of his league? How can he make his current relationship hotter? And here's the most important question of all: How can he do it in an open, honest, *healthy* way—without the male tendency to feel embarrassment and shame?

Tough one. That's why this chapter exists. Have some fun with it. In here, you'll find some of the most immediate, helpful, and yes, hot information about building a better sex life. Most of the research was done on male-female relationships, but a lot of these tips work with same-sex couples, too. It's important, and not just about having sex. Men who aren't satisfied with their sex life are more likely to develop coronary heart disease, according to research in the *European Heart Journal*.

The Fast Five for Better Sex

Simple stuff to do right now (or tonight!)

1

Try something new.
As couples move from the honeymoon phase to the fart-in-front-of-each-other phase, sex can become less exciting and less fun. But it doesn't have to. To restore heat, ask yourself: *How did I tease her at the beginning of our relationship?* Work that back into your repertoire. Then add a toy, a position—anything that injects creativity into what's become routine. Don't be intimidated by

vibrators: They're linked to positive sexual function, such as desire and ease of orgasm. Translation: More fun for both of you. Or just add lube: Research from Indiana University links lube use with greater sexual pleasure and comfort.

2 Cultivate communication.

Research shows that emotional intimacy is more important than any physical factors for predicting sexual satisfaction. So no matter how many new toys and tricks you try, they won't work that well if you and your partner haven't had a meaningful conversation in a while. How do you open up? Men tend to say what they think, but your lady wants to know how you feel—especially how you feel about her. So don't say you think things are "going well." Say you feel happy when you think about her. Or talk about being excited, nervous, even scared—whatever's in your gut at the moment. Expressing your vulnerability will give her a better sense of your mental state and help you two grow closer.

And when you want to broach a sex-related topic, like your needs in the sack? Keep it full of compliments, but also acknowledge what hasn't worked. Then ask her how it felt for her and what she wants you to try again. Want to make a special request to spice up your bedroom romps? Place your order before you two are between the sheets, or she may feel uncomfortable. Start the conversation by acknowledging that it's hard for you to admit. Then explain your interest—that she'll look really sexy or you'll bond more. If the answer is still no, back off for at least a month. Too soon and she'll feel you're badgering her—which will only reduce your odds of realizing your kinky fantasy in the long run.

3 Listen for her feelings.

If your partner is upset, she may not communicate clearly. For instance, the subtext of "You never kiss me when you come home" is "I crave more affection." To make sure you really hear her, give her your full attention: Switch off the TV, ditch the phone, and set up a private time to talk. The worst thing you can do is to shut down when she opens up. Many men might seem like bad listeners because they unintentionally clam up during emotionally charged conversations—the very exchanges that tend to be most important to their partners. It feels bad to see your girlfriend or wife become emotional, and that fear and anxiety can block listening. Another common pitfall: In an attempt to make her feel better, you may subconsciously redirect the talk away from upsetting topics. While your intentions may be good, this comes across as if you're not listening or caring (or both). So when your girlfriend starts venting, take a deep breath and focus on each word that comes out of her mouth. This will keep you grounded and ease anxiety. When she's done talking, let her know that you're sorry she's feeling (fill in the negative emotion). Then say something like, "I want to help. I don't quite know what to do, but I care and I'll be here for you."

4 Exercise together.

Sweating together is sexy: University of Texas researchers found that vigorous exercise activates a woman's sympathetic nervous system, which is also activated during sexual arousal. Both her body and her brain are in the mood! Plus, exercise activates apocrine glands, the site of pheromone release in primates. That might make her want you even more. For bonus points, try a new workout. Novelty sparks hormones in the brain similar to those released when you were falling in love, concluded a study at SUNY–Stony Brook.

5 Multitask in bed.

A national survey from Indiana University found that doing at least four or five sexual acts at each session was a strong predictor of orgasm. That could mean the couples studied just spent more time having sex—or that variety is exciting. Investigate what works for you. Don't jump right to penile–vaginal intercourse. Try partnered masturbation, deep kissing, breast play, erotic massage, manual sex, oral sex, and more. According to a study in the *Journal of Sexual Medicine*, fewer than 1 in 10 women reports always having an orgasm during intercourse. So we asked more than 2,000 *Women's Health* readers which combo moves were most likely to help them climax. Here are your playbook moves, in order of popularity.

33 percent: Manual stimulation + intercourse

30 percent: Oral sex + intercourse

18 percent: Kissing + manual stimulation

10 percent: Vibrator + intercourse

9 percent: Oral sex + vibrator

Want to turn up the heat even more? The next pages include useful tips from our sex and relationship experts.

Before You Get to the Bedroom

MAKE A WISH LIST. A University of New Brunswick study revealed that after 15 years together, couples knew only about 62 percent of what their partner liked in bed, and 26 percent of what their partner disliked. Start a *Yes*, *No*, *Maybe* list for what the two of you would like to try together. Whether you end up getting kinky or not, you should both find this exercise enlightening and empowering.

TURN HER FANTASIES INTO REALITY. In a *Men's Health* survey, one in three women said that during foreplay, they're fantasizing about something they're dying to try but are too scared to bring up. A great way to figure out what she's into is to surprise her with a book of erotic stories and ask her to read her favorite passages out loud.

BE CAREFUL ON CALLS. Don't make your phone the lifeline for your love life. Sharing emotions over the phone could threaten your relationship, a Purdue University study found. When far-apart couples revealed feelings, they were less likely to idealize each other, which can lead to dissatisfaction. One reason: If self-disclosure isn't accompanied by body language, it can be hard to convey understanding and to feel understood, the researchers say. If she unloads over the phone, describe your physical reaction ("I wish I could hug you").

MAKE A COUPLE OF NEW FRIENDS. Boredom is a big contributor to relationship dissatisfaction, according to a study in *Psychological Science*. So get out more: People feel more passionate about their partners when they hang with other couples, say Wayne State University researchers. "We tend to be at our best around others: happy, engaged, and telling stories," says Geoffrey L. Greif, Ph.D., a professor of family therapy and the coauthor of *Two Plus Two: Couples and Their Couple Friendships*. "Seeing other people who value your opinions and respond to your thoughts will also make her appreciate you more, and vice versa." Go on a double date with a fun-loving couple and feed off their excitement.

PUT THE PHONE AWAY. Couples who converse while carrying smartphones—even if they're not using

TRY THIS!

A Sex-Fast

Make all forms off-limits—oral, manual, intercourse, even masturbation. (And no peeking at porn!) It can be for a day, a week, a month, whatever—as long as you both commit. Experts say that self-denial can boost desire and help you rediscover the thrill of the chase.

them—report feeling less empathy from their partner and experience a lower-quality relationship overall, a British study found. The couples also said the phones diminished closeness and trust. One reason may be that these devices act like megaphones to broader conversational audiences. Figuratively, we're never alone.

DITCH THE CALENDAR. Scheduling sex can sap the fun from it. Instead, sneak some R-rated fun into stolen moments. Squeeze her butt in the morning as she makes coffee. Kiss her deeply—for 5 seconds or so—when you come home from work. And build tension . . . always.

SAVE THE DATE. But do schedule a date night: In a study from Australia, couples encouraged to spend 90 minutes a week wooing each other became increasingly satisfied with their relationship. So we asked more than 500 women what thrilled them about the fire starters suggested by the study authors. Here are a few that scored well.

→ Giving her flowers for no reason
→ Tucking a love note into her lunch
→ Taking her on an unexpected date
→ Leaving a hot towel outside her shower
→ Visiting a new city together
→ Reading erotica together
→ Giving each other massages

WASH THE DISHES. As modern as we think we are, a lot of us are still old-fashioned about housework. Studies show that many women bear the brunt of chores. Ladies say it's a turn-on when their partner pitches in.

MASTER THIS BALANCING ACT. Can you walk a tightrope? Canadian research finds that complimenting her traits and abilities while also being realistic about them leads to a more secure relationship. Translation: She'll see right through empty praise. In the study of 55 couples, people rated themselves on 10 qualities and then were told (falsely) how their mates rated them. If the partner ratings matched their own—and were positive—they judged their relationships as the most intimate and secure. Those shown dissimilar ratings said their relationships were on shaky ground.

BECOME A DREAM COUPLE. Here's some worthwhile pillow talk: Telling her about your dreams may help you bond. In a 2013 Swedish study, couples who consistently shared their dreams reported feeling closer to each other than those who didn't. Such private revelations may deepen mutual trust, so try to open up to her at least once a week. One caveat: Don't bother describing the dreams about, say, sex with a coworker. That's oversharing.

KISS OFTEN. Sure, smooching after sex is key, but Oxford researchers found that women in longer-term relationships put higher value on pre-coital kissing. Kissing is emotional upkeep. In fact, locking lips—even outside the sack—was more important to relationship quality than frequent sex was.

WAKE UP YOUR RELATIONSHIP. Don't let sleepiness sabotage your bond with her. A study from UC Berkeley found that sleep deprivation can leave partners too tired to appreciate each other. Commit to a curfew and hit the sack together an hour early. You'll score more quality time between the sheets—and probably net more sleep.

TAKE A YOGA CLASS. Yoga may boost your satisfaction in the sack, a Malaysian study suggests. When men did a stretching and breathing routine three times a week, their sexual fulfillment increased. This type of exercise remaps your brain's perception of your body—you move the way you're designed to, the researchers say. That, in turn, may raise your confidence during sex. Work your lungs while you limber up: Exhale as you begin a pose, hold the pose until your muscles relax, and then release the pose and inhale. (Bonus points if you practice together. You just might end up in a pretzel pose.)

MAINTAIN SOME MYSTERY. Tried something new last night? In the morning, tell her how amazing you thought the night was, and leave it at that. In the meantime, just allow the memory to simmer—it will leave both of you wanting more. Patience will lead to your payoff.

REV HER UP. Laziness may be to blame for a dying sex life. In a British study, women said men taking sex for granted was a major cause of sexual boredom. That's when duty sex begins—and her libido fades. If you amp things up, she'll want to pursue you. So give her a massage, go out dancing, tell her when you fantasize about her—all are powerful cues for her arousal, a University of Texas at Austin study found.

SMART ADVICE
FROM *MEN'S HEALTH* RELATIONSHIPS ADVISOR **DEBBY HERBENICK, PH.D.,**
CODIRECTOR OF THE CENTER FOR SEXUAL HEALTH PROMOTION AT INDIANA UNIVERSITY IN BLOOMINGTON

"Emotional intimacy is a key predictor of a couple's sexual satisfaction. Men unconsciously crave affection-kissing, touching, cuddling—as much as women do, but they tend to initiate it only when they're looking to have sex. Snuggle on the couch while you watch TV. Kiss her on the way out the door. Call her to say you can't wait to see her. These things make a big difference."

Inside the Bedroom

TALK DIRTY. Dirty talk is deeply personal; one person's turn-on is another's mood killer. But once you find the courage to speak up, it won't just cement your bond—it could also lower her inhibitions in the bedroom. So try it. It might feel a little weird at first, but you'll get comfortable. Try practicing dirty talk while masturbating, or watching porn together and mimicking what the actors say—even if it's in a silly, self-conscious way. Become comfortable with it. Something that usually works? Give her honest, graphic compliments. When we surveyed women about dirty talk, they said the hottest things they can hear are:

→   "You feel amazing."
→   "You taste so nice."
→   "I want you."
→   "I wake up hard just thinking about you."
→   "I didn't know you had that in you."

RECHARGE FASTER. It's a common dilemma—you climaxed, but she wants to keep going. Your penis needs a breather. Every time you ejaculate, your pituitary gland produces a surge of oxytocin and prolactin, hormones that make you relax. These hormones suppress dopamine, the neurotransmitter responsible for arousal. Scientists suspect that lengthened refractory

Your Toolbox

VIBRATING PENIS RINGS

These little things can really shake things up in bed. They fit around the base of your shaft, keeping the blood in your penis longer. This can delay ejaculation and also help you stay erect longer after ejaculating—both of which can take your sack session from a sprint to a marathon. Plus, while the ring buzzes her clitoris, it also stimulates your scrotum, an area that's often overlooked during sex. Buy a soft, flexible ring and a bottle of lube; apply the lube and slip the ring over your erect penis before penetration. Now invite your mate into the cowgirl position—while she's on top, she can control how much vibration she feels.

periods are caused by age-related changes in the pituitary system that disrupt the balance of oxytocin and prolactin and suppress dopamine. One natural solution: Raise your dopamine level by eating more foods rich in vitamins B_6, B_{12}, and folate, such as chickpeas, tuna, and asparagus.

MAKE SURE SHE COMES FIRST. Her biggest aphrodisiac might be humble pie. Penn State scientists found that arrogant men may give women less-satisfying orgasms. Women in the study were less likely to climax first—a sign of intense pleasure—if their partners rated themselves as highly masculine and dominant. Self-satisfied men may be less attentive lovers, the researchers say. Put her first in bed and you'll both be satisfied.

REVAMP THE CLASSICS. British researchers found that the missionary, doggy-style, and woman-on-top positions are all conducive to her orgasm. But even the old standbys can be upgraded. Try these variations that will satisfy both of you.

IN MISSIONARY POSITION

→ She places her legs over your shoulders. Legs up = more G-spot stimulation. Plus, the acrobatic element is mentally arousing.

→ Try the coital alignment technique. Start in the missionary position, but rest on your elbows and have her wrap her legs around your thighs. This shifts the angle of her pelvis so that the base of your penis presses against her clitoris. Then rock your hips back and forth instead of thrusting in and out.

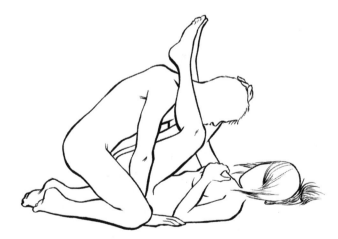

IN DOGGY-STYLE

→ She drops down to her forearms instead of using her hands for support. This positions her butt higher than her head and helps you penetrate more deeply, potentially stimulating her cervix.

→ Have her lie on her stomach with a pillow under her hips, pelvis angled upward. Enter from behind, extending your arms to limit the weight on her. In this position, you can kiss her neck or talk dirty.

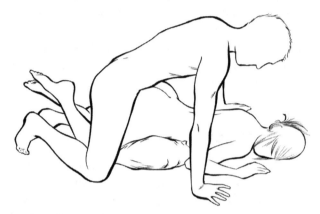

IN WOMAN-ON-TOP

→ She leans forward, bringing her face close to yours. You can kiss and lock eyes, and leaning forward increases friction against the sensitive front wall of her vagina.

→ Sit with your legs extended. Lift your knees, and have her bend her knees so they're next to your chest. Lean back on your arms for support. She'll have total control over the thrusts and movements. You'll enjoy the view and the ride.

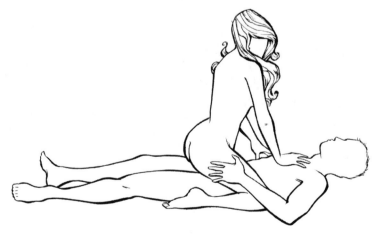

DO SOME GRUNT WORK. Nonverbal communication during sex is more essential to satisfaction than talking is, a Cleveland State University study found. When people described how they communicated in bed and rated their sexual satisfaction, nonverbal cues—touching, eye contact, moaning, gesturing—emerged as predictors of pleasure. Make a game out of wordlessly guiding each other's hands.

TOUCH HER HERE. Quickly zeroing in on her hot spots can derail her arousal. Take your time with light kissing and gentle touching of nongenital areas. Pay attention to these hot spots, from top to bottom:

TRY THIS!

Text-ual Healing

Texting excessively with your girl can diminish relationship satisfaction, but texts of affection ("Thinking of you") do the opposite—they can bolster your bond.

Source: Journal of Couple and Relationship Therapy

→ **HER TRESSES**

Lots going on here. Gentle tugging stimulates nerve endings around hair follicles, and it just feels good; it could also remind her of being pampered at a salon. Playing with her hair may also satisfy her need to bond. In a University of New Hampshire study, partners who "groomed" each other—played with each other's hair, exchanged massages, soaped up together—had higher levels of trust and satisfaction.

→ **HER EARS**

Inside and out, her ears are packed with supersensitive nerve endings. Open your mouth to gently breathe warm air into her ear, and then purse your lips to blow cool air around the outside. Massage her earlobe with your lips or fingers, gently tugging downward. Every so often, enhance her pleasure by working your way up and down her entire ear.

→ **HER NECK**

Neck nibbling is super hot. When we survey women about where they want to be touched, it always rates high. Maybe that's because the neck is a vulnerable spot. Nuzzling a woman's neck connotes intimacy, not eroticism, so it may heighten arousal more than overtly sexual moves do. Kiss the nape of her neck, moving from bare skin into her hair, and flutter the tip of your tongue over her hair follicles.

→ **HER BREASTS**

Some women love nipple stimulation; some don't. But on one thing they all agree: Watching you suck, nibble, and savor her body is damn sexy. The idea of being devoured arouses her mind—which is,

(continued on page 184)

● **HAIR** After massaging her scalp, wrap a lock of hair around your finger and pull gently to send tingling pleasure down her back.

● **FACE** Massage above her eyebrows with your thumbs to relax her face. When she's aroused, her lips will part.

● **EARS** Graze the ridge of her outer ear with your nose. Just hearing your breath will turn her on.

● **NECK** Brush your lips along the thin skin between her throat and chin. You'll engage sensory receptors and trigger an emotional response.

● **ELBOW CREASE** Technically called the antecubital fossa, this area is super-sensitive to differences in temperature. Lick here, then blow softly to create a cooling sensation.

● **BREASTS** The top and underside of the breasts are oft ignored nerve-rich erogenous tissue. Pay attention here before going to the nipple. Your technique should be so light it barely dents the skin.

● **BACK** During sex, take a back-rub break to delay ejaculation. She'll think, "Wow, he's caring and considerate and not just all about sex."

● **BACK OF THE KNEES** Graze the skin here using the full length of three fingers; a firmer touch will please her without tickling.

● **THIGHS** Stroke in the direction of her vagina, but pull away before reaching it. Women want to wonder, "What's he going to do next?"

● **STOMACH** Run your penis across her bare skin. The feel of your erection across her stomach will give her goosebumps.

● **BUTT** Gently caress with fingertips while praising her glutes with a soft voice. Then firmly knead.

● **FEET** When you rub the arch of her right foot, you stimulate an area about 30 inches higher and a little to the left.

Her Pleasure Points

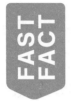
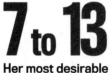

7 to 13

Her most desirable length of time, in minutes, for actual intercourse per sack session

Source: Journal of Sexual Medicine

after all, her largest sexual organ. In fact, women are 19 times more likely to rate sex as "very or extremely pleasurable" if they're emotionally satisfied, according to researchers at Maimonides Medical Center in New York City. Nipples are, well, a sensitive subject: We know you guys love 'em, but too many men land there and never leave. Instead, focus on pleasuring her whole breast, says Yvonne Fulbright, the author of *Touch Me There!* Run your fingers across her breast, edging closer to her nipple, and swirl around the edges of her areola—you're building anticipation. Finally, while cupping her breasts, slip the very tip of her nipple between your lips. Blow. Lick. Tease her with firm, circular motions. Vary your speed and intensity so they don't lose sensation.

→ **HER ANTECUBITAL FOSSA**

That's the technical name for her elbow crease, an area where blood vessels are very close to the surface of her skin, making it supersensitive. This is also a place where the nerves become a ganglion, a cluster of sensitive nerve cells. Hold her hand and slowly straighten her arm. Then gently kiss along the crease on the inside of her elbow. Next, flutter your tongue across her skin and breathe warm air onto the spot.

→ **HER HANDS**

The palm has about 40,000 nerve endings, and stimulating them all will make her whole body feel good. Most people also have light hairs between the bases of their fingers and the knuckles above, making that area extra sensitive. Interlock your fingers with hers, and then use your thumb to massage her palm and the bases of her fingers in a circular motion. It's intimate, but you can still do it in public, which gives it more erotic power.

→ **HER STOMACH**

Think of her belly as a double-points zone. That's not only because many women feel self-conscious about their abs, but also because the upper part houses her solar plexus, a powerful nerve cluster. Start just below her breasts and move toward her belly button, caressing and kissing her softly. By soothing her mentally and relaxing her abs, you'll help increase bloodflow to her clitoral complex, exciting her with the prospect of being touched there later.

→ **HER THIGHS**

Many guys rush over the thighs so they can zero in on what's in between them. Slow down. You're so close to her playground but still far away, which will drive her up the wall. First, tease her with your fingers: Move up her leg, but pull away at the last minute or just graze her mons with your fingertips. Repeat with your tongue, going close enough for her to feel your breath.

→ **HER KNEES**

The backs of her knees harbor nerve receptors known as Pacinian corpuscles; these are especially sensitive to pressure. Plus, the skin here is extremely ticklish. Start at her ankles and gently run your fingertips up the backs of her calves until you reach the soft area behind her knees. Tickle there with your fingertips or tongue, avoiding the bonier, less sensitive parts on the sides.

→ **HER BUTT**

In public, keep your paws off her butt (although covert brushing can heighten the mood for later) and explore subtly sexy spots, like the inside of her wrist. But don't be shy about praising her glutes as if you're her personal trainer. In bed, start by kissing your way down her spine while gently caressing her butt with your fingertips. When your lips reach her cheeks, kiss and nibble softly, and firmly knead her buns. Attention is flattering.

→ **HER FEET**

Foot play can make a so-so session stellar. The part of the brain that processes sensory input for the feet is right next to the part that processes genital stimulation. Some women may have some cross wiring between these two parts of the brain.

USE YOUR FINGERS. The oft-repeated instruction for finding the famed G-spot involves inserting your finger about 2 inches inside her vagina and making a come-hither motion with that finger, pressing it against the top of her vaginal wall. Instead of trying to push a single button, so to speak, think about broadening your coverage. The sensitive area can be higher, lower, or to the side, and its size can vary from woman to woman. You should also tailor your technique—speed, pressure, and angle of approach—to the woman you're with. Some women might like a massaging motion, others a tapping motion. Try this: Put your index and middle fingers in the area and rock them back and forth. Keep your fingers flat and straight, and vary your pressure. Pretend you're playing two keys on a piano, but without curving your fingers. The more time you spend warming her up, the more likely she is to experience "tenting," when muscle contractions pull her uterus upward, helping her vagina expand from about 3 to 4 inches to about 5 to 6 inches long. This ultimately makes for more comfortable and pleasurable sex for both of you.

ADD VARIETY TO ORAL. Perform oral sex on each other while standing against a wall. If she's on the receiving end, have her drape her leg over your

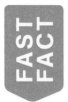
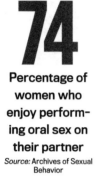

74

Percentage of
women who
enjoy perform-
ing oral sex on
their partner
Source: Archives of Sexual
Behavior

shoulder to help ease your access, and if your tongue gets tired, use your fingers and lips, and even your nose. And don't be too aggressive right off the bat. Start gently in the beginning, with teasing and sensual sucking. Spread her vaginal lips with your hands. It gives you easy access to her clitoris—and shows you're enthusiastic. Base your tongue play on her go-to mode of orgasm. If she usually uses a vibrator, she'll like a more pointed tongue, but if she's more used to intercourse, she'll prefer a softer, flatter tongue. Another good technique: Imagine a clock face on her clitoris and lick outward toward every hour. Try 10 and 2—you'll drive her wild. When she starts writhing, it's not time to try your crazy figure-8 technique. It's a common mistake. You might think, *I want to excite her even more.* So you move—and her O evaporates. Instead, stick with your current move for at least 3 minutes, 10 max.

LOVE GLOVE. Using protection doesn't have to be a barrier to intimacy: Introducing a condom at the end of a foreplay session can make it feel more romantic, according to a study published in the *Archives of Sexual Behavior.* The researchers asked women and men to rate the romanticism of various protected-sex scenarios and found that when guys initiated condom use, women preferred when men verbally suggested it just before intercourse. Grabbing a glove too early (especially without asking her first) presumes sex and may suggest you're overly afraid of contracting a sexually transmitted infection, the researchers say. The scenario both sexes found most romantic? When the woman introduced it. If she's not budging, wait until sex is imminent, and then say, "I want you so bad. Do you mind if we grab a condom?" Covering up should be associated with desire, not disease prevention.

ASK HER TO TOUCH A NEW SPOT. Your prostate is a hidden source of pleasure that can invite a total-body orgasm, says Herbenick. Ask her to stimulate it externally by massaging your perineum, the spot between your testicles and anus. But don't just point at your perineum and say, "Rub it." Start in missionary position, and then angle your body 30 degrees so your butt is tilted toward her lap and she can reach around more easily. Have her massage the area gently with her fingers—your prostate will feel like a nut—and then shift to a firmer, steadier, up-and-down or circular motion. If at first you feel the urge to urinate, don't freak out. Be patient and the sensation will transition from "Oh, no" to "Oh yeah!"

BRING OUT A MIRROR. Sure, mirrored ceilings are a sexual cliché—but for good reason. During sex, mirrors let you occupy two perspectives: the voyeur and the exhibitionist, since you're viewing yourself. Fooling around in front of mirrors also offers you a new view of her: You can see aspects of your partner's body that may be lost from other angles—how she sweats or flushes in certain areas, the way her back arches. If seeing her in action is what excites you, ask her to masturbate while you watch indirectly through a mirror. This adds another voyeuristic layer.

DON'T RUSH THE EXIT INTERVIEW. If she's chatty after sex, consider it a compliment. Her desire for pillow talk may be a sign that she's satisfied, a UC Santa Barbara study found. When women climaxed, they were more likely to make personal disclosures after sex, possibly due to a surge in oxytocin, the bonding hormone. Testosterone can dampen your own desire for bonding, but don't roll over: Pillow talk may boost relationship satisfaction for both sexes.

MASTURBATE—TOGETHER. Letting someone else in on your solo sex life can be nerve-racking for both men and women. It can also be enlightening and intensely intimate. You see your partner at the height of pleasure, without having to worry about how you're performing. She may feel self-conscious at first, so suggest masturbating at the same time under the covers while

COUNTER-INTELLIGENCE

The Sensitive-Jerk Appeal

Sometimes women like jerks—but not guys who are too insensitive. And if you're too nice, that can hurt your chances, too. We surveyed women to find out what's over the top.

UGH—YOU'RE DEFINITELY A JERK!

→ You break up by ignoring calls and texts
→ You're consistently late by half an hour or more
→ You joke by insulting her and then say, "Just kidding!"
→ You describe other women in overly sexual terms
→ You text during dates
→ You wait a week to follow up after a first date
→ You invite friends to meet you during dates

UM—YOU'RE WAY TOO NICE!

→ You say "I'm sorry" for no reason
→ You're a frequent, affectionate poster on her Facebook wall
→ You say "I miss you" when apart for only a few hours
→ You always let her choose the date spot
→ You're too eager to meet her family
→ You send a gushing text 10 minutes after a date
→ You prefer a night in over a night out with the boys

maintaining eye contact. Reinforce how arousing she is, and eventually she may become comfortable tossing the sheets aside. Then, you'll see exactly how she likes to be touched. Take notes.

LAST LONGER. To extend your sack session, use a condom that contains benzocaine, a topical anesthetic that reduces sensation in your penis. Second, use the stop-start technique (pause just before the *ah* moment to cool your jets) and sample positions in which the top side of your penis, which is less sensitive than the underside, receives the most stimulation. For instance, try the sidewinder (spooning from behind) and reach around to caress her clitoris to speed up her orgasm.

LISTEN TO MUSIC. A pulsating musical beat can help the two of you establish a mutual rhythm. So make a foreplaylist that lasts about 20 minutes. As you swap spit, you exchange feel-good chemicals like serotonin and dopamine, which helps your bodies sync up and build excitement.

COMPLIMENT HER DOWN THERE. A woman who feels good about how her parts look is less anxious about sex and finds it easier to reach orgasm, according to an Indiana University study. Our sex and relationships advisor, Debby Herbenick, Ph.D., says: "Many women have insecurities about how their hips, thighs, genitals, or whole body looks naked. Just before you perform oral sex on her, say, 'I love the way you look.' It goes a long way. Many women's conceptions of their bodies have changed entirely in an instant because a partner told her he thought she was beautiful down there." Do you want to be that guy? We thought so.

FOCUS ON FOREPLAY. In a study published in the *Journal of Sex and Marital Therapy*, 60 percent of women said foreplay was their favorite part of sex. So how do you make it awesome? Start building excitement beforehand. Tell her that her butt looks great in that skirt—but don't say it only when you're rushed and on your way out the door, late for work, in an "I love you and you look hot" kind of way. At a party or work function, catch her eye from across the room and smile at her flirtatiously. Make eye contact, and then look her up and down, sending her a nonverbal *Damn, you're sexy.* Another idea? Sext with specifics. Send a flirty text about where on her body you'd like to kiss her later, and see how she responds. If she flirts back, ratchet it up a notch with each text, growing more passionate or explicit—but only if she texts back in kind. Then, when you're in bed, eliminate all distractions. The Kinsey Institute found that one of the biggest turnoffs for women is noticing something messy or dirty around the house. Make sure you're the only thing on her to-do list!

TRY YOUR HAND AT SOMETHING NAUGHTY. Since *Fifty Shades of Grey* became a worldwide phenomenon, more men and women have found themselves curious about bondage. It's natural for men to fantasize about

Better
INSTANTLY
↓

Linger over her earlobes and the back of her neck, typically neglected parts that scored high in a study of erogenous zones by U.K. and South African researchers.

giving up power and control, because it's cathartic and stress relieving. So how do you turn your partner into a dominatrix? Put yourself in a submissive position; encourage her to be on top. Then tell her how hot it would be if she held down your wrists. Emphasize the emotions behind your request—hot, horny, powerless—not specifics of what you want her to do. That makes it exciting for her. She'll take things from there.

CRANK THE SPANK. Bare butts simply scream to be spanked, but if either of you swings too hard your first time at bat, the move may be summarily ejected from your kink repertoire. That'd be a pity, because spanking can hurt so good. She may balk at first, so ease into it. Start gently with your open hand, which offers a wide range of sensations, has a built-in feedback mechanism, and feels more intimate than implements. Don't assume you can just spank her during intercourse and that's enough to turn her on. You'll add to the spanking experience if you actually have her over your knee. Start very slowly with light smacks that just barely sting, and build gradually. If she's enjoying the experience, her breathing should sound smooth and sexy and her butt should be pushing up toward your hand instead of flinching.

TIE EACH OTHER UP. Some people want to be tied up so they can feel controlled. Some enjoy being teased and denied. The appeal for the dominant player, of course, is being in control. But be careful about how you do it. For instance, using cable ties as wrist restraints is a really bad idea. Some other bad ideas: leaving your partner alone while bound, tying her up in a way that restricts circulation, or putting something over her nose and mouth and obstructing her breathing. Instead, start out by loosely tying her wrists, and maybe her ankles, with something that won't be abrasive to her skin, such as silk scarves or ties, and watch that they don't become too tight. There are fleece-lined wrist cuffs that close with buckles, bondage tape, over-the-door suspension cuffs, or under-the-bed restraints that can be employed when the mood strikes. All of these items can be purchased at Amazon.com.

TRY ROLE PLAYING. It's a great kink-starter. But unless you were a drama major, pretending to be someone else is going to make you feel silly and require you to suspend your disbelief. That can be tough, but not as tough as you might think. Skip the elaborate script and period garb and make it easy on yourself. For instance, you could arrange to meet at a nightclub that neither of you has been to before. Arrive in clothes you haven't seen each other in, and after some fleeting eye contact, start chatting as if you are perfect strangers just starting to flirt with each other. From there you can take it in any direction you want. Perhaps one of you can play hard to get while the other portrays the wolfish seducer. You can be an entirely different person, exaggerate a specific facet of your actual personality, or just reconnect with the feeling of meeting your partner for the first time.

Find the Right Partner

GO WHERE THE HOT, FIT WOMEN ARE. If you're on the hunt for a new partner, volunteer at a local triathlon. It's a 1-day commitment and an easy way to meet and impress fit women. In a Cornell University study, women favored altruistic guys for both relationships and 1-night stands.

DRESS SMART. Women zero in on clothes, subconsciously looking for signs of status. Rework your wardrobe. She'll notice shoes instantly, so buff them and swap out the laces with a more daring color, like red or green. Next, invest in a pair of dark jeans. Focus on fit—they should be neither too

Your Toolbox

Lube makes sex hotter–that is, if it doesn't dry up or give her hives. Find the lube that suits your scenario.

WATER-BASED LUBE WITH GLYCERIN
PROS: Inexpensive; won't stain fabrics
CONS: May dry out quickly; can cause irritation
Best for your budget

GLYCERIN-FREE WATER-BASED LUBE
PROS: Lasts longer than lubes with glycerin do; won't stain
CONS: May taste bitter
Best for sensitive skin

SILICONE LUBE
PROS: Waterproof; lasts longer than water-based lubes
CONS: Often pricier than water-based lubes; must be washed off with soap and water
Best for sex in the shower

SALIVA
PROS: Feels more natural and is less irritating than other impromptu lubes (such as Vaseline or massage oil)
CONS: Can increase her risk of a yeast infection
Best for spontaneous sex

loose nor skintight, and the waistband should sit at your actual waist (1 inch above your hipbones). Above the belt, mix things up. Try combining a solid, a pattern, and a texture—like a navy jacket with a plaid dress shirt and a solid knit wool tie.

POUR A HOT CUPPA SEX APPEAL. Starbucks may be the ultimate pickup spot. Pleasant smells could help you score her number, according to research from France. Women were more likely to give men their phone numbers when approached at delicious-smelling places—bakeries, coffee shops, pastry shops—than when they were chatted up in clothing stores or banks. Enticing scents may lift her mood, making her more receptive to your advances.

MAKE SURE SHE'S NOT ALL TALK. Red flag: She prefers Facebook chat to coffee talk. Women who regularly use instant messaging on social media sites tend to be more disagreeable and less empathetic than infrequent chatters, a University of Alabama study found. Facebook flirting is fine, but if she wants to have all your major conversations online, she may be trying to hide unattractive traits, the scientists say.

MASTER MATCH.COM. Talk about unfair: Good-looking men also tend to write the most appealing online-dating profiles, say Villanova University scientists. They had women rate men's photos and profiles separately, and as it turned out, the hottest guys had also written the most enticing profiles. Good-looking men tend to have more self-confidence, which is probably conveyed in their writing, the researchers say. To catch her eye online, don't simply list your interests and skills—use playful language and have fun.

TRY A COMIC COME-ON. So three French guys walk into a bar—seriously: The men went on to prove that making your buddies laugh can catch her eye. In the study, three men went to sidewalk bars in France and sat near a woman who was alone. One of the trio told jokes, the other two laughed, and then one of them asked the lady for her digits. While they took turns being the joke teller, the guy hitting on the woman was the same each time. After 54 women, his success rate was 43 percent when he was the jokester, but only 15 percent when he was one of the guys laughing.

TRY THE VOICE OF SEX. Ben Stein, ladies' man? Men with monotone voices have more sex, a new study in the *Archives of Sexual Behavior* reports. Researchers told males they were competing with a man in another room for a date and then recorded them as they addressed him. The less a man's pitch varied, the more sex partners he reported. A monotone may intimidate other men, giving you a better shot. Give yourself a pep talk. Confidence can steady your voice, the scientists say.

MASTER TABLE MANNERS. At the risk of sounding stodgy, a few words about manners: Use them—always and as naturally as possible. Good composure at the table indicates good composure elsewhere. A few key principles: Offer her the more comfortable seat and the better view. Invite her to taste the wine (before or after you do) when the server presents it. Don't get drunk, or at least noticeably so. As for dinner, offer her a bite of your dish, but don't eat off her plate unless enthusiastically invited. Say "excuse me" before standing to head to the restroom. And yes, be respectful to the service staff. If something is wrong with the food, address the problem immediately and politely. (Coarse confrontation is hard to digest.) Dessert? It doesn't matter if you've saved room or not: She wants some.

TRY A BETTER OPENING LINE. A study in the *Journal of Social Psychology* shows what women really like to hear. If you want to show her that you're funny or sociable:

→ "Do you have any raisins? No? Well then, how about a date?"
→ "Shall we talk or continue flirting from a distance?"
→ "Can I get a picture of you so I can show Santa what I want for Christmas?"

If you want to show her that you're smart and trustworthy:

→ "I feel a little embarrassed about this . . . but I'd like to meet you. What's your name?"
→ "Hi, I saw you and thought, 'I'm going to kick myself all night if I don't at least say hi.' So . . . hi. What's your name?"
→ "I saw you across the room and knew I had to meet you. What's your name?"

BE FUNNY—FOR REAL. There are many paths to a woman's digits, but only one shortcut: humor. Now, you may be thinking, *I try to be funny, and it never works.* There's your problem: The more you try for laughs, the fewer you receive. The fix? Building off something you have in common, such as a hot topic in the news or an event you both just witnessed. But if you just saw, say, the bartender spill a drink, resist the urge to turn him into a punch line: Research shows that the best flirtation strategy is affiliative humor—warm, low-key, playful joking—rather than mean-spirited quips.

FIND YOUR GROOVE. Does your "Thriller" thrill her? Women judge how hot you are by your dance moves, say researchers in Germany. Two groups of women watched men dance and scored them on either attractiveness or risk-taking propensity. The most adventurous men, the study found, were also rated the hottest. Killer moves may signal desirable traits such as status and competitiveness, so bust out some signature steps with confidence. Imitating others is obvious—and unattractive.

TRY YOUR BEST ANGLE. Keep your chin up. Women find you more masculine and attractive if you tilt your chin upward, according to a study on photo preferences in *Evolutionary Psychology*. Conversely, men find women who tilt their chins down to be more feminine and attractive. Researchers think these preferences may have evolved because men are typically taller than women.

CALL HER BLUFF. Her tease is your test: Women play "hard to get" not only to boost their sex appeal, but also to assess your level of commitment, a study in the *European Journal of Personality* revealed. They want to know if you're in it for more than casual sex. The more you show your willingness to accept the challenges of the chase, the more likely she is to think you're seeking a serious relationship. So don't be discouraged by these tactics: She sounds busy, she's hard to reach, her availability is limited, her initial interest seems to fade, or she seeks your attention and then ignores it. Now . . .

SHOULD YOU PLAY HARD TO GET, TOO? Maybe. Women are more attracted to men whose feelings about them are a mystery, the journal *Psychological Science* reveals. In a study using online profiles, women were told that men liked them, rated them average, or had unknown feelings. The women rated the mysterious guys as most attractive. Being inscrutable makes her think about you more, the study authors say.

SHOW HER A GOOD TIME. Looks like the fun guys win at love: In a Penn State study, women rated "playful" and "fun-loving" as highly desirable qualities in men—more than good looks and intelligence. Playfulness is the opposite of aggression, so it gives women a sense of safety. So work more lighthearted stuff—sports, games, fun foreplay—into your downtime.

IMPRESS WITH LESS. Leaving your phone out during a date could ruin your odds of connecting, a study in the *Journal of Social and Personal Relationships* reports. Seeing it primes you (and probably her) to think about your broader social network and can distract you from the here and now. Turn off the cellphone and pocket it before you meet her.

EARN HER TRUST. Maybe you flash a Rolex and look like Clooney. But women somehow manage to look past all that. For a long-term relationship, women care more about whether you've cheated in the past than about financial stability, good looks, or common interests, a study from Oakland University found. Women hate sharing: Having a history of cheating suggests that you may divide your assets—financial or otherwise—among other women, which reduces their value to a potential partner. This may have been an evolutionary adaptation. Want to prove you'll be faithful? Just be a dependable guy—call when you say you will, for example, and she'll likely assume you're reliable in other ways too.

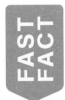

FAST FACT

52

Percentage of women whose sexual fantasies include both male and female partners
Source: Archives of Sexual Behavior

GRAB A REBOUND. She just went through a breakup? Don't wait. Now's the time to make your move. People who quickly rebound trust their next partner more, a study in the *Journal of Social and Personal Relationships* reports. They also feel more confident and desirable. That's great news for you (in bed). But before you put yourself out there . . .

ASSESS HER EX FACTOR. If a woman says a breakup with her ex was mutual, that's good news, a study in the *Journal of Social Psychology* concluded. Calling a split mutual and dating others means a woman is less likely

TRY THIS!

Diffuse Her Jealousy

If your lady has a jealous streak, here's how to talk her down.

WHAT HAPPENED

She noticed that you noticed a beautiful woman.

DEFUSE IT

Don't deny your wandering eyes. Instead, say you were looking at something specific, such as the woman's legs, but then add that your honey's gams are even hotter. By paying her a compliment, you eliminate the threat.

WHAT HAPPENED

You were hanging out with a female friend.

DEFUSE IT

Resist the urge to say, "Why don't you trust me?" A better response: "It's nice to know you care about me enough to be jealous." Then plan something unique with her that shows your relationship is unlike those you have with other women.

WHAT HAPPENED

She accuses you of being a flirt—all the time.

DEFUSE IT

Ask for a few recent examples and then invite her to share how they made her feel. Listen, and then when she's finished, assure her that you don't want to hurt her. Talking about emotions will bring you closer and repair your bond.

WHAT HAPPENED

You mentioned an ex.

DEFUSE IT

Reassure her that there's a reason your ex is your ex. Tell her the truth—and what she needs to hear—that your ex was once part of your life, but there's a reason you've moved on.

to go back to her former partner, researchers found. However, if she has a hard time defining her relationship with her ex, she may be more likely to reunite with him. Another warning sign: venting about their last fight. Frustration that stems from isolated events rather than the relationship itself may lead to impulsive—and temporary—breakups.

HIT THE STRINGS. Is this John Mayer's secret? A guitar may boost your sex appeal, a French experiment reveals. When a man asked a random woman for her phone number, she was more likely to oblige if he was carrying a guitar case than if he was empty-handed or toting a gym bag. Musical talent may signal qualities like intelligence or commitment to hard work, the researchers say. But don't brag about your skills. Invite her to hear you play in a casual setting.

SCORE A SECOND DATE. Women value a good listener, but they also want to hear what you have to say. Focusing entirely on her side of the conversation may hurt your second-date chances, according to research in the *Journal of Experimental Social Psychology*. When strangers engaged in back-and-forth conversation, they felt closer, liked each other more, and thought they had more in common than when one dished while the other listened. It's best to keep the talking and listening equal. Caution: Simply returning her questions is boring. So if she asks about, say, your favorite travel spot, you might ask her about a childhood trip.

SAVE YOURSELF. If you're looking for a lasting relationship, don't rush into bed with her. The longer you wait to have sex, the higher your likelihood of having a better marriage, say researchers at Brigham Young University. They surveyed 2,035 spouses on such topics as communication, relationship satisfaction and stability, and sexual timing and quality. Partners who'd held off on sex for at least a month into dating had more positive responses than those who didn't wait.

FAST FACT

40

Percentage rise in women's reported sexual attraction to guys in red shirts

Source: Journal of Experimental Psychology: General

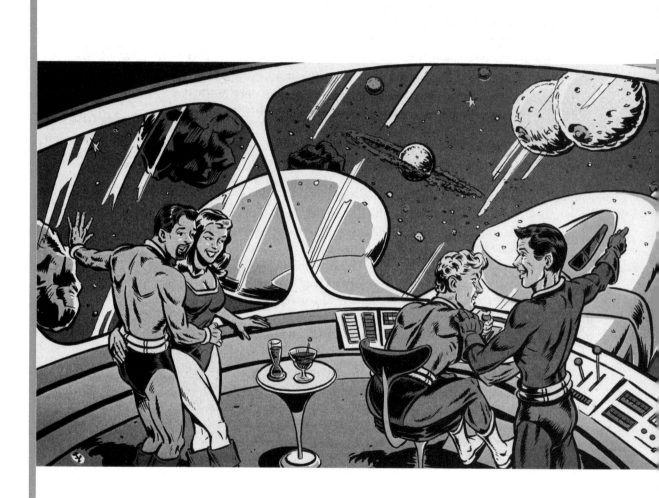

Love Lessons from Gay Guys

Same-sex couples are happier and more sexually satisfied than everyone else. What can you learn from them to improve your hetero hookups?

BY MICHAEL CALLAHAN

A FUNNY THING HAPPENED WHEN GAY COUPLES WERE TOLD BY judges that they couldn't tie the knot: They invented a whole new kind of relationship blueprint. And then researchers checked it out and found that it seemed to be working better than the other one.

A landmark study published in the journal *Developmental Psychology* followed gay couples for 3 years and found that by nearly every metric, they reported higher-quality relationships and felt more satisfied than straight married couples did.

This wasn't exactly news to me. As a gay man, I know we defy the expectations for typical relationships.

And while one study doesn't mean we have all the answers, it does mean we could have something to teach you. After all, we date guys like you—we are guys like you. Here are some things that homosexual guys can teach heterosexual guys.

Gay Guys Make Sex an Adventure

That study in *Developmental Psychology* found that gay couples have higher levels of affection and intimacy compared to heterosexual couples. That's partly because we access a greater number of sensual tools in order to enjoy sex to the fullest. People in same-sex relationships tend to be more satisfied with things like deep kissing, touching, and undressing their partners than people in heterosexual relationships are, according to a study in the *Journal of Sex Research*. Of the four groups studied—straight men, straight women, gay men, and lesbians—straight men actually scored the lowest sexual satisfaction from those same things.

Where do they go wrong? A more narrow-minded approach to sex could be partly to blame. "Sometimes straight men undervalue sex play other than intercourse," says *Men's Health* sex and relationships advisor Debby Herbenick, Ph.D. "It's the variety of sex—kissing, touching, breast stimulation, toys, and oral sex—that adds a much-needed dimension to a couple's sex life. Gay men often have a larger menu of things to choose from." Which seems counterintuitive, since men have matching parts. But gender roles, Herbenick says, can be more flexible among gay men, so there's less stigma attached to things like the use of sex toys. Gay porn also eroticizes behaviors like mutual masturbation, which you don't see much of in straight porn.

Straight couples also often struggle to be blunt about what they want from sex, says therapist Rik Isensee, a counselor based in San Francisco and the author of *Love Between Men*. "It can make some men feel vulnerable to admit that they could learn anything new about how to please their partner."

When you have that talk, start with simple requests, Herbenick says. If you normally have sex at night, see if she's game first thing in the morning, or head to the basement and christen the pool table. Spontaneity and unpredictability are thrilling, and the residual excitement will leave her wanting more. Then follow up the next day, Herbenick says. Try something like, "Wasn't that fun last night? Here's what I'd like to try next . . . " and give her a chance to respond. You'll likely wind up with new material to fuel your sex life for months.

Or you could take a cue from another source of our creativity: porn. Used as fantasy fuel, pornography can actually spark sexual novelty and creativity, which is valuable given that two people in a relationship almost never have identical sex drives.

If you're going to show porn to your wife, though, be careful what you click on, says Herbenick. "Most women don't like mainstream porn, but female-oriented options are becoming increasingly available, like those from Make Love Not Porn, which depict women enjoying sex and being respected during the act."

Admiring Other Guys Is Part of the Fun

Most straight guys can only imagine what might happen if their wife or girlfriend caught them leering too long at the yoga instructor. (The answer: nothing good.) That's why when Drew, 45, and his partner, Ari, 43, check out a hot guy, their straight friends are often baffled when it doesn't lead to a spat. "Straight men always say they wish they could do things like that," Drew says, "and women are shocked that we're so comfortable with it." Ari and Drew are not exceptions. Another study in *Developmental Psychology* explored differences between straight and gay couples and found gay men to be "among the most secure adults" interviewed. Ian Kerner, a sex therapist based in New York City, says much of this comes down to gay men's ability to generally separate love from sex. "Gay couples have often had more experience with open relationships and are more open to talking about it and experimenting with it," he says. A 2010 San Francisco State University study backs him up: The researchers looked at 566 gay male couples and found that nearly half were in open relationships.

This also may be why flirting among friends isn't a big deal for most gay men either. In fact, it's almost a constant: Many of us are fine with the fact that our better halves flirt—in a way a lot of straight couples aren't. "I think, 'Look, he's going home with me every night,'" says Brian, 36, a lawyer in Philadelphia who's been with his boyfriend for 4 years. "I know he loves me, and I trust him completely."

That's easy for my friend Brian to say, right? He's not looking at the silent treatment for an entire week. Commitment and trust are critical to fostering intimacy with women, and flirting openly undermines those qualities.

"Women feel threatened and disrespected when their guy flirts with another woman because it makes them feel unsafe," says Paul Hokemeyer, Ph.D., a marriage and family therapist in New York City. "Sexually, economically, and socially, women are more vulnerable. That's changing, of course, but there's still a ways to go." Herbenick suggests trying simple games, like "Hot or Not" or "Never Have I Ever," which allow you to bring up other people—and your dating past—in a nonthreatening or even self-deprecating way.

Of course, just because gay men might be more comfortable with a little flirting doesn't mean we're free of the insecurities that may keep the average straight woman awake at night. So if you're looking to make her feel more secure in the relationship, here's another thing you should do (please, bear with me): Talk more. My last boyfriend and I instituted a weekly "temperature check" where we just confirmed that everything was kosher between us. And sometimes that's all you need. Just knowing that she has the ability, and a designated time, to air any grievances may save you a world of passive aggression, says Hokemeyer.

While you don't always need to be having The Talk, taking the temperature every so often isn't a bad idea. If that's not your style, there are other easy ways to show her that she's valued and safe in the relationship, says Hokemeyer. One of the simplest: Every time she mentions something small that she likes—a favorite drink, a new TV show, a pizza joint she's been hoping to try—take two seconds and enter it in your phone's notepad. Pick one to spring on her a few days later, and you'll reinforce that she's the only woman on your mind. And another long talk will be the last thing on hers.

Gay Guys Are Cool with Alone Time

Ari recently won an all-expenses-paid trip to Venice and Verona. And he took it—without his partner, Drew. "Having time to myself is never an issue," Drew says. Healthy couples have strong lives together and strong lives apart—which is important, because couples don't thrive when they're joined at the hip. "It's when you ground yourself that you start to feel better, healthier, clearer, and more satisfied with life," says Hokemeyer.

Whether we're traveling alone or with our partners, we're doing a good job of capitalizing on our time off. A survey by Community Marketing and Insights, a market research firm, found that gay and bisexual men average four vacations a year and that almost half have taken one lasting 5 nights or longer. And just 20 percent of gay or bisexual men were motivated by romance with their partner when choosing a destination. Higher on the list: relaxing, and quality time with buds.

Straight couples become more self-focused, especially when kids enter the picture, says sex therapist Kerner. "But gay male couples are more likely to have extended communities of friends who act like surrogate families."

While date nights and "being there" for the other person are key, so is finding the time to disconnect and regroup on your own. Here's what might help: Encourage her to plan at least one getaway that's all hers, too—and to do it in advance. Just looking forward to your vacation can actually boost your happiness levels for weeks or even months before your trip, according to a study in the journal *Applied Research in Quality of Life*.

Such freedom takes some getting used to, admittedly. But it can also offer a lot of breathing room. One of the best relationships of my life was with a guy who lived by one simple motto: "We love each other, and we'll figure it out." Because that's the beauty of blueprints: They can always be altered to fit what you need.

(Some names and details in this story have been changed.)

What Gay Men Say

83 PERCENT

Are grateful they don't have to deal with a straight woman

23 PERCENT

Report having sex three or four times a week

69 PERCENT

Say their straight male friends ask them for relationship advice

Based on a *Men's Health/Out* magazine survey of 3,290 men in gay relationships

CHAPTER

11

Trouble-shooting Your Body

Pain in the Neck?
Rumblings in Your Gut?
Here Are Your Fast Fixes for
Just about Anything.

In the first 10 chapters, you learned about the lifestyle upgrades

that will keep you fit and healthy for (your very long) life. We also showed you how to draft an all-star health care team, docs who can fix any big bumps on the road of life. But don't forget about the little things—the somewhat random,

■
Better
INSTANTLY
↓
Stiffle hiccups by swallowing 2 teaspoons of sugar. The coarse granules will stimulate and reset the irritated nerve that's causing your diaphragm to spasm.

sometimes serious, but always annoying health problems that, if left unchecked, can take you out—or at the very least, make you miserable. Fortunately, you can solve many of those yourself. Heck, we even alphabetized them for you. Try these remedies to common maladies to heal up faster.

Acne

Zits aren't just for teenagers. If you find yourself with a breakout, zap it with salicylic acid and benzoyl peroxide. Using these ingredients in combination eliminates acne better than benzoyl alone, say Harvard scientists. Use a 2 percent salicylic acid face wash, and then apply a 5 to 10 percent benzoyl peroxide ointment overnight. For "bacne," try a salicylic acid body wash. To ward off future breakouts, rethink your diet. Scientists at NYU report that high-glycemic foods, such as rice, potatoes, bread, and sugary snacks and drinks, may contribute to acne. A diet loaded with sugars and starches causes a rise in insulin and blood glucose, which may influence hormones and other proteins that make breakouts worse, the researchers say. For a healthy face (and body), limit your carb intake to no more than 40 percent of your total daily calories and eliminate high-glycemic foods.

SEE A DOCTOR IF . . . OTC methods aren't working. A dermatologist can prescribe something stronger. Your doc might also order an oral glucose tolerance test because pimples may signal insulin resistance, a precursor to type 2 diabetes. In a study published in the journal *Endocrine*, men with acne had fasting insulin levels nearly double those of guys with clear skin.

Alcoholism

Just how much is too much? One early symptom of alcoholism is going over the limits you set for yourself. Another is having a consistent desire to quit or cut down on boozing, but difficulty following through. If you have a family history of alcoholism, pay special attention. You aren't exactly doomed to drunkenness, but studies do show that genetics accounts for up to 60 percent of a man's risk of alcoholism. In addition, guys are more likely than women are to inherit the disease.

SEE A DOCTOR IF . . . you think your drinking is a problem, or you answer "yes" to one or more of these questions, according to the National Institutes of Health. In the past year, have you:

→ Had times when you ended up drinking more or for longer than you intended?

→ More than once wanted to cut down or stop drinking, or tried to, but couldn't?

→ Spent a lot of time being sick from or getting over the aftereffects of drinking?

→ Experienced a strong need or urge to drink?

→ Found that drinking—or being sick from drinking—often interfered with taking care of your home or family? Or caused job troubles? Or school problems?

→ Continued to drink even though it was causing trouble with your family or friends?

→ Given up or cut back on activities that were important or interesting to you, or gave you pleasure, in order to drink?

→ More than once gotten into situations while or after drinking that increased your chances of getting hurt (such as driving, swimming, using machinery, walking in a dangerous area, or having unsafe sex)?

→ Continued to drink even though it was making you feel depressed or anxious or adding to another health problem? Or after having had a memory blackout?

→ Had to drink much more than you once did to get the effect you want? Or found that your usual number of drinks had much less effect than before?

→ Found that when the effects of alcohol were wearing off, you had withdrawal symptoms, such as trouble sleeping, shakiness, irritability, anxiety, depression, restlessness, nausea, or sweating? Or sensed things that were not there?

Allergies

The sniffing, the itchy eyes—allergies are annoying at best, and often debilitating. They're one of the ultimate examples of your body playing tricks on you: Your immune system encounters an invader—such as pollen—and registers it as a threat. Then, it launches a counterattack, which leaves you with a runny nose and itchy eyes. Left untreated, allergies can predispose you to sinus infections, ear infections, and even asthma. One problem that may slow down your recovery: Allergy symptoms can mimic those of other conditions, like colds. So take this test from the American College of Allergy, Asthma, and Immunology:

→ How did your symptoms start? Cold symptoms evolve, but allergy symptoms often strike all at once.

→ How long have you been miserable? Colds typically clear up within a week or two, whereas allergies may drag on.

→ Achy and feverish? Probably a cold or the flu.

→ Itchy eyes? Allergies, most likely.

→ Sore throat or coughing? Generally a cold.

If it is allergies, fight back with loratadine (Claritin). Fexofenadine (Allegra), loratadine, and cetirizine (Zyrtec) are equally effective at fighting allergy symptoms, but Claritin is less likely to make you sleepy. Another option? A corticosteroid nasal spray containing triamcinolone—Nasacort— was approved for over-the-counter sale in 2013. These inflammation-fighting hormones can have fewer side effects than antihistamines like loratadine. The reason? They go right in your nose instead of throughout your body. Studies also show that corticosteroid sprays reduce nasal blockage and discharge more effectively than antihistamines do. Then, boost your results with a few simple drug-free strategies. Start by wearing sunglasses anytime you step out into the pollen zone. Eyes still itching? Use eyedrops and a cool compress. U.K. scientists found that the combo helps allergy-addled eyes. Give each eye a drop of preservative-free lubricating eyedrops to dilute allergens. Then relieve swelling by applying a frozen gel pack for 5 minutes.

SEE A DOCTOR IF . . . your symptoms don't improve within 2 weeks. Your doc may prescribe stronger meds.

Appendicitis

If a sharp pain strikes quickly in your upper abdomen and then hits the lower right side, go to the emergency room. (You might also have nausea, vomiting, or fever.) It may be appendicitis, and the symptoms worsen dramatically over a 24-hour period. If it is left untreated, your appendix can rupture and spread infection throughout your abdominal cavity. Doctors aren't sure what causes appendicitis, but studies do suggest that the disease is less common in people who eat plenty of fiber. Consider that extra motivation to eat whole grains and leafy vegetables.

Asthma

This disease is often the butt of jokes—why is it always the dorky kid who puffs the inhaler in movies? But for people who have asthma, it's not a laughing matter. Asthma inflames and narrows your airways, which can leave you gasping for air, wheezing, and coughing. It can also cause a tight feeling in your chest.

SEE A DOCTOR IF . . . you feel the signature symptoms. You may need an inhaler. While you're there, ask your doc about the Propeller inhaler sensor (propellerhealth.com). The attachment hooks to your basic inhaler to automatically track your usage, which can help people with asthma and

COPD avoid attacks. People in a small study published in *PLOS One* had 38 percent more symptom-free days after 2 months with the device. Another option? Track your triggers and symptoms manually using AsthmaSense Cloud, a free app. It will alert you when you're at risk for an attack.

Athlete's Foot

This foot fungus can latch on to your feet after you walk barefoot on an infected surface. Eliminate it with butenafine (in Lotrimin Ultra) or terbinafine (in Lamisil[AT]); they're two of the most effective OTC antifungals, according to a meta-analysis from Brazil. To prevent infection, dry your feet after swimming and wash them immediately after playing sports. Wear socks if someone at home is infected, and wear sandals in communal areas. And wash your socks in hot water. In a study from Israel, researchers found that when fungus-laden socks were washed in warm water, 36 percent still contained spores, compared with just 6 percent of socks washed in a hot cycle. Worst case: You could re-infect yourself when you don socks laundered at a lower temp.

SEE A DOCTOR IF . . . you follow the directions on an OTC treatment, but your symptoms don't clear up. You may need a prescription for an anti-fungal in pill form.

Bacterial Food Poisoning

Back away from that chicken: Foodborne bugs like the various *Salmonella* species and *Clostridium perfringens* sicken more than a million people per year. Undercooked meats are a common source of these bacteria, so always cook ground pork or beef to an internal temperature of 160°F, poultry to 165°F, and steak to 145°F. Like your burgers rare? Store-bought ground beef can be contaminated by the contents of cows' intestines, so grind beef yourself or ask a butcher to do it. If you end up with the runs anyway, your first instinct might be to run to remedies like Imodium. Skip these if you see blood or slimy, gloppy mucus—signs of bacteria at work. Stifling diarrhea can cause toxin buildup, damaging your intestines. Instead, replace the fluids you're ejecting from both ends by drinking 8 to 10 glasses of water a day. Also, eat potassium-rich foods, such as bananas and potatoes. (Peel the spuds to limit fiber.)

SEE A DOCTOR IF . . . you're still perched on the porcelain after 3 days. Make it sooner if you have severe abdominal pain, see blood in your diarrhea or vomit, or have a fever above 101°F. These symptoms may indicate that bugs have spread outside your GI tract, requiring antibiotics.

Bad Breath

A bar of soap won't fix your filthy mouth. After brushing, use a mouthwash with bacteria-fighting cetylpyridinium chloride (CPC), such as Crest Pro-Health Multi-Protection Rinse. It's alcohol-free, so it won't dry your mouth and wipe out bacteria-fighting enzymes in your saliva. Use the clear version, because CPC can cause dyes to stain your teeth. Now, if bad breath only strikes after you eat garlic and onions, consider this: Onions contain sulfur byproducts that are absorbed into your blood, so the sulfur smell is actually coming from your lungs. After your oniony entrée, snack on a side dish that has parsley, fennel, or mustard seeds. Studies suggest that these foods may help dilute the sulfur byproducts, while chewing stimulates saliva flow. Another option: Munch on an apple. This fruit contains an odor-busting enzyme that makes garlic breath less galling, according to a study in the *Journal of Food Science*. Or drink plenty of water, and chew strawberry sugarless gum. Research published in the *International Journal of Dentistry* found that strawberry gum boosts spit production faster than other flavors.

SEE A DOCTOR IF . . . these remedies don't work. Chronic bad breath can be a sign of a sinus infection, gum disease, or other conditions that might require medical intervention.

Baldness

Two-thirds of men face hair loss by age 35. Blame your parents: Male-pattern baldness is an inherited sensitivity to dihydrotestosterone (DHT, a byproduct of testosterone), which leads to finer hair, a receding hairline, and finally a deserted scalp. If your hair is only on the sides and middle top of your head, the bare areas form the letter M (as in male-pattern baldness). But thinning that spreads across your scalp and not to your crown or temples often indicates an underlying health issue. Hormonal or nutritional deficiencies, such as thyroid problems, low iron, or low protein, can cause shedding. See a dermatologist as soon as thinning begins so you can have a scalp biopsy to rule out worrisome triggers. To find a dermatologist specializing in hair loss, go to aad.org/find-a-derm, enter your zip code, and select "hair disorders" as the specialty. And while they may be tempting, don't succumb to infomercials and ads for hair-growth miracles. The best solutions are FDA approved: finasteride (Propecia) and minoxidil (Rogaine). Propecia works by blocking the conversion of testosterone to DHT, but there's a side effect to consider: It could mess with nerve-signaling pathways to your penis, resulting in ED and a loused-up libido, a study in the *Journal of Sexual Medicine* found.

Most men don't experience these side effects, but if you're uneasy about the

ED risk, skip the Propecia. As for Rogaine, it's thought to stimulate hair growth, although scientists aren't sure how. Use it at least twice a day and for at least 6 months. Finally, switch your shampoo. Ketoconazole, an antifungal used to fight dandruff, may save your mane by reducing production of testosterone (and therefore DHT) in hair follicles, say scientists at the University of British Columbia. In fact, in a Belgian study, balding men who used a 1 percent ketoconazole shampoo two or three times a week for 6 months saw a 17 percent reduction in hair shedding. Try Nizoral A-D, the only nonprescription shampoo that contains ketoconazole. Lather up with a quarter-size dollop two or three times a week; any more than that could dry out your hair and cause breakage. Use nonirritating baby shampoo in between.

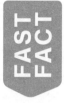

Bunions

Does your big toe look like a boomerang? When your first toe is misaligned (possibly from flat feet or a family history of bunions), it can swing toward the other toes. As a result, the joint that holds your toe loses alignment and bulges out—resulting in a bump called a bunion. To prevent bunions, make sure your shoes fit properly. Don't cram your toes into pointed dress shoes. If you notice that your big toe is angled or your joint is forming a bump, try toe spacers to keep your big toe pointing straight.

SEE A DOCTOR IF . . . the bunion is painful. You might need surgery to correct it.

Canker Sores

Mouthful of misery? You need three key ingredients: numbing benzocaine, cetylpyridinium chloride to keep oral bacteria out of the wound, and benzoin tincture to create a bandage-like layer over your sore. The only OTC product that has it all: Kank-A Mouth Pain Liquid. After applying it, avoid spicy or acidic foods, which may dissolve the protective film. Or try a more natural remedy: bee vomit. In a study from Saudi Arabia, honey reduced the size and pain of these mouth ulcers better than topical steroids did; it also cut healing time by up to 5 days compared with OTC options. Credit the sweet stuff's antibacterial and anti-inflammatory properties.

SEE A DOCTOR IF . . . the sore doesn't heal.

Cataracts

Let's start with a quick primer on your peepers. Your cornea is the clear outer covering of your eye, and it helps you focus on these words you're reading.

Behind your cornea sits your lens, which helps to focus light on your retina. As you age, that lens may gradually become more opaque. Eventually, the cloudiness causes images to appear blurred—typically in your mid-60s. To keep your eyes from going south, try eating more of this soul food: collard greens. They're jam-packed with lutein and zeaxanthin, a dynamic antioxidant duo that can slash your risk of cataracts by up to 42 percent, say scientists in Finland. Other foods with this eye-saving combo? Kale, spinach, turnip greens, and chard. And always wear sunglasses when you're outside, of course.

SEE A DOCTOR IF . . . you notice any changes in your vision.

Celiac Disease and Gluten Sensitivity

If you don't know what gluten is by now, you haven't been paying attention to the TV doctors. Just in case, I'll tell you—it's a protein found in wheat, barley, and rye, as well as in many common food additives. It gives dough its elasticity and baked goods their satisfying chewiness. But for people who have celiac disease—a type of autoimmune disorder—eating foods that contain gluten can lead to a cascade of nasty reactions, including damage to the small intestine, poor nutrient absorption, diarrhea, abdominal pain, bloating, anemia, and fatigue. There is no cure for celiac disease and no drugs can treat it; you can only manage the condition by sticking to a gluten-free diet for the rest of your life. In addition, a rising percentage of people in the United States consider themselves "gluten sensitive." "These people may have a food intolerance or experience many celiac-type symptoms after consuming foods that contain gluten," says Lara Field, M.S., R.D., a dietitian at the University of Chicago's Celiac Disease Center. Some may have a form of wheat allergy. First step: Keep a log of the times that these hangovers hit. What did you eat and when? If gluten is the common factor, go without it for 2 weeks while keeping up with your dietary diary. At the end of this washout period, revert to your old eating habits for 2 more weeks. "If you feel significantly worse in that latter 2-week period," says Mike Roussell, Ph.D., a nutrition consultant and author of *The Six Pillars of Nutrition*, "you might want to rid your diet of gluten permanently." For added confirmation, talk to your doctor about ordering blood tests that can detect some of the antibodies associated with celiac disease. Just be sure to keep eating foods containing gluten before the test—otherwise, your results may not be accurate.

SEE A DOCTOR IF . . . you fail the test above or if you have unexplained symptoms, such as gastrointestinal discomfort, fatigue, or a rash, especially after eating wheat. Your doctor will conduct a blood test to see for sure.

Colds

Read the directions to soothe your symptoms.

→ **COUGH:** See below. For more, see page 213.
→ **SORE THROAT:** See below. For more, see page 233.
→ **RUNNY NOSE:** Try a decongestant nasal spray. Research published in the *American Journal of Rhinology and Allergy* found that people who used a decongestant nasal spray containing oxymetazoline (such as Afrin) three times a day had lower levels of the rhinovirus in their mucus. By wiping out some of the virus, you may be able to slow its spread through your body. But don't spray for longer than 3 days—it can cause swollen blood vessels, leading to more congestion.

Then, cozy up with a cup of tea. A U.K. study found that cold sufferers who slowly sipped a hot beverage for 10 minutes saw drastic reductions in coughing, sore throat, runny nose, and sneezing. Warm drinks soothe the mucous membranes in your nose, mouth, and throat, reducing irritation, the researchers say. Your tea should be hot, but not too hot—you don't want to cause inflammation. Add honey and lemon: The sweetness and acidity can stimulate salivation to clear your throat and sinuses. Then, sync with zinc. Zinc lozenges may reduce the duration of the common cold, a Canadian review concluded. As soon as your throat feels scratchy—often the first sign of a cold—start sucking on zinc acetate lozenges, such as Zicam. This is the form of the metal that's most effective at fighting colds, say researchers in Finland. Aim for 75 milligrams a day, but don't go overboard. Limit yourself to one lozenge every few hours for a few days. (Regular use for 6 weeks or longer could lead to nerve damage.)

SEE A DOCTOR IF . . . you don't get better in 10 days, or if you spike a fever.

Cold Sores

Tongue hitting some rough patches? If you carry the herpes simplex virus, cold sores can strike anytime. Unfortunately, they tend to appear at the worst times: Stress can allow herpes to emerge from its hiding place in your nervous system, say British researchers. Abreva is the only OTC med that contains docosanol, which targets cold-sore-causing herpes. "It strengthens

To the untrained eye–and sometimes to the eye of a physician–the flu can look like a cold. And a case of mistaken identity can mean delayed treatment and extended misery. Enter rapid influenza diagnostic tests, which are often administered at pharmacy clinics and provide results within 30 minutes. Ask the pharmacist if it the test flags influenza A and B and how it's administered. A McGill University review found that nasal swabs may be more sensitive than nasopharyngeal washes or throat swabs, reducing the risk of a false negative.

cell walls to keep the virus from infiltrating healthy cells and shortens the duration of outbreaks," says W. Steven Pray, Ph.D., D.Ph., a professor of pharmacy at Southwestern Oklahoma State University in Weatherford. In a Canadian study, docosanol users had faster healing of oral lesions than a placebo group did. At the first sign of a sore, smear on Abreva. Then, a few hours later, apply numbing benzocaine (Anbesol). Repeat the Abreva five times a day. Chronic stress may impair the function of virus-fighting T cells. Sunlight can also rouse the dormant herpes virus. When UV rays hit your lips, they're thought to stimulate the nerves that run from the site of the original infection back to where the virus sleeps. So cover your kisser with a balm that blocks both UVA and UVB rays. One more: When your immune system is battling a cold or the flu, the herpes virus tries to sneak past your distracted defenses. Stop it by downing a few glasses of green tea every day you're sick. Pakistani researchers noted that EGCG, an antioxidant found in green tea, may turbocharge your T cells.

SEE YOUR DOCTOR IF . . . you experience chronic cold sores. Your doctor can prescribe antiviral drugs, which won't kill herpes but can stop the virus from making the DNA it needs to reproduce. Ask about the antiviral valaciclovir (Valtrex). If you pop 2 grams at the first hint of a cold sore and then again 12 hours later, you may prevent an outbreak. Another option? A prescription topical treatment, like Xerese; it combines the antiviral acyclovir along with hydrocortisone to reduce swelling and promote healing.

Concussion

Think of your head as a big egg: The shell is your skull, the white is your cerebrospinal fluid, and the yolk is your brain. A violent impact causes the yolk to vibrate and sometimes even bash into the shell. If the force is strong enough, you'll end up with a concussion. And yet, for all that trauma, there's often no visible evidence of injury because the damage is on the inside.

SEE A DOCTOR IF . . . any knock to your head results in vomiting, dilated pupils, or loss of smell or taste; you should be checked out by a neurologist. Same goes for headaches, dizziness, or memory loss that persists for longer than 5 days. Don't just assume that if you didn't black out, you're fine.

Conjunctivitis

More commonly known as pinkeye, this eye condition causes symptoms like itchiness, redness, discharge, and tearing from your peepers. It can be caused by bacteria, viruses, allergies, or chemical irritants.

SEE A DOCTOR IF . . . you have these symptoms. You may need antibiotic eyedrops.

Constipation

If your trips to the bathroom are a struggle, consider drinking an extra glass of water with every meal. Too little fluid intake is the biggest predictor of constipation, according to research in the *American Journal of Gastroenterology*. People who consume less water are more likely to suffer constipation than those who drink more. Adding more insoluble fiber to your diet helps too. Your body can't digest this type of roughage, so it passes through your gut and softens your stool. In fact, a U.K. study found that adding at least 3.5 grams of wheat bran, a type of insoluble fiber, to your daily diet can improve constipation and other aspects of digestion in just 2 weeks.

SEE A DOCTOR IF . . . constipation persists, or if you have blood in your scat. Changes in the form or frequency of your poop can indicate a more serious problem, such as irritable bowel syndrome, Crohn's disease, a bowel obstruction, or maybe even colon or stomach cancer.

Cough

Stop your hack track with dextromethorphan (NyQuil, Robitussin DM, Mucinex DM), the most effective OTC cough suppressant. Scientists aren't sure why it works, but it's thought to block a cough center in your brain. Pick a product with 30 milligrams per dose. In the meantime, stash some menthol cough drops in your desk drawer. Menthol's cooling effect seems to interrupt the neural activity involved in coughing, researchers say. For a phlegmy cough, use a product that contains guaifenesin, an expectorant that thins mucus. Still suffering? A spoonful of honey can help by spurring saliva production. (A moist throat may curtail coughing.) Or try this: Make a paste from a tablespoon of honey and another tablespoon of instant coffee crystals; stir it into a glass of warm water. In an Iranian study, people with lingering coughs who drank this three times a day for a week were coughing less than a control group a week later.

SEE A DOCTOR IF . . . you're short of breath. You might have asthma. And if you have a fever, chills, night sweats, and chest pain with your coughs, you could have tuberculosis. (That's right, people still get this disease.) If your coughing is accompanied by unintentional weight loss, rust-colored phlegm, or bronchitis that keeps coming back, you could have a serious problem with your lungs. If you're coughing up pink, frothy mucus, go to the emergency room. You may have fluid in your lungs, according to the American Academy of Family Physicians. You should also drop everything and head to the hospital if your coughing comes with sharp chest pain, a rapid heartbeat, leg swelling, and sudden shortness of breath. Finally, if your cough is the result of inhaled dust or other particles, see a doctor right away.

Dandruff

If it snows wherever you go, you can blame a fungus called *Pityrosporum ovale*. Change the forecast with Nizoral A-D, the only nonprescription shampoo that contains the anti-fungal ketoconazole. Just limit your lathering to once every 3 days; any more can cause irritation. The rest of the time, W. Steven Pray, Ph.D., D.Ph., a professor of pharmacy at Southwestern Oklahoma State University in Weatherford, recommends shampooing with Head and Shoulders, which contains pyrithione zinc, a compound that slows the shedding of skin cells on your scalp. And don't let wet hair hit the pillow. The moist environment encourages the growth of yeast, a dandruff culprit.

SEE A DOCTOR IF . . . this doesn't work. A dermatologist can prescribe stronger stuff.

Diarrhea

Research suggests that the healthiest bowel movements resemble smooth sausage links. If you're producing loose blobs instead of bratwurst or going more often than ever, swallow some Metamucil or Benefiber. In an American Pharmacists Association survey, these were the most recommended fiber supplement brands. "Soluble fiber absorbs water and becomes gel-like as it travels through your system," says T. Lee Baumann, M.D., a medical consultant based in Birmingham, Alabama, and the author of *Clearing the Air: Art of the Bowel Movement*. The result: firmer and less frequent feces.

SEE A DOCTOR IF . . . dietary adjustments don't make a difference, or ASAP if what you see in the toilet looks like thin ribbons or pencil-size strands. These can signal a bowel obstruction or even colon cancer.

Dizziness

This is a symptom you shouldn't ignore. It can signal a concussion, a stroke, and other deadly problems. See a doctor immediately if you're off-balance.

Dry Eyes

Feel like you could use a few more tears? It's common, and you might be able to blame your computer. Using one for long hours may increase your risk of dry eye by decreasing concentrations of mucin 5AC, a protective substance in tears. Choose preservative-free drops to lubricate your eyes without causing further irritation.

SEE A DOCTOR IF . . . the problem gets worse. Specifically, an ophthalmologist. You could have a more severe eye problem or another disease such as Sjögren's syndrome, an autoimmune disorder that causes a decrease in tear production.

Ear Infection

This happens when fluid builds up in your eustachian tube, which runs from the middle of each ear to the back of your throat. Allergies, colds, sinus infections, and other irritants can increase your risk.

SEE A DOCTOR IF . . . the pain in your ear lasts for 7 days. If a doctor's examination shows that the membrane covering your auditory canal is bulging, then the infection might be bacterial. You'll need an antibiotic.

Eczema

Turn to topical corticosteroids. These stop itching from inflammatory causes, like eczema, allergic reactions, poison ivy, or rashes. Use hydrocortisone briefly and for mild itchiness.

SEE A DOCTOR IF . . . you have severe itching. An M.D. can give you a stronger steroid. Just avoid using any steroid for too long—they can actually thin your skin if used chronically.

Fatigue

If you feel drowsy—or sleepy—it could just be that you're out of shape. In a study published in *Mental Health and Physical Activity*, people who exercised for 150 minutes a week had 65 percent less daytime sleepiness than those who exercised for less time. Fatigue is more serious—it involves a lack of energy and motivation, and it can be caused by myriad things. It might just be that your schedule is overwhelming you. You can combat fatigue by cleaning up your habits—getting adequate sleep, eating a well-balanced diet, meditating, reducing stress, and so on.

SEE A DOCTOR IF . . . this doesn't work. Fatigue can also signal other things, like depression, or an overactive or underactive thyroid. It can even be a result of cancer, diabetes, and other major diseases.

Food Allergy

While a child's peanut allergy is nothing to sneeze at, many adults may not need to skip the Skippy after all. A study review in the *Journal of the American Dietetic Association* found that even though 1 in 5 people alters their diet because they fear adverse reactions, fewer than 1 in 10 truly has a food allergy. The tests used for diagnosis are partly to blame: So-called positive results can be wrong nearly half the time, indicating a food allergy where none exists. If the results of your skin-prick or blood test are unclear or inconclusive, your doctor can confirm the diagnosis with a food challenge, during which you eat increasing amounts of a food at regular intervals under carefully controlled conditions.

SEE A DOCTOR IF . . . you suspect you have a food allergy. It can cause a wide range of symptoms, from an itchy tongue and lips, vomiting, diarrhea, hives, and more, according to an analysis from Poland. Sometimes these symptoms can strike within just a few seconds or minutes of eating the food. In that case, seek immediate medical attention—you may be on the way to potentially deadly anaphylactic shock. This is more common with allergies to eggs, nuts, peanuts, fish, and shellfish. A reaction from a food allergy can also cause less-immediate symptoms, such as fatigue, irritability, depression, headache, insomnia, bloating, and more, within a few hours or days after ingestion of the food at fault. That's more common with allergies to milk, chocolate, legumes, citrus fruits, and food additives.

Gallstones

Your liver produces bile, and the gallbladder stores it for release into the small intestine, where it is used to digest things. Bile consists of several different substances in a very delicate chemical balance, and sometimes this balance goes out of whack. You might make too much of certain bile components. Your gallbladder may empty cholesterol too slowly. Result: gallstones. Research in the *European Journal of Gastroenterology and Hepatology* shows that 38 percent of gallstones occur in people with BMIs above 25. A study from India also suggests that people with gallstones eat more saturated fat than those without them.

SEE A DOCTOR IF . . . you have symptoms of a gallbladder attack, which is caused by stones blocking the ducts that lead to the small intestine, such as pain in your upper right or upper middle abdomen, nausea and vomiting, yellowing skin, or clay-colored poop.

Gas

If you have intestinal pressure, bloating, tightness, and sharp stabbing pains, reconsider your eating habits. Low-carb diets may help reduce gas. So may probiotics, which are often found in yogurt. But first you need to determine whether you're lactose intolerant. If dairy products turn your butt into a trumpet, omit them for 2 weeks to see if your gas subsides. When you need something to take the air right out of your balloon, try simethicone. The ingredient breaks the surface tension of gas bubbles so they can combine and more easily (read: stealthily) pass through your system. Take it three or four times a day as needed, in doses of 60 to 125 milligrams. And next time, act preemptively and take Beano right before a big meal. It contains alpha-galactosidase, which breaks down gas-producing carbs. Not sure what qualifies as "normal" when it comes to the gas you pass? According to the National Institute of Diabetes and Digestive and Kidney Diseases, the average guy passes gas 13 to 21 times a day.

SEE YOUR DOCTOR IF . . . dietary changes aren't enough and you still think you're too gassy. Your body could be having trouble processing certain sugars, such as fructose or lactose, or starchy carbs such as wheat or corn.

Gout

This is a disease in which excess uric acid in your blood forms crystals around your joints. The result is joint inflammation and pain, most commonly felt in your big toe. The ache manifests as severe, sudden swelling, known as a flare. To prevent it, drink less alcohol and lay off heavy animal fats. A diet rich in purines—chemicals commonly found in red meat and seafood—can raise your gout risk, since your body metabolizes these compounds to make uric acid.

SEE A DOCTOR IF . . . you have symptoms of a flare.

Gum Disease

The spaces between your gums and your teeth should be snug. But if you have gum disease, those spaces turn into germ-filled pockets. It's the top

■
Better
INSTANTLY
↓
Take 2 teaspoons of vinegar with a carb-heavy meal and you may reduce your body's glycemic response by 20 percent, say scientists at Arizona State University. The acetic acid in vinegar slows stomach emptying, reducing the rate at which carbs are absorbed. The easiest way to indulge: salad dressing.

reason adults lose teeth, and it's bad for the rest of your body, too. A study from the United Kingdom shows that one common oral bacterium can trigger blood clots. The bug, *Streptococcus gordonii*, can enter your bloodstream through bleeding gums and make a molecule that mimics a clotting protein. To reduce your risk, stock up on seafood. Harvard researchers found that consuming DHA (a type of omega-3 fatty acid) can lower your risk of developing periodontitis, a common gum disease, by 20 percent. The scientists believe DHA may discourage the growth of bacteria that attack gum tissue, and may also reduce inflammation-related tissue loss. To reap the benefit, eat 3 ounces a week of canned albacore (white) tuna, the amount used in the study.

Your oral hygiene routine can also help you avoid gum disease. If you haven't already, upgrade your toothbrush. Electric toothbrushes help reduce plaque and prevent gingivitis better than manual brushes do, according to a recent Cochrane Collaboration review. Grab one with a built-in timer. Brushing for 2 minutes removes 26 percent more plaque than brushing for 45 seconds, which is how long the average American's brush session lasts. In addition, don't be frugal with floss. You need at least 18 inches in order to grip it properly and always have a clean, unshredded segment. Also, make sure your hands are no more than 2 inches apart for better control; the farther apart they are, the greater the likelihood that the strand will snap in the middle and gouge your gum.

SEE A DOCTOR IF . . . you suspect you have gum disease. Red gums, bleeding gums, even chronic bad breath can signal gum disease. Your best bet for recovery is to schedule frequent professional cleanings at your dentist's office.

Hammertoe

If your toes look like they're permanently bent, you might have this condition. It happens when the middle joint of one or more toes bends due to an imbalance between the muscles and tendons that hold it straight. Over time, the tendons tighten up and the toes stick in a bent position. Ill-fitting shoes can increase your risk of this condition, so make sure you have about a thumb's width of space between your longest toe and your shoe. Already have it? Hammertoes can become painful and require surgery, but you may be able to avoid the scalpel if you keep the tendons loose with foot exercises. Lay a towel on the floor and pick it up using your toes. Then drop it and repeat.

SEE A DOCTOR IF . . . your pain interferes with your daily life. Surgery may be required.

Hangover

These are the stuff of legend. And hit movies. But what really happens on your trip to hangover town? Here's the story: Your body metabolizes booze into acetaldehyde, which is turned into acetate, which is then processed into a neurochemical called adenosine. Acetaldehyde is toxic to brain cells, and adenosine dilates blood vessels in your brain. The effect is a pounding headache. But it doesn't stop there: Alcohol can lead to a drop in blood sugar, which creates a power shortage for your mental machinery. When your blood sugar is low, your brain cells can't produce enough energy and can't work properly, which slows your thinking. Your best bet to expedite recovery: Eat high-fiber carbs, like oatmeal, to slowly raise your blood sugar; drink lots of water to combat dehydration; and sip caffeinated coffee to thwart the effects of adenosine metabolism. Don't attempt to head off a headache with aspirin, which can further irritate your already inflamed stomach lining. Acetaminophen is worse: To process this chemical, your liver makes an enzyme called cytochrome p450—the same one it uses to break down alcohol. Since your liver can produce only a limited amount of p450 at once, you risk damaging the organ with unprocessed alcohol and acetaminophen. Ibuprofen is the lesser evil, but frequent use may also cause ulceration in your GI tract. So go drug free: Place an ice pack or a warm, moist cloth—whichever feels better—on your head and neck. To relieve lingering nausea, stay hydrated and eat eggs—they contain cysteine, a compound that helps clear acetaldehyde from your system. Or make an omelet with a cysteine-rich cheese, like Swiss. Or, for a hit of hydration, electrolytes, and cysteine, blend cold chocolate milk with a scoop of whey protein powder and drink up.

Headaches

First, let's determine what kind of headache you have.

Tension headaches deliver dull and typically steady pain, often across your forehead. They can be brought on by stress, which throws your brain's pain processors out of whack. Studies find that relaxation techniques can reduce headache frequency by 50 percent or more.

Migraines involve severe, throbbing pain, often on one side, and are sometimes accompanied by nausea. Common triggers include changes in sleeping patterns, skipped meals, particular foods, and exposure to bright lights or loud sounds. (A hangover headache is actually a mild migraine.)

Cluster headaches usually strike one side of your head. Scientists can't figure out what causes these doozies—which our readers have rated as one of

Outsmart Your Headache

To ease your agony, first figure out what's rockin' your noggin.

TENSION HEADACHE

FEELS LIKE . . . your skull is in a vise. Stress can cause brain chemicals to flatline, activating pain pathways, says Jessica Ailani, M.D., a headache specialist at Georgetown University.

DO THIS: TAKE A HIKE. A 10-minute walk can bring your neurotransmitters back to healthy levels, says Dr. Ailani.

MIGRAINE

FEELS LIKE . . . a railroad spike in one side of your head. As with tension headaches, migraines tend to be triggered by a dip in brain chemicals. Light and noise increase the ache, says Dr. Ailani.

DO THIS: DRINK UP. Follow two Tylenol with Gatorade and coffee, says Dr. Ailani. Hydration and caffeine will boost relief.

SINUS PAIN

FEELS LIKE . . . intense pressure in your cheeks and brow. When sinus cavities become inflamed, the mucus inside can't drain, says rhinologist Martin Citardi, M.D., of the University of Texas.

DO THIS: BURN IT OUT. Spritzes of capsaicin nasal spray can ease the ache, according to University of Cincinnati scientists.

CLUSTER HEADACHE

FEELS LIKE . . . only the worst pain ever (hence the nickname "suicide headache"). Eye redness and a droopy lid are other tells. Brain abnormalities may be to blame, says Dr. Ailani.

DO THIS: HIT THE OXYGEN. If it lasts longer than 20 minutes, get a ride to the E. R. "Oxygen can stop the pain," says Dr. Ailani.

the most painful health problems ever—but one theory is that the pain is related to a sudden release of histamine, the same chemical released when you have allergies. Cluster headaches may feel like the area behind one eye hurts. Sometimes, this causes that eye to water or your nose to run. They might last just 15 minutes; they might last 3 hours. No matter what, they're no fun.

When a headache strikes, your first inclination is probably to grab some ibuprofen. That might be fine—if you only have a headache once a year. Trouble is, if you use over-the-counter pain relievers too often, you can actually make your headaches worse by reducing your pain threshold. Limit pill popping to twice a week; if you need more meds, see a doctor. For pill-free relief, apply ice for 10 to 15 minutes every hour. It will calm the inflamed, irritated nerves and muscles on the outside of your head. Acupressure can also reduce pain from chronic headaches, a Taiwanese study found. Some people find relief by using their right index finger and thumb to gently squeeze the muscle between their left index finger and thumb.

If you experience cluster headaches, talk to your doctor. You may need prescription medication to stave off future attacks. To prevent future tension or migraine headaches, hit the gym on a regular basis. Regular exercise may help prevent migraines as well as drugs do, according to a new Swedish study. People who exercised for 40 minutes three times a week had the same reduction in migraines as people who took the prescription migraine drug topiramate (Topamax). Acupuncture may reduce the frequency of tension headaches and can also be an effective treatment, according to a recent review from the Cochrane Collaboration. And a separate Cochrane review concluded the same for migraine sufferers. Myofascial release, which is a special tissue-stretching technique, can help prevent tension headaches when performed on a person's back, neck, and face, a study in the *Journal of Bodywork and Movement Therapies* found. Participants' headache frequency fell by more than half.

SEE A DOCTOR IF . . . these remedies don't help.

Heartburn

This condition—known formally as acid reflux—causes a burning sensation to move up your chest. It's caused by stomach acid backing up into your esophagus. If your heartburn is infrequent and responds to antacids, don't sweat it. But if it hits more than twice a week, you could have gastroesophageal reflux disease (GERD), a condition in which food or acid from the stomach rises into your esophagus, possibly damaging it over time. Some studies even suggest that GERD might increase your risk of esophageal cancer. Weight loss and a sensation of food "sticking" on the way down can indicate GERD or something more serious; see your doctor.

If you've tried acid reflux medications but still have heartburn, you may be bringing a garden hose to a four-alarm fire. "The medications may not be blocking enough stomach acid, leaving it to flow continually into your esophagus," says John Clarke, M.D., clinical director of the Johns Hopkins Center for Neurogastroenterology in Baltimore. If you're taking a proton pump inhibitor, such as esomeprazole (Nexium), ask your doctor to increase your dosage or add a nightly hit of a histamine receptor blocker, such as ranitidine (Zantac). At the same time, take a good look at your eating habits to see whether you're inadvertently fanning the flames. Researchers in Japan recently found that heartburn sufferers were more likely than healthy people to eat dinner within 2 hours of bedtime and to munch on midnight snacks more than three times a week.

SEE A DOCTOR IF . . . modifying your meds and eating earlier in the evening doesn't extinguish the fire. Ask your doc for an esophagogastroduodenoscopy (say it three times fast and your procedure is free!). This test lets the doctor sneak a peek at the lining of your esophagus and stomach to check for growths, ulcers, or inflammation. Your doctor may also order formal reflux testing (which requires a catheter or wireless system) to find out if some fluid other than stomach acid, such as bile, is causing the conflagration.

Hemorrhoids

An itching, stinging, or burning feeling on your backside could mean that you ate too many hot wings last night. But when spicy foods aren't to blame, the most likely cause is hemorrhoids: swollen veins in your anus or rectum. The veins can become inflamed from constipation, straining on the john, or sitting for too long during the day. If constipation is the culprit, start with our advice on page 213. Then, soothe the inflammation with hemorrhoidal suppositories containing phenylephrine, such as Preparation H. Suppositories are better than creams because your anal canal extends into your body, and it's, er, hard to reach in there with cream.

SEE A DOCTOR IF . . . you're still wincing after 5 days. Ask for Proctofoam, an easy-to-apply foam containing hydrocortisone and pramoxine. And don't procrastinate: You could also have a tear in the lining of your anal canal, caused by straining or passing hard stools. Or, your pain could signal Crohn's disease. This autoimmune disorder can spur the formation of small tracts in your colon or rectum that extend through the skin near your anus, causing pain and bleeding.

Hernia

These happen when an internal organ or fat tissue pokes through a weakened muscle. Yuck. They most often occur in the gut, when a portion of the intestine or the bladder pokes through the abdominal wall. Bear down as if you're having a bowel movement and feel the area in question. "A lot of times you can feel a soft protrusion where intestines have poked through the abdominal muscles," says Travis Stork, M.D., *Men's Health*'s emergency-medicine advisor and the author of *The Lean Belly Prescription*. That's a hernia.

SEE A DOCTOR IF . . . the area suddenly becomes more painful, particularly after you cough or lift something heavy. You could have a strangulated hernia, which happens when the muscle cuts off bloodflow to the intruding organ. That's a medical emergency.

Pop Chart
Your cheat sheet for over-the-counter pain pills

	IBUPROFEN	NAPROXEN	ASPIRIN	ACETAMINOPHEN
Best for	Toothache, headache, postworkout soreness, sprains, back pain. Ibuprofen (e.g., Advil) blocks enzymes that produce inflammatory compounds called prostaglandins.	Tendinitis or bursitis, headache, body aches. Like ibuprofen, this Aleve ingredient is a nonsteroidal anti-inflammatory drug (NSAID), which limits the production of prostaglandins.	The same aches you'd use ibuprofen and naproxen to treat. This pill blocks production of both prostaglandins and cyclooxygenase, a precursor in the inflammatory process.	Headache, fever, or any minor aches without swelling–acetaminophen (e.g., Tylenol) doesn't ease inflammation. It may work by blocking an enzyme in your nervous system.
Take	200 to 400 mg every 4 to 6 hours but no more than 1,200 mg in 24 hours.	One or two 220 mg tablets every 8 to 12 hours but no more than 660 mg in 24 hours.	One or two 325 mg tablets every 4 hours but no more than 4,000 mg in 24 hours.	325 to 1,000 mg every 4 to 8 hours but no more than 3,900 mg in 24 hours.
Beware	It suppresses inflammation so well that it may impede cold or flu recovery. A chronic imbalance of prostaglandins and other chemicals can raise your heart attack and stroke risk.	Naproxen and ibuprofen increase sun sensitivity. And like other NSAIDs, they may cause GI side effects. Cardiac risk is uncertain, but check with your doctor if you have heart issues.	GI risks include stomach ulcers. Aspirin also blocks a clotting compound, making bleeding hard to stop. Watch for swelling or trouble breathing; 1 percent of people are allergic.	Don't use it for a hangover or if you regularly have two or more drinks a day; it can damage your liver. Read the labels of cough and cold meds–many contain acetaminophen.

Influenza

We already talked about how to prevent the flu back on page 40. But if you still get sick, keep your nose clean. When flu patients squirted a saline solution into their nostrils three times a day for 8 days, they recovered about 2 days faster, a recent study in China found. Why? Nasal irrigation may rinse out the virus as well as inflammatory molecules. Use a saline solution, but be careful because two deaths have been linked to irrigation with amoeba-contaminated tap water administered using a neti pot. Use only distilled water or H_2O you boiled first. When you're done, clean the container with fresh disinfected water and let it air-dry.

Ingrown Toenail

This condition might seem trivial, but if infection sets in, it can cause you some serious pain and suffering. An ingrown toenail forms when the corner or side of a toenail grows into the soft flesh. To prevent it, always cut your toenails in a straight line. File the sharp edges. If an ingrown strikes, soak the foot in soapy water for 15 minutes a day to soften the nail, then dry it and apply an antibiotic ointment.

SEE A DOCTOR IF . . . the nail needs to be separated from the skin. That's not a DIY situation.

Irritable Bowel Syndrome

Researchers aren't exactly sure what causes irritable bowel syndrome (IBS), but people who have it know that it's literally a pain in the butt. IBS can cause diarrhea, constipation, urgency, and other symptoms that make pooping a stressful experience. One way to soothe your symptoms? Eat more soluble fiber. In a study in the *British Medical Journal*, IBS patients who ate 10 grams of soluble fiber a day for 12 weeks reduced their symptoms by 54 percent. Soluble fiber may relax your bowel, the researchers say.

SEE A DOCTOR IF . . . your symptoms really disrupt your life; Rx medications are available. Plus, if your symptoms are really severe, there's a chance IBS isn't the culprit. You could have something more serious, such as an inflammatory bowel disease, which requires closer monitoring by your doc.

Itchiness

Make that itch your bitch: A Mount Sinai Hospital study found that hydrocortisone combined with the numbing agent pramoxine hydrochloride rapidly reduced itching. You won't find an OTC product with both, so simultaneously smear on Cortizone-10 Maximum Strength and Caladryl Clear Lotion. It should do the trick for mosquito bites as well as for rashes from poison ivy, oak, or sumac.

SEE A DOCTOR IF . . . the condition doesn't improve.

Jock Itch

We all get a case of itchy balls once in a while, but this version is a bona fide medical condition caused by a fungus. To determine whether you have it, scratch the irritated area. If skin flakes off, or if the area becomes warmer and itchier after a sweaty workout, you probably have jock itch, and it will likely get worse over time. Jock itch typically stays in the folds of your skin and can be treated with an over-the-counter cream such as Lamisil.

SEE A DOCTOR IF . . . you follow the package directions and the problem doesn't resolve.

Kidney Stones

Every guy I know who's had a kidney stone says it's the most painful thing he's ever encountered. In pain studies, it tends to rank up there with childbirth. (For perspective, it's worse than a penile fracture—ouch!) To dodge it, start with weight control. Heavy men may have more stone-promoting substances, such as calcium and oxalate, in their urine as a result of overeating. But even if you're lean, don't assume your world can't be rocked: A poor diet, a family history of stones, and medical conditions such as an overactive thyroid can raise your odds. To dilute your urine and reduce your risk of stones, drink more water. A study in the *Clinical Journal of the American Society of Nephrology* found that men who drink more than 2½ liters of fluid a day are 29 percent less likely to form stones than those who drink less. Whatever you do, don't quench your thirst with soda—in a study published in the same journal, people who drank a can of sugar-sweetened cola per day increased their risk of kidney stones by 23 percent.

SEE A DOCTOR IF . . . you have symptoms of kidney stones, including having a persistent urge to urinate or pain when you do; seeing pink-, red-, or brown-colored urine in the bowl; or having a sharp pain in your back or lower abdomen.

Low Bone Density

Aging does a number on everyone's bones, not just the skeletons of little old ladies. One recent Mayo Clinic study found that the thickness of a bone's trabecula—the spongy, supportive material inside—shrank in men by almost 30 percent from ages 24 to 48. Then, at around age 65, your bones begin shedding more of the mineral building blocks that make them strong, a process that causes even faster degeneration. Fortunately, the go-to fruit of grandparents may be the secret to younger bones. Florida State University research has shown that men who add prunes to their diets can boost their bone density by 11 percent. The researchers say that may be because prunes have unique antioxidants that fight osteoporosis. Plus, the dried fruit may increase the magnesium content in bones, making them stronger and denser.

Better INSTANTLY

↓

Switch seats. If you find a chair that you can sit in with both feet flat on the floor and set your computer monitor at eye level, 75 percent of your neck and back problems will improve, according to the Texas Back Institute.

YOUR BODY DISSECTED
BY T.E. HOLT, M.D.

WHY DOES THE SOUND OF FINGERNAILS ON A CHALKBOARD DRIVE ME NUTS?

The high-pitched sound is similar to a predator's shriek, a noise that can trigger your fight-or-flight response. When U.K. researchers had people listen to a variety of unpleasant sounds, MRI scans showed that the nails-on-a-chalkboard screech lit up the participants' amygdalae. This brain control center governs the body's automatic response to stress. Plus, a sound like this falls within the 2,000- to 4,000-hertz frequency range, where the ear is most sensitive.

Shoot for three prunes a day, with a glass of water to keep the fiber and sugar alcohol from dehydrating you. (Try adding diced prunes to trail mix or oatmeal.) For extra insurance, eat two medium apples or 2 ounces of fresh blueberries a day—both promote bone growth by reducing the amount of calcium lost in your urine. One more thing: Weight-bearing exercise is good for your bones. Use those dumbbells.

SEE A DOCTOR IF . . . you're over 50 and have risk factors for osteoporosis, such as low body weight, low testosterone, at least one bone fracture during your adulthood, or a history of smoking.

Lyme Disease

You've probably heard the standard advice about Lyme disease—see a doctor if you spot a bull's-eye-shaped rash. And you should! But don't dismiss strange marks that don't follow the pattern. Even skin reactions that don't look like a bull's-eye can signal Lyme disease, according to a study published in the journal *Emerging Infectious Diseases*. Of people in the study who were infected with Lyme bacteria, 71 percent had rashes that appeared to be spider bites, immune reactions, or common skin infections.

SEE A DOCTOR IF . . . you notice any unusual rash 2 inches or larger, paired with symptoms such as fever or body aches. Your physician may order an enzyme immunoassay test for Lyme disease.

Macular Degeneration

This disease is a top cause of vision loss in the United States. It happens when cells in your macula—part of your eye that helps you see fine details straight ahead—deteriorate. Back on page 210, we told you how important the antioxidants lutein and zeaxanthin are for your macula. Running may also reduce your risk of age-related macular degeneration, although researchers aren't sure why. People who averaged just over a mile to 2 miles a day had a 19 percent lower risk of developing the condition than those who ran less, according to a study from the Lawrence Berkeley National Laboratory.

SEE A DOCTOR IF . . . you notice any changes in your vision. Any disruptions in this sense can indicate a serious problem.

Memory Loss

Only your fittest brain cells survive your 20s—and Jell-O shots and Jägermeister aren't entirely to blame. During that decade, your brain starts to shrivel, and its white matter becomes less efficient at nerve signaling. The effect: Your working memory—your short-term ability to reason, comprehend, and retain information—may gradually begin to slip. Playing with balls may help your brain bounce back. In a 2009 British study, people who practiced juggling for 6 weeks strengthened the structural integrity of their white matter. It didn't even matter if they dropped the balls; the benefit was linked to time spent training, not proficiency. The reason? Practicing a new skill may encourage the formation of myelin, the white matter that helps conduct nerve impulses, the scientists say. Start with the three-ball cascade—this was the basic juggling skill the study participants practiced. Work on it for at least 30 minutes a day, 5 days a week. Or try another pursuit that combines learning with physical activity, such as archery, surfing, or bowling.

SEE A DOCTOR IF . . . you answered "yes" to the memory questions on page 22.

Motion Sickness

When you're traveling by land, air, or sea, your stomach may decide it's time to show everyone what you ate for lunch. Motion sickness isn't a well-understood phenomenon, but some doctors think it's evolutionary—when the room starts to spin, your body thinks you've ingested something harmful and tries to expel it. To reduce your symptoms, sit where there's minimal motion—in the front seat of a car, over the wing of a plane, or in the front or middle of a ship near water level. Then stare at the horizon. This helps your body distinguish between the motion of the vehicle and that of your body, say University of Minnesota researchers. At the same time, set your Spotify to a

Coldplay station. Researchers in Germany found that listening to relaxing, pleasant music helps stave off motion sickness better than jamming to livelier tunes or sitting silently. You can also snack on gingerroot—a dose of 2 to 4 grams has been shown to ease motion sickness, perhaps because a compound called 6-gingerol slows nerve transmissions that tell your guts to rumble. If you're willing to spend more cash, try the ReliefBand. A study in *Military Medicine* found that this device relieves motion sickness by delivering electrical signals to an acupressure point linked to nausea.

SEE A DOCTOR IF . . . it becomes a chronic condition.

Nail Fungus

If your nails are frail and crumble like chalk when you trim them, you might have nail fungus. Fungal invaders also make it so your nail lifts easily, leaving a gap between the nail and the nail bed, unlike with a runner's toe. One other telltale sign is a foul smell caused by bacteria or the fungus.

SEE A DOCTOR IF . . . you have symptoms. You'll probably need an Rx antifungal to fix this.

Osteoarthritis

The condition can announce itself with swelling, but it usually starts with nagging joint pain that can progress from minor to severe. The knees are a common spot, but osteoarthritis can strike other joints, too, and is often seen in the hips, hands, and spine. One way to reduce your risk, and ease pain if you already have arthritis, is to warm up before you work out. An injury from your 20s can resurface as osteoarthritis pain in your 40s. And stay slim. If you're heavy, your joints have to work harder to carry your weight, and fat cells promote joint inflammation. If you already have arthritis, try a natural remedy—curcumin. Researchers in Thailand found that 1,500 milligrams taken daily for 4 weeks can relieve knee pain from osteoarthritis as well as 1,200 milligrams of ibuprofen can. Then ask your doctor about cutting-edge treatments.

The ultimate solution may be hip or knee joint replacement surgery. It's effective, but it does have a few drawbacks—several weeks of recovery time, for one. Plus, the average artificial joint only lasts 15 to 20 years, so if you're young, you could end up needing follow-up surgeries to replace them. That's why your doctor might recommend some temporary treatments first.

Some docs may also suggest prolotherapy for osteoarthritis, in which an irritant solution is injected into a joint. In a University of Wisconsin study, people who received three to five monthly treatments reported 25 percent improvement in knee stiffness, pain, and function after 24 weeks. Visit aaomed.org/prolotherapy-doctor to find an orthopedist with proper training in the field. Another option is platelet-rich plasma therapy, where doctors take a small amount of your blood, spin it to concentrate the plasma, and then re-inject it into your knee to promote healing. One study in the *Clinical Journal of Sports Medicine* suggests that it can delay osteoarthritis progression. Insurance may not cover the treatment, so read the fine print on your policy and inquire about prices before you take the plunge.

SEE A DOCTOR IF . . . you are in pain during movement for several weeks, have stiffness, or feel a grating sensation when you use the joint. Your doctor will order x-rays and look for signs of deterioration of the cartilage that cushions the ends of the bones in your joints. Eventually, the cartilage may wear down to the point where you are left with bone rubbing on bone.

Peptic Ulcer

This is a sore in the lining of your stomach or small intestine. In the stomach, it's called a gastric ulcer, but the intestinal type is called a duodenal ulcer and is more common in men. It can cause nausea, hunger 1 to 3 hours after eating, or a steady, dull pain. Antacids can soothe the irritation in the short term, but you should see a doctor. Because most ulcers are caused by *Helicobacter pylori* bacteria, you may need antibiotics.

SEE A DOCTOR IF . . . you have symptoms. Don't ignore this—you risk internal bleeding and perforation.

Phobias

There's nothing to be afraid of. It's just your brain, anticipating. Healthy alarm in the face of a threat lasts a moment; inordinate anxiety can spiral into a chronic disability. If phobias affect you, a psychologist or psychiatrist can help you work on the specific trigger. If you suffer from a common phobia, you can try these strategies.

HEIGHTS: People whose visual perception is off—that is, they tend to overestimate distances—may be more likely to latch on to that fear, a California State University study suggests. To work on it, start by looking out of a second-story window until you become comfortable with it over time, then repeat the process at a third-story window, then a fourth-story one, and so on. When you're ready, progress to balconies.

FLYING: Coach yourself through a faux flight, imagining as many details (sights, sounds, smells) as possible. Lieutenant Commander Eric Potterat, Ph.D., a clinical psychologist with Naval Special Warfare Command, preps

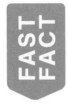

FAST FACT

4,000

Number of American men who stagger into the ER each year with a scrotum injury.

Source: The Journal of Urology

Navy SEALs with mental walk-throughs of different operations. "Your mind thinks, 'Hey, I've done this before,' transforming an unfamiliar situation into a controlled environment," he says.

PUBLIC SPEAKING: Before you step on stage, suck in several gut-filling breaths, counting 4 seconds with each inhale and exhale. You'll decrease your blood pressure, slow your heart rate, and—most important—distract yourself from thoughts of failure. "When you focus away from your fear," says Potterat, "you begin to control it."

SNAKES: This one's probably in your DNA: Ancestors with a strong fear of dangerous animals were more likely to survive. Repeated exposure helps, but take it easy at first. Start by watching videos (try nationalgeographic.com). When you're comfortable with that, visit a zoo to look at a real snake, and eventually visit a pet store to touch one, says anxiety specialist Richard Zinbarg, Ph.D., a psychiatry and behavioral sciences professor at Northwestern University in Evanston, Illinois.

INJECTIONS: Most people with injection phobias have a history of passing out, a French study found. Blame a "biphasic cardiac response": Your BP shoots up, then drops when you see blood, predisposing you to passing out. Getting pricked? Press your thighs into the chair till your face flushes. That's a sign you're pumping more blood, and by counteracting the BP drop, you prevent fainting.

SEE A DOCTOR IF . . . a phobia stops you from enjoying life.

Plantar Warts

These nasty warts on the bottoms of your feet caused by the human papillomavirus, grow inward. It's probably a plantar wart if it has black specks, feels painful when you press from side to side, and disrupts the fingerprint-like lines across your sole. Plantar warts are persistent—they can last months or even years, and there's no one foolproof way to eradicate them. But this strategy is a good bet: Use a pumice stone to remove the dead skin covering the wart. Then, apply Forces of Nature Wart Control ($30, forcesofnatureusa.com), which contains several natural extracts with antiviral properties, including *Thuja occidentalis* and tea tree oil.

SEE A DOCTOR IF . . . the warts don't improve within a month. A dermatologist can bring out some additional weapons in the wart arsenal. He or she may apply trichloroacetic acid

TRY THIS!

Brush Away Razor Bumps

Extra-sharp whiskers can curl and actually penetrate back into your skin, giving you irritating pimple-like bumps. After shaving, use a soft-bristled toothbrush to rub your neck in small circular motions. This will extract hair coils from your skin before they irritate you.

and liquid nitrogen and then inject the warts with a small amount of candida fungus to encourage the immune system to launch an attack. Once your wart is wiped out, prevent a re-infection by wearing flip-flops when you walk around germy zones, like public pools or gym locker rooms.

Poison Ivy, Oak, or Sumac

Leaves of three, let them be. If it's too late, and you find yourself in a patch of poison ivy, oak, or sumac, wash with soap and water as soon as possible to get the urushiol oil off your skin. Even better, use a product like Tecnu Extreme Medicated Poison Ivy Scrub. It has ingredients that remove the plant's oils and usher them off your skin when you rinse. If you develop the rash, try a hydrocortisone cream such as Cortaid to decrease the swelling that causes the itch. Just don't use it on areas bigger than the size of your palm, because too much could be absorbed into your bloodstream and further irritate the skin. Large tracts of oozing rash can be soothed and dried using calamine lotion. Tame your itch with the remedy on page 224.

SEE A DOCTOR IF . . . the rash is extensive or has infiltrated your eyes. A steroid shot will clear it up quick.

Razor Burn

If your mug looks like it has rug burn, dip a clean washcloth into a bowl of cool milk and dab it on the irritated areas. (The coolness can help reduce swelling, and milk's lactic acid has anti-inflammatory properties.) Next time, use pre-shave cream or oil to prep your face. These products reduce drag and moisturize your skin, minimizing razor burn. A razor with glide strips will also help. Most of them contain polyethylene glycol or a similar compound that hydrates hair, making it more pliable and easier to shave.

Receding Gums

Your hairline isn't the only thing that recedes as you age. Your gums can pull back, leaving more of your teeth exposed and leaving you vulnerable to sensitivity. Gum disease can cause it, but so can vigorous brushing. If you brush too hard, you can push your gums away from your teeth. So go soft—use about one-tenth of the pressure you'd need to crack an egg.

SEE A DOCTOR IF . . . you've noticed that your teeth look longer. You might have gum disease; even if you don't, a dentist may be able to help you halt the recession.

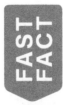

Percentage reduction in arm soreness reported by lifters who took 3 grams of an omega-3 supplement every day for a week

Source: Journal of Sports Science and Medicine

Rheumatoid Arthritis

This is an autoimmune disorder in which your body attacks healthy joint tissue. It tends to affect the small joints in your hands and feet first, and then it attacks larger ones like the shoulders and elbows. Research from South Korea showed that the people who consumed the most vitamin D were 24 percent less likely to develop rheumatoid arthritis (RA) than those who consumed the least D. There's no cure for RA, but doctors can prescribe anti-inflammatory medicines that will ease your symptoms.

SEE A DOCTOR IF . . . you think you have RA.

Sinus Infection

Sinuses are like balloons in your skull. They sit behind your forehead, nose, cheeks, and eyes. After a cold or allergy attack, they can become clogged with mucus, irritated, and inflamed. You might have a sore throat and phlegm in your throat. You might have a headache or tenderness in your face. Cough, fatigue, fever, a stuffed-up nose, and a decrease in your sense of smell can also indicate that you have a sinus infection. Saline nasal spray can curb the swelling. Then rest your head: A study from China reveals that you can clear a chronic sinus infection faster just by resting your head. Of sinus patients on medication, some sat down in a chair, bent at the waist, leaned forward, and placed their head on a flat surface twice a day for 20 minutes. Within 6 weeks they had less congestion, postnasal drip, and sinus pressure than participants who just took medication. That's because fluid pools below the drainage tubes in your sinuses. By changing the angle of your head, you let gravity draw mucus out, the researchers say.

SEE A DOCTOR IF . . . your symptoms haven't improved within 10 days or have worsened after 5 to 7 days. If your doctor determines that the infection is bacterial, you may receive an antibiotic.

Sore Muscles

Aching after exercise? These strategies really work.

→ Wear compression pants: Marathoners who wore the tights (such as those by 2XU) for 24 hours after their races felt less sore, U.K. research revealed.

→ Foam-roll your legs: Rolling your stems for 20 minutes after a leg session can help lessen pain for up to 72 hours, a Canadian study found.

→ Sip pickle juice: Downing 2½ ounces after a sweat session can help you recover from cramps 37 percent faster than drinking water can.

→   Drink some java: Drinking the caffeine equivalent of 2½ cups of coffee 1 hour before a workout and daily thereafter reduces soreness.

Sore Throat

Spritz your throat with numbing, pain-fighting benzocaine, like Cepacol Ultra Sore Throat Spray. Once the tenderness subsides, take a dose of ibuprofen to tamp down your throat inflammation.

SEE A DOCTOR IF . . . you have a fever, white streaks or pus on your tonsils, and tender lymph nodes. Your doctor may perform a throat culture or rapid antigen test to see whether you have strep throat. If you do, you'll need an antibiotic.

Staph Infection

Staphylococcus aureus is one nasty bacterium. It can infect many parts of your body, from your intestines in a case of food poisoning, to open wounds or cuts. A course of antibiotics can easily clear some cases, but some forms of staph, like MRSA, don't go down so easy. More people in the United States die each year from this antibiotic-resistant form of staph than from AIDS or emphysema, according to CDC data. The predominant MRSA strain, USA300, can secrete a toxin that attacks white blood cells, making it an especially dangerous menace. To protect yourself, regularly wipe down hard surfaces in your home with a disinfectant that includes MRSA on its list of targeted germs, such as Clorox bleach. (Dilute ¾ cup of bleach in a gallon of water.) A Simmons College study found that 26 percent of American homes tested were contaminated with MRSA, most commonly found on dish towels and kitchen faucet handles. At the gym—also a major MRSA hot spot—steer clear of worn-out equipment, since damaged surfaces can easily harbor bacteria, the CDC warns. For extra insurance, place a towel between you and the exercise machine's seat, yoga mat, and locker room or sauna bench.

SEE A DOCTOR IF . . . you have any sores that are red, swollen, and pus-filled. These infections are serious business.

COUNTER- INTELLIGENCE

Don't Pull a Puncture

Nail in your thigh? Pull it out. But if you get impaled by anything more significant, don't remove the sword/knitting needle/wooden stake/ballpoint pen because that could actually worsen the bleeding. Try to control it by applying direct pressure around the wound with your fingers, according to our friends at the American College of Emergency Physicians. Then bring your shish-kebab'd self to the ER.

Sunburn

Look like a lobster after too long in the sun? Stop by a home store and grab an aloe vera plant. The juice in the leaves contains more than 75 active components—including vitamins, minerals, and enzymes. While bottled aloe is convenient, it's less potent than the fresh stuff because some helpful compounds deteriorate while the gel sits on a store shelf. Plus, the fragrances, preservatives, and fillers in bottled products dilute the aloe's natural potency. So just cut a leaf from an aloe plant, split it open, and apply the gel to your burn twice a day. If you're traveling, the next best option is an organic gel. A washcloth soaked in cold milk is another soothing home remedy that can cool the burn.

SEE A DOCTOR IF . . . a bad sunburn is actually the cooking of proteins in your skin. Large areas of blistering require a doctor's care to avoid infection. Also, fever, light-headedness, or confusion due to sunburn could be a sign of possible deadly heatstroke.

Temporomandibular Joint Disorder

Open your mouth. Now close it. Does your jaw pop, click, or snap? If the noise is loud and sharp, your temporomandibular joint—the hinge and/or cartilage of your upper and lower jaw—may be out of alignment. Generally, if you're having problems, baby your jaw: Avoid gum and chewy foods like bagels, taffy, and (sorry) steak.

SEE A DOCTOR IF . . . your jaw locks or won't open or close all the way. And if you're a nighttime jaw clencher, ask your dentist about a mouth guard or splint. That will limit jaw stress and keep your problem from getting worse.

Tendinitis

Tendons attach muscle to bone. With tendinitis, that tissue becomes inflamed and sore. You might feel nagging pain at night. You can blame wear and tear due to sports, hobbies, or your job. To reduce your risk, avoid trying to go from slug to stud too fast. If you're looking to get more fit, you should gradually increase your exercise. Shoe inserts called orthotics can help correct many of these imbalances and support your tendons and ligaments. While a custom pair from a podiatrist can cost up to $750, it's still cheaper than knee or hip surgery later.

SEE A DOCTOR IF . . . you're struggling with chronic tendinitis. You can discuss additional treatment options, including pain-relieving injections. In the short-term, naproxen, the active ingredient in Aleve, can provide relief for a few days by limiting your production of inflammatory compounds called prostaglandins. But don't take this—or ibuprofen, acetaminophen, or aspirin—on a long-term basis unless your doctor tells you to.

Thyroid Problems

Your thyroid gland is only 40 to 60 millimeters long, but it's the ringleader of your endocrine system. From its position just below your Adam's apple, your thyroid creates and stores hormones that control everything from your metabolism to your growth rate. The essential chemical for all these functions is iodine. Without enough of this element pumping through your thyroid, you may begin to experience fatigue, depression, lethargy, cloudy thinking, and weight gain. Make sure you consume at least 150 micrograms per day—unless you've already been diagnosed with a thyroid problem and your doctor has given you other guidelines. Good sources include kelp, cod, yogurt, iodized salt, milk, bread, shrimp, and eggs. Now, if your thyroid is out of whack, your body will notice. The problem is that you might not know what's wrong. Many of the symptoms of an overactive thyroid, such as anxiety, weight loss, and heart palpitations, or an underactive thyroid, such as fatigue, watery eyes, and dry skin, can be confused with symptoms of other diseases.

SEE A DOCTOR IF . . . you have strange symptoms. Ask your doctor to check your thyroid hormone levels.

Tinnitus

Soft ringing, buzzing, hissing, and other so-called phantom noises that only you can hear. They occur when your auditory nerve fibers and the neurons that decode noises fall out of sync, causing you to become aware of sound being processed. It can come and go or be a constant sensation. It's often due to irritation of the inner ear from exposure to loud noise, earwax blockage, or stiffening of the bones of your middle ear as you age. It could also be caused by abnormal inner ear fluid pressure (Ménière's disease), trauma to the head, and in rare cases high blood pressure.

SEE A DOCTOR IF . . . your tinnitus is continuous and only in one ear. This could signal an infection or inner-ear disorder. Tinnitus is not a disease per say but a symptom of a problem. It can be very frustrating because in many cases no cause can be identified. Your doctor may recommend counseling or strategies to help you live with the noise. Also see a doc if you experience hearing loss or dizziness, which could be signs of Ménière's disease, a hearing and balance disorder, or even a tumor.

(continued on page 238)

Refrigerator Fixes
16 home health remedies for do-it-yourselfers

When common health glitches strike, you can run to the drugstore for some overpriced relief. Or you can open your refrigerator or pantry. Seems like a no-brainer to keep your slippers on and stay at home. Try these natural first-aid fixes.

APPLE CIDER VINEGAR

It aids digestion and can ease heartburn by neutralizing excess acid. The pH in cider vinegar is more natural and won't damage the stomach like antacids can. Mix 1 teaspoon apple cider vinegar with 8 ounces of water and 1 teaspoon honey. Take once in the morning and once at night or after a meal for indigestion.

BACON

Use it to staunch nosebleeds. Take a piece of uncooked bacon and fold it in half lengthwise. Then fold it in half again lengthwise over a section of string, letting an inch or so of it hang out either side. Mold the bacon into a small pencil like shape and put it in the freezer. When your next nosebleed strikes, place a slightly defrosted pork plug in your nose (allowing the string to hang out of your nose). Gently tug on the string to remove when the bacon gets soft. Compounds in the bacon called *leukotrienes* will stop the bleeding.

BAKING SODA

A paste of baking soda and water takes away the sting of most bug bites, especially bee stings, since the baking soda neutralizes the acidity of bee venom.

BANANAS

Potassium-packed bananas are useful for relieving diarrhea and muscle cramps and lowering blood pressure.

COFFEE

If you feel an asthma attack coming on and you are far from home or anywhere else you can get an inhaler, have 2 cups of coffee. Caffeine is chemically related to theophylline, a bronchodilator that was used for many years in asthma treatments. Use coffee only in an emergency because inhalers are much more effective.

CORNSTARCH

It works great for preventing chafing and as relief from rectal itch. Sprinkle cornstarch on a cotton ball and dust around your anus to keep it dry and alleviate itching.

FROZEN PEAS

Whether it's an arthritis flare-up in your knee or a twisted ankle, a bag of frozen peas molds nicely around a joint to reduce swelling and pain. Keep it there for 20 minutes each hour to bring down inflammation.

GARLIC

Raw garlic has natural antifungal properties that work wonders against athlete's foot. Put several crushed garlic cloves in a basin of warm water and a couple shots of rubbing alcohol. Soak your feet to relieve itching and burning between your toes.

GINGER

Shave some slices and steep in boiling water for a soothing tea. Its anti-inflammatory properties make it useful to people with arthritis, bursitis, or tendonitis. It can also help relieve gas, nausea, motion sickness, allergies, and bad breath.

HONEY ON TOAST

Before or after drinking alcohol, eat a piece of toast or a cracker slathered with honey. Honey supplies fructose, which helps the body metabolize alcohol ingested and reduces hangover symptoms.

HORSERADISH OR WASABI

Eating an eighth to a quarter teaspoon of horseradish from a bottle (or wasabi paste) will clear up a stuffy nose.

LEMON

Use the juice to soothe wasp stings or get rid of body odor. Squeeze it into hot water to relieve a cough, a sore throat, or bad breath. Lemon water is also good for triggering bowel movements.

OLIVE OIL

Use it to soothe razor burn.

PAPAYA AND PINEAPPLE

To beat indigestion that's causing excessive belching, eat papaya, pineapple, cantaloupe, or peaches. The juices from these "neutral-based" fruits can soothe your stomach and keep the bubbles at bay.

PEANUT BUTTER

One of many home remedies for hiccups, a spoonful of Jif will often do the trick. Swallowing a teaspoon of creamy peanut butter will stimulate the vagus nerve fibers in the throat.

VINEGAR

Dandruff flakes on your blazer? After shampooing, rinse your hair with a mixture of 1 tablespoon vinegar and 1 quart of water. The rinse normalizes the scalp's natural pH balance, reducing the flakes.

Tooth Discoloration

If you have a set of pearly yellows, start with a good whitening toothpaste. Watch out, though: Many contain harsh abrasives that will wear on your tooth enamel. Skip those and opt for a paste that contains peroxide. Supersmile and IntelliWhite are two examples we've tested and recommended at *Men's Health*. The nice thing about this strategy is that you already brush—hopefully—so this won't take up extra time. However, the results won't be as dramatic as what you'll see with some other strategies. Over-the-counter strips and trays with peroxide also work. Once you've whitened, defend yourself against future stains. The fibrous flesh of crunchy vegetables and fruits, like apples, celery, and carrots, acts like a high-grit scrub brush to remove stains. Greens like spinach and broccoli contain minerals that form a protective film over teeth, helping to block stains. Finally, drink more water. Make sure you chase sips of coffee with water to prevent dark pigments from lingering.

SEE A DOCTOR IF . . . you want brighter results. In-office treatments contain stronger formulations—such as 18 percent peroxide versus the 3 to 10 percent usually found in DIY kits. If you have sensitive teeth, a dentist can also help you pick a formulation that won't sting.

Urinary Tract Infection

Most women pee after sex, and you should too. A postcoital trip to the toilet can help flush out bacteria and possibly prevent a urinary tract infection—the most common type of infection among people who end up in the ER after having sex, Swiss researchers report. Yes, men can get them too—and left untreated, a UTI can spread to the kidneys, which can cause a more serious infection.

SEE A DOCTOR IF . . . you have bloody or cloudy urine or if it hurts when you pee.

Viral Stomach Bugs

Although they travel incognito as "stomach flu" and stow away on cruise ships, norovirus and its cousins have nothing to do with influenza. As they release toxins that send your GI tract into panic mode, your intestines push water, sodium, and potassium into your gut, leaving you with watery diarrhea and a serious electrolyte shortage. Just one brief encounter with an infected person or a contaminated surface is enough for norovirus to turn your world—and your stomach—upside down, so it's hard to avoid this. Still, you can lower your odds by washing your hands regularly before and after handling food or performing any, um, toilet-related tasks. Scrub with soap and warm water for 20 seconds, especially if someone you know has been sick with a stomach bug. When these illnesses strike, it can feel as if your butt will never leave the bowl: Your body may need 2 days to clear these viruses. As you wait, it's safe to slow the flow with loperamide (Imodium). And drink 8 ounces of clear liquid after every toilet trip. Stick with water or a hydration drink for diarrhea, like Pedialyte. (It works for adults too.) You can also try a low-sugar sports drink, but avoid the regular kind—sugar will pull more fluid from intestinal cells, worsening diarrhea.

SEE A DOCTOR IF . . . you lose more than 5 percent of your body weight within a day—you may need IV rehydration to prevent serious complications such as brain swelling, seizures, and even kidney failure.

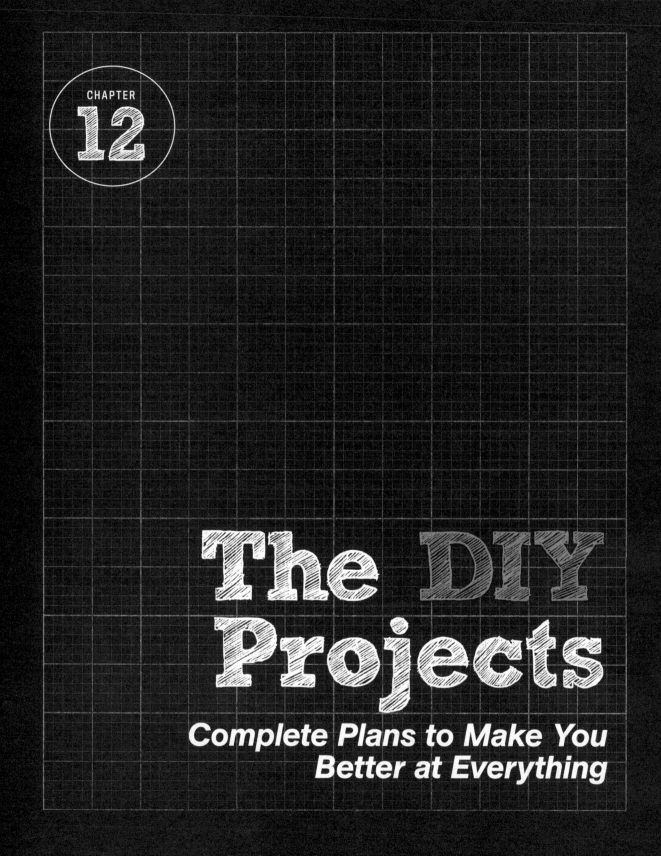

The DIY Projects

*Complete Plans to Make You
Better at Everything*

Whether you're ice fishing for walleye, fixing a toilet, carving a Pinewood Derby car for your Cub Scout, or building your biceps, you get better results when you have the right tools and an intelligent set of instructions.

It's fair to say that most men who have accomplished anything meaningful in life didn't just wing it. They had a plan (and the smartest of them, a plan B). So, here are yours—blueprints for 35 do-it-yourself projects that'll make you much better at everything.

And unlike that Lil' Homemaker Kitchen Set you tried assembling (from 500 lil' pieces) on the living room floor last Christmas, the instructions here are quick and easy to follow. Plus, the finished product can last a lifetime.

LOWER YOUR BLOOD PRESSURE BY 16 POINTS

A lot of men in this land are high. Nearly one in four American men between the ages of 35 and 44 has hypertension, as well as 9 percent of men between 20 and 34, says the American Heart Association. Reducing sodium intake is the first step in the right direction, but you may not know why. Here's the dangerous mechanism: Sodium causes you to retain water in your blood, which adds volume and boosts pressure. Constant high pressure on your arteries, in turn, exposes you to a greater risk of heart attack, stroke, and even penis problems. That's why lowering BP through natural means makes a nifty DIY project for a lot of guys. How 'bout you?

1 Start with salt

You should consume about 1,500 milligrams of sodium daily, but the average American takes in more than double that. To reduce the amount, toss the saltshaker over your shoulder and start seasoning your food with spices, herbs, lemon, and salt-free seasoning blends. For the greatest impact, however, avoid processed foods, the source of most dietary sodium.

2 Tea up

Australian researchers found that people who drank 3 cups of black tea every day for 6 months saw a 2-point drop in both diastolic and systolic blood pressure. Tea flavonoids may reduce concentrations of endothelin-1, a protein that constricts blood vessels, the researchers report. Less than 3 cups a day may work too.

3 Grab a bunch of grapes

Men with metabolic syndrome (a set of conditions that can lead to heart disease) who ate the powder equivalent of about 2 cups of grapes daily for a month lowered their systolic blood pressure by 6 points, according to a study from the University of Connecticut. The polyphenols in grapes may help relax blood vessels and improve their function, the scientists say.

4 Breathe slowly and deeply

Slow breathing and meditative practices such as yoga decrease stress hormones, which elevate renin, a kidney enzyme that raises blood pressure. Try 5 minutes in the morning and at night. You can even do it on your commute. Inhale deeply and expand your belly. Exhale and release tension.

5 Breathe quickly and deeply

Three days a week, do a cardio workout at 60 to 65 percent of your maximum heart rate for 40 minutes. Exercise helps the heart use oxygen more efficiently, so it doesn't have to work as hard to pump blood. Does "workout" sound too much like work? Then walk. In a study, hypertensive patients who went for walks at a brisk pace lowered their pressure by almost 8 mm Hg over 6 mm Hg.

6 Beet it

Drinking 17 ounces of beet juice can yield a 5-point drop in blood pressure in just 6 hours, according to a 2012 Australian study. The crimson root veggie is rich in nitrates, which converts into nitric acid, which is thought to relax blood vessels and improve bloodflow.

7 LOL

Laughing at a funny movie causes blood vessels to dilate by 22 percent, according to a study from the University of Maryland. The physical act of laughing causes the tissue forming the inner lining of your blood vessels to expand, increasing bloodflow and reducing blood pressure.

8 Try a DASH

The acronym stands for Dietary Approaches to Stop Hypertension, a plan developed by the National Heart, Lung, and Blood Institute to provide guidelines for people wanting to lower their BP. It involves keeping total calories to 55 percent carbs, 27 percent fat, and 18 percent protein and your sodium intake under 2,300 milligrams a day. A typical DASH menu focuses on fruits and vegetables, whole grains, and protein from poultry, fish, beans, and nuts while minimizing added sugars and salt. And it works. A study in the *Archives of Internal Medicine* found that it can lower systolic blood pressure by up to 16 points in 4 months in people with high BP.

FAST FACT

7

Pounds in 10 weeks you can lose if you pair a reduced-calorie DASH diet with resistance training. You can also gain muscle and decrease body fat mass by 11 percent.

Source: University of Rhode Island

LOSE 10 POUNDS

Losing weight is a numbers game. It involves not only eating fewer calories and burning more, but also eating the right quantities of certain types of foods and strategizing ways to rev up your metabolic rate. All of this is construction material for a nifty DIY project that most of us could use. Here are simple steps to take that'll help you lose either the first 10 or the last 10.

1 Assess your protein needs

Protein stokes your body's inner fire (metabolism) more than fat or carbohydrates do. To ensure you're getting the right amount, multiply your target weight by 0.7 to 1 gram. So, for example, if you want to get down to 170 pounds, you should eat 119 to 170 grams of protein spread over the course of each day.

2 Eat more plants, less processed crap

Fast foods, baked goods, snacks, and stuff that comes in boxes or cans tend to be high in calories and fast-burning carbohydrates. Eliminating these foods from your diet is good, but because of the calorie trim, it can also dial down your metabolism. Reduce that effect by getting your quota of protein and also filling up on high-fiber carbs. Ideally, you should get 38 grams of fiber per day. (See Project 5.) A quick way to ballpark that: Aim for five servings of produce daily, plus two of beans (lentils, black beans, hummus) or whole grains (quinoa, popcorn, oatmeal).

3 Outsmart cravings

This isn't as hard as it seems. Just do this: Plan out what you are going to eat for the day and eat something every 3 hours to keep your blood sugar level and your hunger at bay. Also, make sure you are working toward your protein quota every time you have a meal or snack. This really works to stifle cravings for high-calorie crapola.

(4) Master your metabolism

First, understand how your body burns calories. Fifteen to 30 percent of your calories are burned through your activity; 10 percent of your daily energy is used to turn food into fuel, and 60 to 70 percent of calories burn away through your body's cells and organs functioning to keep you alive. You're already working toward increasing calories burned through digestion by eating more protein and nonstarchy carbs. So now turn your effort to boosting calorie burn through activity. Any exercise can help you shed fat. But to see the biggest results in the last time, do intense interval training, which can boost your burn rate for up to 36 hours. Combine that style of training with weight lifting, and you're likely to blast more fat, according to Italian researchers. In their study, one group of men did 32 minutes of interval-style lifting (heavy weights, periodic 20-second rests, longer rests between sets). Another did 62 minutes of lighter lifts using a more traditional approach (3 sets of 12 to 14 reps, shorter rests between sets). Over the next 22 hours, the heavy lifters burned an extra 363 calories. Your muscles work harder with intervals, so they have to do more postworkout rebuilding. That burns calories and lifts levels of metabolism-boosting hormones.

(5) Think before you drink

It's not a food group—for most guys—but alcohol can make or break your efforts to lose your gut. First of all, it's a source of liquid calories, which aren't satiating. A report from the National Center for Health Statistics shows that the average American adult consumes about an extra 100 calories per day from alcohol, which can add up. Even worse, men eat more calories and make unhealthier food choices on days they drink alcohol, according to a study in the *American Journal of Clinical Nutrition.* As you might know, even a slight buzz can make you focus on immediate gratification (pizza) rather than achieving long-term goals (weight loss). So eat a snack rich in protein and healthy fats, such as nuts, before that first sip. That will keep your blood sugar level steady and slow the absorption of alcohol, which can help fend off postdrinking pig-outs. In any case, limit alcohol or, better yet, eliminate it altogether if you're really set on seeing your abs.

SCULPT 6-PACK ABS

If you're wearing a roll of flab over your abs, complete Project #2 before attempting this one. It'll make it much easier. Once you've shed that layer of fat, you might be able to see the beginnings of a six-pack poking through. To really make 'em pop, do ab exercises that also trigger other regions of your core, such as your obliques.

Here's an abs workout project that'll do the trick. Add it to your regular workout or do it on rest days when you aren't lifting weights. There are three levels that get progressively more difficult; each workout includes three exercises. Start with Level 1. Do two sets of each move consecutively, resting between sets and between exercises. For side planks, you will perform the move on your left and right to complete one set.

Do the Level 1 workout four times in a week. After one or two weeks, move to Level 2 and so on. When a level becomes easy, add the extra exercises Stir the Pot and Rolling Planks.

LEVEL 1

EXERCISE	SETS	REST	DURATION
1 Plank	2	30 s	30 s
2 Mountain Climber with Hands on Bench	2	30 s	30 s
3 Side Plank	2	30 s	30 s

LEVEL 2

EXERCISE	SETS	REST	DURATION
1 Plank with Feet Elevated	2	30 s	30 s
2 Mountain Climber with Hands on Swiss Ball	2	30 s	30 s
3 Side Plank with Feet Elevated	2	30 s	30 s

LEVEL 3

EXERCISE	SETS	REST	DURATION
1 Extended Plank	2	30 s	30 s
2 Swiss-Ball Jackknife	2	30 s	15 reps
3 Single-Leg Side Plank	2	30 s	30 s

1 Plank

Assume a pushup position, but with your elbows bent and your weight resting on your forearms. Your body should form a straight line. Now brace your abs as if someone is about to punch you in the gut. Hold for 30 seconds. Rest 30 seconds. That's 1 set.

2 Mountain Climber with Hands on Bench

In a pushup position with your hands on a bench, brace your abs and slowly lift your right knee toward your chest. Pause for 1 or 2 seconds, lower it, and then raise your left knee. Alternate for 30 seconds, rest 30, and repeat once.

3 Side Plank

Lie on your right side and prop your upper body up on your right forearm. Raise your hips until your body forms a straight line from ankles to shoulders. Now brace your abs and hold for 30 seconds. Roll over onto your left side and repeat. Rest 30 seconds. That's 1 set. Do another.

Extras

STIR THE POT: Assume a pushup position, but place your elbows and forearms on a Swiss ball. Move your elbows in a circle, making sure that your core doesn't rotate. Circle clockwise and counterclockwise until failure.

ROLLING PLANKS: Hold a side plank for 10 seconds, rotate to a plank for 10 seconds, and then hit the other side for 10 more seconds. That's 1 set. Do 6. (See illustration on page 307.)

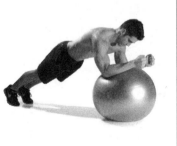

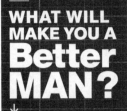

WHAT WILL MAKE YOU A Better MAN?

↓

"Beach-worthy abs," say 95 percent of respondents to a Men's Health *survey.*

DO STUFF FASTER

There's never enough time in the day to get it all done. You wish you had a 25th hour, right? Well, maybe you're a tortoise and need to be more like the hare. Being quicker and more efficient doesn't take a lot of time if you know how to speed past common time sucks. Make this your next project.

→ **COOK ANY MEAL QUICKER.** Lay out all the ingredients before firing up the stove. Do the dishes whenever there's downtime.

→ **DEFUSE AN ARGUMENT.** 1. Select a predesignated safe word to signal a 30-minute time-out. The first step is getting both of you to a calmer place. 2. Set your phone alarm for 25 minutes and use that time to distract yourself from the argument with something you enjoy doing, like playing a video game or going for a run. 3. Be a bigger man. Spend 5 minutes of your time-out thinking about how you can be the first to take a little responsibility.

→ **NAVIGATE YOUR PHONE.** Most people don't use voice commands as much as they could, says Yahoo Tech founder David Pogue. For instance, saying "Call Chris at the office" is a lot speedier than scrolling through your contacts.

→ **LOCATE IMPORTANT E-MAILS.** For vital details like confirmation codes when traveling, screen-grab the message. It'll be easier to spot in your photo gallery than in your inbox.

→ **LOSE FAT IN 20 MINUTES FLAT.** Incinerate calories faster by combining burpees and pushups (shown), says trainer Jonathan Amato, C.S.C.S. Make it even harder (not shown): Do 40 seconds of burpees; rest 20 seconds; then do 40 seconds of lunges, rotating your torso 90 degrees in the direction of your forward leg at the bottom of the move. Rest for 20 seconds. Repeat for 8 minutes. Then rest a minute and do it again. If you can. It's freaking hard. But efficient.

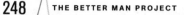

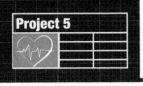

EAT 30 GRAMS (OR MORE) OF FIBER EVER YDAY

Nutrition experts recommend eating about 38 grams of satiating, cholesterol-lowering, dump-improving fiber a day. The average guy gets less than half that—15 grams. Becoming better than average when it comes to fiber intake may sound tougher than snaking out a hairball clog in a shower drain, but you can make it pretty easy on yourself if you simply boost your consumption of plant foods. What constitutes a good source of fiber? Anything over 2.5 grams per serving. Just pick your daily seven servings from the following:

FOOD	SERVING SIZE	FIBER (G)
All-Bran cereal	½ cup	9
Lentils, cooked	½ cup	7.8
Spinach, frozen, cooked	1 cup	7
Chickpeas	½ cup	6.2
Kidney beans, cooked	½ cup	5.7
Pear	1 medium	5.5
Apple	1 large	5.4
Orange	1 large	4.4
Popcorn, air popped	3½ cups	4.1
Edamame, shelled	½ cup	4
Raspberries	½ cup	4
Strawberries, sliced	1 cup	3.3
Banana	1 medium	3.1
Pearled barley, cooked	½ cup	3
Plums, dried (prunes)	3 medium	2
Blueberries	½ cup	1.8
Rice, brown, long-grain, cooked	½ cup	1.8

HAVE SEX 8 TIMES THIS WEEK

Consider this extra-credit work for your blood pressure project. Yes, many studies have linked sex with lower blood pressure—sexual intercourse, that is; masturbation doesn't have the same effect. So, send her the study and this calendar created by one of the magazine's female staffers. It's totally doable.

① Monday: Anti-stress sex

The first day of the week has her tension level skyrocketing. Ease her into sex by waiting until an hour after dinner, when she's had time to unwind. Begin rubbing her temples, neck, and shoulders until you see them drop and the tension fall out of her face. Let your hands slide down to her quads, and rub her thighs until they relax completely. At this point, she'll welcome your fingers on her clitoris.

② Tuesday: Before-dinner quickie

Lean in for a long, wet, romantic kiss before you both have bellies full of food. Let the makeout session linger on (and on and on . . .) as you press her back up against the kitchen cabinets. When she melts in your arms, push her skirt up and lift her up onto the counter.

③ Wednesday: The dry hump

What better for Hump Day than rediscovering the joys of dry humping? This is perfect for that moment when the DVD ends and you're both lying on the couch. Roll on top of her, and target her neck and collarbone with your mouth while slowly grinding your crotch against hers. Increase the pressure until she's worked up and is reaching for your zipper.

④ Thursday: Lazy sex

Spoon her when you're curled up in bed. Run your hand along the side of her torso, hip, and thigh several times before letting your fingers wander between her legs. When her breathing deepens and she starts to sigh, slide in from behind and proceed with minimal energy and fuss.

Friday: Post-going-out sex

Don't wait to get settled. Start kissing at the door, unbutton her blouse in the hallway, then lay her down on the living room carpet. Don't be shy about getting a little aggressive.

Saturday: Shower sex

Head out together on a bike ride or run in the hot afternoon sun so a shower is a must when you get back home. Soap her up, wash her hair, and run your hands all over her body to help rinse off the suds. When you both step out of the tub, instead of handing her a towel, get down on your knees and put your tongue to work on her fresh, clean body.

Sunday: Morning sex, times two

Spend the morning in bed—but not the way you did as a kid. After you've slipped out of the sack to brush your teeth and grab a glass of water, climb back in and coax her into a sleepy a.m. romp. Afterward, use pillow talk and cuddling to keep her between the sheets until you feel something stirring again. Let your second go-round be about exploration. Lick and touch every inch of her. Kiss places you've neglected for months. This one isn't about reaching your peak or hers—it's about savoring every sensation.

NAIL THE SINGLE-ARM PUSHUP

For building strength and a big chest, there's really no reason on earth to do one-arm pushups. But it's impressive as hell. To learn to conquer one of the most awe-inspiring muscle-man feats, follow this strength and coordination plan suggested by Zach Even-Esh, owner of Underground Strength Gym in Edison, New Jersey.

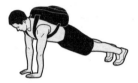

① Build strength

Four days a week, wear a heavy backpack and do pushups to failure. Next do offset pushups, with one hand on the floor and the other on a small box. After 5 to 10 reps, switch hands and repeat. Lastly, get rid of the box and do close-hands pushups to failure. Rest. Do 5 sets of each.

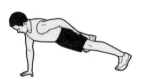

② Master balance

Static holds improve muscle memory and core strength. To do them, assume a top pushup position with your feet twice shoulder-width apart. Raise one hand and place it below your butt; hold for at least 15 seconds, or until failure. Then rest. Do 3 to 5 sets, 4 days a week.

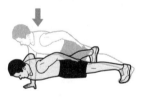

③ Practice it

Spread your feet wide. Place one hand on the floor under your shoulder and the opposite hand by your butt. Tense your body. Lower yourself to the floor, turning your elbow, shoulder, and palm in toward your body. As you reach the ground, push yourself up.

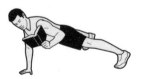
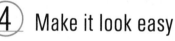

④ Make it look easy

Ugly first attempt? Practice several times a day, 4 days a week, to increase strength, stability, and muscle memory, until you can do this.

BUILD A MEDICAL HISTORY CHEAT SHEET

Anytime you visit a new doctor, whether a GP or a specialist, you are asked to answer a mess of questions about your personal health history. Don't rely on memory. Bring a cheat sheet with you to speed through the process and provide your doctor with the most accurate info.

Fill this out as best you can, call doctors' offices for results, and bring it with you to your next appointment.

RECENT TESTS	DATE	RESULTS
Digital rectal exam		
Prostate exam		
PSA		
Test for blood in stool		
Colonoscopy		
Resting EKG		
Stress EKG		
Nuclear stress test		
Chest x-ray		
Blood pressure		
Eye exam/eye pressure		
Cholesterol (HDL, LDL, triglycerides)		
Hemoglobin A_{1c}		
Urinalysis		

List all current medications, including dose and frequency.

_____

_____

_____

_____

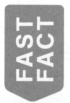
List all supplements, including dose and frequency.

_____
_____
_____
_____
_____

List all surgeries and diagnostic procedures you have had.

PROCEDURE	DATE	REASON

List all questions you have for the doctor (so you remember to ask them).

_____
_____
_____
_____
_____

Take notes from your visit.

_____
_____
_____
_____
_____

FAMILY HEALTH HISTORY

CONDITION	FAMILY MEMBER	CONDITION	FAMILY MEMBER
Anemia		Arthritis	
Cancer		Osteoporosis	
High blood pressure		Memory problems	
Heart disease		Alzheimer's disease	
Heart attack		Parkinson's disease	
Diabetes		Stroke	
Endocrine disorders		Prostate cancer	
Lung disease		Depression	
Liver disease		Other mental health problems	
Allergies		Substance abuse	

FAMILY MEMBER	ALIVE OR DEAD	AGE/HEALTH CONDITION/ CAUSE OF DEATH
Father		
Mother		
Child		
Sibling (Male)		
Sibling (Female)		
Maternal Grandfather		
Maternal Grandmother		
Paternal Grandfather		
Paternal Grandmother		

APPROACH ANY WOMAN

There are a slew of ways to land dates and dodge having an actual conversation with a woman—Tinder, OkCupid, Snapchat, Twitter, texting in general. And as Internet dating becomes the new norm, guys are slowing losing their social skills, including their ability to woo women without their iPhone as a wingman. Don't miss your chance with her because you're too busy swiping through your phone. Nothing beats the thrill of *actually* winning a woman's heart with your own words. "Women are attracted to men who go after what they want," says R. Don Steele, author of *Body Language Secrets: A Guide During Courtship & Dating*. "It's just up to you to make it happen."

Worried you'll fumble without auto-text? If you're even a little confident (*and relaxed*), women will talk to you. But just like riding a bike or learning to swim, you're going to need a little push into uncomfortable situations to learn how to come out like looking like Clooney. Here are three steps to catching her gaze and charming her heart:

1. **WORK THE ROOM.** Pocket your smartphone, play pool, chat with the bartenders, hit the jukebox. Women will see you as social, confident, and competent—all factors that will contribute to their first impression of you when you approach them.

2. **WATCH FOR CUES.** Before you make a big move, make sure her body language is inviting. Note if she's blushing, constantly making eye contact, and tilting her head playfully—it could mean she's interested, says Steele.

3. **MAKE A STATEMENT.** Don't lead with "Hi, my name is _____." It's invasive and too open-ended. A better angle is to make the conversation situational. For example, if you're at a concert start the conversation by asking her something about the warmup band. After some banter, roll out the introductions.

Here's how to make your move in different scenarios.

She's your barista

Be friendly, initiate small talk, leave a tip, and *always* address her by her name, explains Renee Piane, author of *Love Mechanics*. "Women respond best to men they're comfortable with." After you've visited a few times, you can make your move, and ask her out for coffee—outside of the cafe.

She's your M.D.

Be discrete. "Since this is a private setting—most likely involving just the two of you in her office—you don't want to come on too strong," says Steele. The best time to make your move is on the way out. "Be direct and give her your business card," says Steele. "Dragging the moment out can be awkward."

You go to the same gym

Don't be creepy. Be friendly with other people in the gym, too, which will make her feel less threatened by your advances. As she sees how you treat others in the gym, she'll feel more comfortable around you. Ask her to grab a bite after a workout. Bonus points if you casually mention a healthy restaurant.

She's a receptionist

Be charming. No guy is at her workplace to meet with the receptionist; he's there to meet her boss. So make her feel important. Stick out your hand, introduce yourself, flash a smile, and try and make her laugh. Don't make her feel uncomfortable in the waiting room. Just leave your card on the way out and say you'd like to see her again.

*Never ask a yes-no question. It limits her involvement in the conversation and makes it too easy for things to stall out. So instead of asking her if she likes to go out dancing, ask her, "What kinds of things do you like to do when you're out with your friends?" Then shut your mouth, smile, and nod as she opens up to you. Women appreciate when a guy's a good listener.

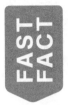

62

Percentage of men who consider it immoral to read confidential documents left by an office printer or fax

Source: Men's Health reader poll

ADD INCHES TO YOUR BICEPS AND CHEST

If your workouts aren't producing the results you want no matter how much time you put in, you're probably going about it all wrong. Tackle this project aimed at fixing mistakes and creating muscle mass.

1 Stop focusing on the mirror muscles

Most guys' workouts are top heavy, focusing on the chest and arms. "Guys get too obsessed with little muscles and not obsessed enough with the big muscles," says *Men's Health* training advisor Mike Boyle, M.A., A.T.C. "You can't see your glutes, you can't see your lats, your spinal rectors, you can't see a lot of the really important, valuable muscles in the mirror." A sign of true fitness is a muscular backside. Your largest muscles, including the glutes, are in your lower body, and training them releases hormones that build size and strength everywhere else. Try the elevated-back-foot split squat. Hold a bar across your upper back using an overhand grip. Assume a staggered stance, with your left foot forward and your right foot back and on a 6-inch step or box. Lower your body as far as you can and then push back up to the starting position. Do 10 reps, switch legs, and repeat. That's 1 set; do 3.

2 Lift faster

Explosive lifting leads to fast gains because it activates more fast-twitch muscle fibers, which have the greatest growth potential. You'll also crank up your heart rate, increasing your calorie burn. Do the lifting phase of each exercise as fast as possible. (The speed of the lift itself doesn't matter. As long as the movement is explosive, your body will recruit fast-twitch fibers.) Then take at least 2 seconds to lower the weight.

3 Warm up the right way

There's a reason why sprinters hop a few times before stepping into the starting blocks: Jumping kick-starts the central nervous system, helping to activate more muscle fibers. "The name for this neuromuscular priming is post-activation potentiation [PAP]," says Tony Gentilcore, C.S.C.S., co-owner of Cressey Sports Performance in Hudson, Massachusetts. "And it's a key to greater strength both in and out of the gym." Consider this: Separate studies published in the *Journal of Strength and Conditioning Research* show that inducing PAP through jumps can help you leap more than 7 percent higher and squat nearly 18 more pounds. For an immediate boost prior to a lower-body exercise, do three quick countermovement jumps: Push your hips back, bend your knees, and leap vertically. For upper-body moves, do a single, extra-heavy rep at the beginning of an exercise. It fires up your nervous system and makes the subsequent reps feel significantly lighter.

(4) Keep your workouts fresh

Think back over the past 30 days. "It's time to switch things up when you lose motivation or if your lifts have not increased for 4 weeks," says Bret Contreras, M.A., C.S.C.S., who trains Olympic and professional athletes. Make subtle changes so that your strength and coordination continue to improve. For example, change your grip, substitute dumbbells for barbells, or adjust your number of reps. By varying your movement patterns slightly, you increase your chances of sparking continuous gains, which will also stoke your motivational fire. This approach leads to better results than experimenting with a fad called muscle confusion, which is constantly doing new exercises so your muscles don't adapt to a routine. Use Contreras's 3-week workout plan to hit "refresh" on your regimen.

Pick a variation of each of the following: squat, deadlift, bench press, chinup, shoulder press, and row. Do these moves on the days specified below for 3 weeks.

MONDAY: 3 sets of 8 to 12 reps
WEDNESDAY: 4 sets of 6 to 8 reps
FRIDAY: 4 sets of 4 to 6 reps

Go for a record in each lift on the third Friday. Then pick new variations for the next 3 weeks.

(5) Pull more weight

Do at least 3 sets of pulling exercises—rows, pullups, and pulldowns—for every 2 sets of chest and shoulder presses you perform. Chances are you've been doing just the opposite, so this approach can help you build the muscles you've been neglecting. The result: Improved posture, better overall muscle balance, and faster gains.

DODGE DIABETES

1 Get in shape

People who have pre-diabetes (a fasting blood sugar level between 100 and 125 milligrams per deciliter, or mg/dl) can reduce their risk of developing full-blown diabetes by 58 percent with moderate physical activity for at least 150 minutes a week and a 5 to 7 percent reduction in body weight, according to findings from the CDC's Diabetes Prevention Program study.

2 Play D against diabetes

If your vitamin D level is adequate, you may be less likely to have high blood sugar. In a study in the journal *Diabetes Care,* people with lower blood levels of vitamin D were 47 percent more likely to have pre-diabetes than those with the highest numbers. Vitamin D may help cells recognize insulin, the researchers say. Boost your D intake by eating more fatty fish.

3 Ditch sugary drinks

People who drink one or two sugary beverages a day have a 26 percent higher risk of diabetes compared to people who drink 'em less than once a month, according to a study published in the journal *Diabetes Care.* Drink coffee instead. In a study published in the *American Journal of Clinical Nutrition,* people who drank at least 4 cups of caffeinated coffee a day were 23 percent less likely to have type 2 diabetes later in life. According to the authors, the polyphenols in coffee may reduce oxidative stress linked to the development of chronic diseases.

4 Know the symptoms

Do you feel thirsty all the time? Do you pee so often that your friends make fun of you? If so, you may already have diabetes. The Centers for Disease Control and Prevention estimates that there are 8 million undiagnosed cases of diabetes in the United States. Have your blood sugar level checked with one of the diagnostic tests on page 105.

BUILD A WORKOUT YOU CAN DO ANYWHERE

If you drive a truck for a living or you seem to be forever on the road, learn a total-body workout routine that you can do anywhere, even in as small a space as a hotel room. We learned it by interviewing a bunch of truckers. Choose two to four of the following standing moves and two to four of the ground moves from the following lists. Do the exercises at 75 percent to 85 percent of your maximum heart rate for 20 seconds apiece interspersed with 10 seconds of rest. That's 1 cycle. Do up to 4 cycles with 60 seconds of rest between them. (*Note:* The boldfaced exercises are among the most metabolically taxing.)

STANDING

1. Squat
2. Jumping jack
3. Running in place
4. Shadowboxing (with a kick)
5. Lunge
6. **Lunge jump**
7. **Squat jump**
8. Side-to-side toe touch jump
9. Hop
10. Stepup

GROUND

1. Pushup
2. **Spiderman pushup**
3. Crunch
4. Bicycle crunch
5. Hand-to-toe crunch
6. **Burpee**
7. Plank
8. **Side plank with leg lift**
9. Mountain climber
10. Bird dog

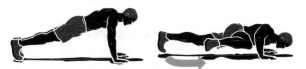

SPIDER MAN PUSHUP

LUNGE JUMP

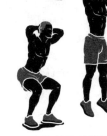

SQUAT JUMP

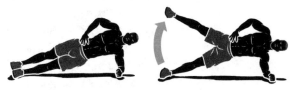

SIDE PLANK

LOWER YOUR LDL; BOOST YOUR HDL

Your lifestyle has a huge impact on your good (HDL) and bad (LDL) choles-terol numbers, so raising the good and lowering the bad makes for a terrific DIY project. A general goal to shoot for is lower than 100 mg/dl for LDL and more than 60 mg/dl for HDL, and you should try to achieve both through natural measures, although statin drugs are effective backups to consider if the numbers aren't where you'd like them to be.

Cholesterol is a waxy substance that can build up on the walls of your arteries and lead to clots and inflammation that can cause heart attacks. Cholesterol is made by your body and also comes from food. The cholesterol you get from food isn't a big worry. However, when you eat a diet high in saturated and trans fats, your liver produces more cholesterol. Stands to rea-son, then, that lowering your intake of certain foods can reduce your LDL. Here are 12 lifestyle changes for a healthier cholesterol profile.

1 Boost your bean count

Canadian researchers conducted an analysis of numerous studies that included more than 1,000 participants and found that people who ate one daily serving—equal to ¾ cup—of legumes for 3 weeks averaged a 5 percent decrease in their LDL level. The researchers pointed out that a decrease of that magnitude has been shown to result in an equal decrease in cardiovas-cular disease risk. You can easily work them into your next meal with these suggestions from Mike Roussell, Ph.D., a *Men's Health* nutrition advisor.

CHICKPEAS: Also called garbanzo beans, these legumes pack equal amounts of protein and fiber (5 grams) per serving. For a meal, add chick-peas with cumin, onions, tomatoes, and diced chicken breast, says Roussell. Chickpeas are also the main ingredient in hummus. Grab a container at the store to use as a dip for baby carrots.

LENTILS: In addition to helping with your cholesterol, lentils are fiber wunderkinder. (Boiled, they have about 16 grams of fiber per cup.) "Once lentils are cooked, they go great on salads or mixed with brown rice and sautéed onions," says Roussell.

BEANS: Your goal is to make these less boring. Try mixing black beans with rice and salsa for a simple dip for your nachos, says Roussell. At break-fast, provide an extra protein punch by adding any variety of beans and cumin to your scrambled eggs.

PEAS: Peas pack protein as well—one serving contains 16 grams. Try substituting mashed peas for mashed potatoes. "Peas can be pureed and eaten with a steak, or you can get them frozen with carrots for a fast side dish to any protein source," says Roussell.

② Eat more nuts

In an analysis of 25 different studies on walnuts, pecans, almonds, peanuts, pistachios, and macadamia nuts, researchers at Loma Linda University found that eating 67 grams of nuts per day—that's a little more than 2 ounces—increased the ratio of HDL to LDL in the blood by 8.3 percent. And Australian scientists found that when men replaced 15 percent of their daily calorie intake with macadamia nuts—12 to 16 nuts a day—their HDL levels went up by 8 percent. Walnuts are also powerhouse HDL boosters. Researchers found that they can raise HDL by 9 percent. Try crushed walnuts mixed into yogurt for a quick breakfast.

③ Quit smoking

Doing so can increase your HDL cholesterol by up to 10 percent.

④ Lose weight

Extra pounds take a toll on HDL cholesterol. If you're overweight, for every 6 pounds you lose, your HDL may increase by 1 mg/dl.

⑤ Boost your endurance

Researchers in Japan found that exercising for 20 minutes a day increases your HDL by 2.5 mg/dl. That's not much, but for every additional 10 minutes per day you keep huffing in the gym, you add an extra 1.4 mg/dl to your HDL. It doesn't matter whether you pull a rowing machine or power through a tough barbell routine, just keep your activity level at a point where you're panting but not out of breath.

⑥ Build killer quads

Ohio University researchers discovered that older men who did lower-body work—squats, leg extensions, leg presses—twice a week for 16 weeks raised their HDL levels by 19 percent. For legs and HDL levels that are something to look at, follow the lead of the men in the study: Do 3 sets of 6 to 8 repetitions of the half squat, leg extension, and leg press, resting for no more than 2 minutes between sets. Use a weight that's about 85 percent of the amount you can lift just once.

⑦ Take a calcium supplement

In a study published in the *American Journal of Medicine*, people who took a daily 1,000-milligram calcium supplement saw their HDL cholesterol level rise by 7 percent. Choose a brand that contains calcium citrate (not coral calcium) and 400 international units of vitamin D for maximum absorption.

⑧ Go fishing

When Canadian researchers compared a steady diet of whitefish with regular consumption of lean beef and chicken, they found that the fish-eating folks experienced a 26 percent increase in HDL2, a particularly protective form of HDL.

⑨ Eat oatmeal cookies

In a University of Connecticut study, men with high LDL cholesterol (above 200 mg/dl) who ate oat-bran cookies daily for 8 weeks dropped their levels by more than 20 percent.

⑩ Switch your spread

Buy trans fat–free margarine, such as Smart Balance Buttery Spread. Researchers in Norway found that, compared with butter, no-trans margarine lowered LDL cholesterol by 11 percent.

⑪ Eat grapefruit

One a day can reduce arterial narrowing by 46 percent, lower your LDL cholesterol by more than 10 percent, and help drop your blood pressure by more than 5 points.

⑫ Take the Concord

University of California researchers found that compounds in Concord grapes help slow the formation of artery-clogging LDL cholesterol. The grapes also lower blood pressure by an average of 6 points if you drink just 12 ounces of their juice a day.

IMPROVE YOUR FLEXIBILITY WITH YOGA

Every man needs to stretch more, which makes yoga an ideal activity that not enough men do, either because they find it too difficult or don't like how they look in Lululemon crops. Philadelphia-based mixed martial arts expert Phil Migliarese understands this and has lured men into the practice with a class called Yoga for Fighters, a tough name for a serious stretch series designed for the masculine body and mindset.

"Normal yoga studios do poses that average guys just can't do," says Migliarese, a fifth-degree black belt in Brazilian jujitsu and master-level yoga teacher. He combined key moves from his 20-year study of both jujitsu and Ashtanga vinyasa practices to create his own unique hybrid. "Men also have issues like tight hips and hamstrings that everyday yoga just doesn't address properly."

Migliarese fixes that with a method based on Sun Salutation. It mixes dynamic movement, stretching, and focused breathing to build strength and power, enhance mobility, and hone focus and endurance. "Most guys have never tried anything like it, so they make across-the-board athletic improvements extremely fast," says Migliarese. "They're also surprised to discover that it's as challenging as an actual fight. It's a grappling match with yourself."

Sun Salutation

Move through these poses in the order shown, breathing in and out through your nose the entire time. Hold each pose for three deep breaths. Inhale on upward movements (even numbers) and exhale on downward movements (odd numbers). Complete the sequence 3 to 5 times.

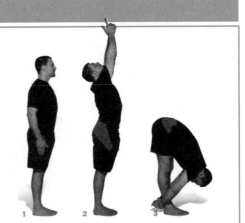

1. Stand tall with your feet together, your chest up, and your arms by your sides. **2.** Raise your hands above your head, interlocking all your fingers except your index fingers. **3.** Hinge forward, keeping your legs straight as you bring your face as close to your shins as possible.

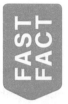

Sun Salutation

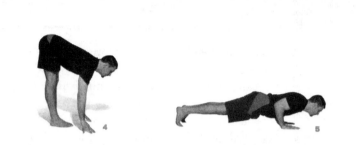

4. Lift your head and torso, keeping your back flat. Support yourself with your hands on your shins or the floor. **5.** Bend your knees, put your palms on the floor, and kick back into a pushup position. Hold your chest a few inches off the floor.

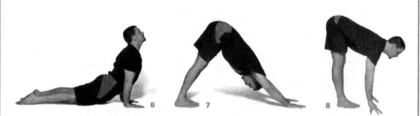

6. Without raising your hips, straighten your arms and stretch your upper body toward the ceiling. **7.** Lift your hips and try to touch your heels to the floor. Keep your back flat and your legs straight. **8.** Step forward and lift your head and torso. Keep your legs and arms straight. Place your hands on your shins or the floor.

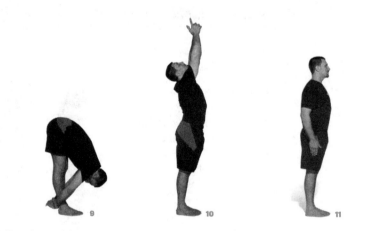

9. Hinge forward, keeping your legs straight as you bring your face as close to your shins as possible. **10.** Raise your torso and stand tall. Bring your palms together above your head, interlocking all your fingers except your index fingers. **11.** Slowly sweep your hands down to your sides. Repeat the entire sequence.

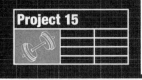
IMPROVE YOUR ENDURANCE

Remember the Beep Test on page 27? To increase endurance, simply repeat it once a week. On two other days each week, do sprint intervals. Sprint at 85 percent of your maximum effort for 1 minute and then rest for 2 minutes. Do that 5 to 8 times total. Intervals are the best way to improve your VO_2 max, the maximum amount of oxygen your body can process at once, which is a powerful indicator of your aerobic fitness level. Here are some other steps to take for a second wind.

① Go the extra mile

Set an ambitious mile time—say, 30 seconds under your personal best—and then head out for intervals. If your goal is 6 minutes, run a half mile in 3 minutes and walk 3 minutes. Do this 4 times, adding an interval each week so by week 3 you're at 6 intervals. By week 4, try to run your goal time.

② Build core endurance

Endurance isn't just for runners—you need endurance in your core to maintain proper form during pushups and other exercises that engage this system. Try these to build a better middle.

→ **THREE-POINT TENNIS BALL TOSS:** Hold the top position of a single-arm pushup (feet slightly beyond hip width, body straight from head to heels, weight supported on one hand) and bounce a tennis ball off a wall. Catch the ball and immediately bounce it back against the wall. Do 2 sets of 15 reps with each arm.

→ **PLANK PUSH/PULL:** Assume a plank position on the floor with a weight plate between your forearms. Lift your right arm, push the plate forward as far as possible, and then pull it back. Do 2 sets of 10 reps with each arm.

③ Give yourself a pep talk

A recent study from the U.K. showed that repeating motivational mantras can improve endurance by 18 percent. Participants chose four motivational mantras—two for the middle phase of a workout and two for the end. Start with upbeat ones: "Feeling good!" "You're a winner!" When your E light starts to flash, unleash the fatigue blasters, like "Dig deep" and "Push it."

RIDE YOUR BIKE 100 MILES

It doesn't matter whether your bike tires are thin and smooth or fat and knobby—finishing a century (a day-long 100-mile endurance ride) is a rite of passage for anyone who owns a bicycle. Use your endurance plan in Project 15 on page 267 to get your body ready and then sign up for one of these events. There are more than 425 century rides each year in the United States, so you have lots of opportunities. Start investigating at bikeacentury.com. Or plan on one of these killer 100-milers:

① Go off-road

The Leadville Trail 100 MTB is a real slog: The elevation profile of this Colorado event looks like a shark's maw: six peaks with a total of 12,612 feet of climbing forest trails and mountain roads through the Rockies. You're never below 9,200 feet, and the altitude makes all the climbing even more difficult. Elite riders finish in about 6 hours; the stragglers cross the line in closer to 13. Get more info at leadvilleraceseries.com/mtb.

② Take the pavement

For a sizzling good ride, try the Hotter'N Hell Hundred: This midsummer blast in Wichita Falls, Texas, is the nation's most popular century ride, drawing more than 12,500 riders each year. The relatively flat course is fast—top riders finish in 4 hours. You'll barely notice the triple-digit temperatures, until you stop for fresh fruit and Gatorade at the rest stops dotted every 10 miles along the way. Get more info at hh100.org.

PAMPER HER WITH THE PERFECT BATH

The goal of this run-her-a-soothing-bath project shouldn't be to achieve your pleasure, but hers. If you become a better man in the romance department, don't worry, the good stuff will follow. This DIY is all about making your sweetheart feel appreciated and pampered. The message it sends is that you are paying attention and are aware of her stress level and her feelings. Women find that incredibly sexy in a man—and you haven't even turned on the tap. There's an art to pampering with a proper bathtub soak, so take some cues from an expert, Dee Patel, assistant general manager and bath concierge at the Hermitage Hotel in Nashville.

① Bring the heat

Make sure the bathwater is hot enough; 92°F is ideal for most people. If you have no thermometer, use the inside of your wrist to make sure the water is not scalding. Your calloused fingers aren't as sensitive to temperature.

② Use good scents

Studies have linked the scent of lavender to a relaxation response, so reach for some lavender bath oils and salts to add to the hot water as it's filling the tub. Try Ahava Lavender Bath Salt ($22, ahavaus.com). In a pinch, try 2 tablespoons of olive oil. Add half of it while the water is running.

③ Remember the robe

Fill the tub to within 6 inches of the top so she can submerge herself from the neck down. Set out a bath pillow (a rolled hand towel works, too) along with a bath mat, a dryer-warmed towel and robe, and pair of slippers.

④ Set the stage

Dim the lights and light some unscented candles—you don't want the fragrances to clash. Skip the clichéd rose petals and set three orchids, water lilies, or gardenias adrift instead. Offer her water and wine. And have the bathrobe nearby for her. Then leave her to enjoy the peace.

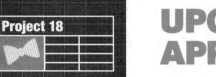

UPGRADE YOUR APPEARANCE

Face it. No matter how cool and confident you act in your Prada suit, if your eyebrows look like Leonid Brezhnev's, nobody will take you seriously. Is it time to clean up your act? A grooming and style makeover is always a great DIY project that can reap beaucoup rewards in the human resources and finance departments.

1 Eliminate wrinkles

The kind on your shirt, not your face. (We'll get to those later.) Because nothing says "I don't care about how I look" quite like a frumpy button-down. Commit to a cleaner, more professional look—it's easier than you think. For a quick solution, put aluminum foil under the ironing board cover. "The foil reflects the heat back, which eliminates creases faster," says Linda Cobb, author of *Talking Dirty with the Queen of Clean*. Still won't come out? Your clothes might be too dry. Try ironing while they're still damp.

2 Get the perfect haircut

Pick the right cut for your face rather than choosing a hairstyle that looks good on guys on TV and in magazines, says Craig the Barber, CEO of the Grooming Concierge.

OVAL: Symmetrical, with eyes evenly spaced and one eye-width distance between them. "They can pull off any haircut," Craig says, "because the eyes, nose, and mouth are well proportioned."

ROUND: A full and round jawline and, in many cases, a round hairline. "Styles with height will help lengthen the face," Craig says.

PEAR: Narrow forehead, broad jawline. Opt for a "round" haircut with the sides equal to the top, which will help balance the face.

TRIANGULAR: Wide hairline, broad jawline, and narrow chin. "Keep your hair short so the top of your head isn't the focal point," Craig says.

SQUARE: If your cheekbones, forehead, and jaw are the same width, you can pull off most hairstyles—except for flattops, which will make your face look even squarer.

Shave closer

Start with a hot shower. The warm water will soften your facial hair, and showering before you shave will ensure at least a modicum of alertness on your part. Use less shaving cream. Too much will gunk up your razor and cause you to miss spots. Or try a shaving oil, which some men find provides the closest, smoothest shave. As for shaving against the grain, most experts, predictably, think you shouldn't fight nature. Making the hairs stand up will allow your blade to catch a little skin, even if you don't bleed. Finish with an alcohol-free aftershave. A moisturizer with sunblock is best, as it traps moisture and provides other, obvious advantages.

Whiten your teeth

When picking an at-home whitener, use common sense: Stronger bleach concentrations work faster. If you want a complete overhaul from a home kit, look for a carbamide peroxide concentration of at least 10 percent. In a German study, in-office trays whitened teeth six shades in three sessions ($500 to $1,000), and the at-home variety required seven uses ($300 to $600). Whitening strips required 32 applications ($20 to $150).

But you can't just suck a strip and forget it. Use a whitening toothpaste to keep the shine from fading, and a whitening floss—the plaque-heavy areas between your teeth soak up colors. And watch the coffee, juice, and wine; they're oral-bling killers.

Clean up your beard

In general, your beard should not be any longer than the hair on your head. Maintain a 1:1 ratio. Never shave to the jawline. End your beard an inch above your Adam's apple. Create a natural fade there by setting a trimmer to 2 or 2.5. Use a mild, nonlathering face wash. Apply conditioner to your beard. If you've trimmed enough to see skin through your beard, exfoliate.

6 Frame your face

Look to Johnny Depp and Justin Timberlake for inspiration. Both of those men know the transformative power that a great set of specs can hold. "Wearing different glasses is the easiest way to switch up your look," says Lauren Solomon, a professional image consultant and president of LS Image Associates. "People notice your face first and will note the difference immediately."

7　Bag eye wrinkles

Steep two teabags, let them cool, wrap each in a clean dishcloth, lie down, and place a bag over each closed eye for 5 to 15 minutes. Green, black and chamomile teas have astringents that constrict blood vessels and pull skin taut.

8　Clean your nails

Extend a clean, professional-looking hand at your first big meeting of the year. "You can easily eliminate discoloration with whitening toothpaste," says Mona Gohara, M.D., assistant clinical professor of dermatology at Yale University School of Medicine. "The same ingredients and abrasives that brighten your teeth will brighten your nails." Rub a small amount on the top of each digit and leave it on for 1 minute.

9　Look more refreshed

Leave your white and blue button-ups on the shelf and opt for shirts in pastel colors. "A pop of color around your face will make you look brighter," says image consultant Solomon. "And the colored collar will bring focus to your face."

10　Add layers

Sometimes the key to great style is as easy as adding one more thing. Layers not only make you look better, they're also more functional, allowing you to easily transition into an after-work outfit, or stay warm when the temp dips at night. If you're normally a T-shirt-and-jeans kind of guy, add a chunky sweater, a leather jacket, or a scarf to brighten up your look.

11　Belt it

Dress shoes should be matched with a slim belt, while casual shoes call for a wider belt. Suede shoes? Wear a suede belt.

12　Grow instantly

No human growth hormone in the fridge? Lengthen the look of your legs. Match your socks to your pants, not to your shoes.

⑬ Don't hide behind a bulky sweater

A fine-gauge knit for sweater-cardigan, crew, or V-neck—offers a better fit than a thick sweater. With just a T-shirt underneath, you'll look muscular, sleek, and relaxed.

⑭ Dry brush

Next time you reach for your toothbrush, do a dry run first. Studies show that dry-brushing your teeth before a regular brushing cuts tartar by 60 percent. Use a soft dry brush, first, then rinse, then follow up with toothpaste and water.

⑮ Get the perfect suit

Your clothes are almost always too big. If you can only afford to tailor one thing, make it your Sunday best. "Every man needs at least one good suit that fits well and conveys confidence," says Michael Andrews, founder and CEO of Michael Andrews Bespoke, a custom-tailor shop in New York City. Just know that all tailors aren't created equal, so look up reviews on consumer-friendly sites like Yelp. "Older English and Italian tailors make a good suit, but their styling might not be current, while others may focus on style and less on construction," Andrews says.

⑯ Get the right shoes

You don't need different kicks for every outfit, but you should have more than one dress pair, one gym pair, and one casual pair. Shoes are an easy place to be creative, so experiment with styles and colors. Find a great monk strap that you can wear with a suit or dark jeans. Cognac- and burgundy-colored shoes also offer tremendous versatility.

⑰ Install a full-length mirror

When it comes to fashion, men tend to focus solely on what's happening from the waist up rather than the whole package. For starters, you'll get a better sense of how colors work together and other details you might typically ignore—like whether or not it's finally time to replace those hand-me-down loafers. You can get a good mirror for as little as $30, and even if you're not inclined to use it, the woman in your life most certainly will.

WHAT WILL MAKE YOU A Better MAN?
↓
"If you look good, you feel good. If you feel good, you do good. If you do good, you smile."

—Actor/comedian Kevin Hart

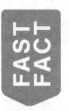

90

Percentage of men who say they would run up the "Rocky steps"–the steps of the Philadelphia Museum of Art–if given the chance

18 Fight the effects of aging

Ninety percent of the signs of aging—like wrinkles and sun spots—come from everyday sun exposure. Wear a moisturizer that has an SPF of 30 or higher—even in winter. Wrinkle-inducing UVA rays are present year-round.

19 Tame chest hair

Hey, Chewbacca, the ideal chest-hair length is just under an inch. To get your fur perfect, use your electric shaver with a number 6 setting.

20 Add flair to your suit

Don't think of it as a mere jacket, shirt, tie, and pants, but as a complete look. If you've got a basic navy suit, look for shoes that carry a subtle hint of gold. Wear a belt and a tie with the same gold tint, or a blue-and-gold patterned shirt.

21 Add flair to your sports coat

A pocket square can make a sports coat look extra special. But you don't have to go all origami on it. Just pinch the middle fabric with your thumb and forefinger and let the sides fall, grab the hanging square like a banana with your other hand, and fold over once. Insert. It'll look great rather than like you were trying too hard.

22 Dry up

If your sweaty pits make you look like an extra from Cool Hand Luke, ask your doctor for a prescription product called Drysol, which contains 20 percent aluminum choloride, a chemical that will decrease sweating by closing off the sweat ducts.

23 Buy a pair of black cap-toe shoes

The kind with a slightly matte finish (not mirror-shines) will strengthen your best suit but still work with casual pants on Fridays. Give your tired wing-tips to the former congressman in the mailroom.

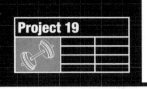

BANISH BACK PAIN

It's estimated that up to 80 percent of Americans will experience debilitating back pain (usually lower-back pain) at some point in their lives. The good news is that, in most cases, the pain will ease up within 6 weeks with little or no medical treatment. Better news: You can avoid pain altogether with a little preventive medicine, the kind that's in this DIY project.

① Strengthen your core

Your abs and other middle muscles support your spine, so doing the ab exercises on page 246 will be a great start. Plus, our sports medicine advisor, Jordan D. Metzl, M.D., swears by the cat camel: Get down on all fours and gently arch your lower back. Then lower your head and round your upper back. That's 1 repetition. Move back and forth between cat and camel positions slowly for 3 minutes. Repeat once a day. Two more great lower-back strengthening exercises:

THE BIRD DOG

Get on your hands and knees, with your hands on the floor directly below your shoulders and your knees directly below your hips. Keep your back flat throughout the exercise. Slowly lift your left leg straight backwards and your right arm out straight in front of you so that both limbs are parallel with the floor. Hold for 10 seconds, then return them to the floor and repeat with the right leg and left arm. Continue alternating for 12 reps.

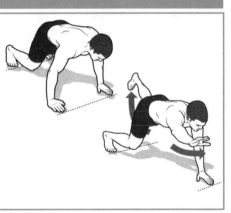

Lie on your back with your knees bent and your feet flat on the floor. Hold your arms out a foot from your hips, palms up. Keeping your upper back and shoulders on the floor, raise your hips until your upper legs and torso form a straight line from your knees to your shoulders. Squeeze your glutes as you hold the top position for a second. Lower your hips to the floor and repeat 11 more times. To make it harder, elevate your feet on a bench and support your upper body with straight arms and hands on the floor, as shown. Then raise your hips.

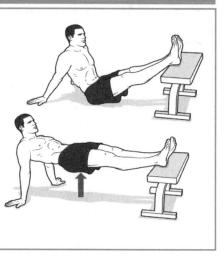

② Protect your back as you work out

When you do core work, tense the muscles of your midsection and then try to make yourself as tall as you can. This helps keep your spine's highly flexible lumbar section stiff so it's naturally arched, not rounded or overarched. During overhead work, pull your shoulders down and back so your shoulder blades can't move. (In other words, flex your lats the way a bodybuilder does.) The strong muscles that control your shoulder blades originate on your upper spine, so this helps brace your upper back. Then, during pushups and planks and while rising from deadlifts, squeeze your glutes. Contracting your butt muscles "locks" the hinge between your sacrum and lumbar regions, making your lower back and hips move as one unit. That's what to do. Here's what to avoid:

A ROUNDED BACK. Your lumbar spine is the most vulnerable spinal structure because the posterior ligaments surrounding it are weaker. Lifting weight with your hips too high puts a lot of stress on these ligaments; that can lead to muscle spasms and lasting lower-back pain.

LOOSE SHOULDERS. When you don't stabilize your shoulders, your back is more likely to round. The pressure then shifts the fluid in the center of the lumbar disks, resulting in bulges or disk herniations.

HYPEREXTENSION. By overarching your lower back, you overload the lumbar area. The result isn't good: stiffness, progressive arthritic changes, pain, or even stress fractures. So when you stand up, make sure you squeeze your glutes to avoid hyperextension.

③ Stay off the couch

Lounging in front of the TV won't cure a bad back. Lying down for a prolonged period of time is one of the worst things you can do for lower-back pain because it makes your back muscles stiff and weak. That makes them prone to injury and pain. If you have back pain, you can exercise—just do it smarter. Opt for low-impact activities, such as walking or swimming, which target muscle stiffness without jolting your joints. That said, if even these activities are unbearable or if the pain doesn't let up in 5 to 7 days, schedule a doctor's appointment.

④ Don't wreck it while you drive

Car trips can accelerate back pain. The fix: Pay as much attention to the curve of your spine as you do to the curves in the road. When you stand, your lower back has a natural arc, one you need to maintain as you sit. The trouble is that most automobile seats are designed for short-term comfort, not long-term support. A plush seat can cause your spine to slump; this puts pressure on your disks, resulting in pain. To take the pressure off, start by adjusting the back of your seat so it's perpendicular to the floor, and then recline it back about two clicks. The ideal position is different for each person, but the angle between your thighs and torso should be about 110 degrees and your hips should be relaxed. Next, if your seat has a built-in lumbar adjustment, set it for softer in the morning when your disks are swollen with fluid, and firmer at night when they're less hydrated. No lumbar adjustment? Use an inflatable support or lumbar roll. If after these tweaks you still find yourself aching on the interstate, stop for a few stretch breaks. Raise your arms overhead and inhale deeply. This lifts your rib cage off your pelvis, restoring the curve in your lower spine. Repeat 3 to 5 times at each break, or until you feel less pain.

⑤ Give your lower back a healing massage

If you've been sitting for a long while and your lower back aches, try this quick self-massage that can be done anywhere. Place a tennis ball between your right side (a few inches above your hip) and a wall. Shift your weight to your left leg and bend your right knee. Turn away from the wall so the ball rolls toward your spine. Turn back. Repeat 5 times. Move the ball an inch lower and repeat. Once you reach your tailbone, work on your left side.

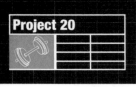
INJURY-PROOF YOUR KNEES

(1) Rethink running

You might have heard that running is bad for your knees. That's true for some people who have had injuries, but recent research suggests that running may not increase your risk of chronic knee problems like osteoarthritis. Just run smart: If you hit the trail, be careful on steep or uneven terrain. These conditions increase your risk of runner's knee, a problem where your thighbone rotates too far inward, putting pressure on your kneecap. You feel dull pain under your kneecap, especially when you sit for a long time with a bent knee or take stairs.

(2) Strengthen your hip muscles

They control your thighbones, and the motion of your thighbones affects your knees. Try these two moves, doing 1 set of 10 reps and working up to 3 sets a day.

→ **MOVE 1.** Stand with one foot in the loop of a resistance band and the other foot on top of the band (adjust the length to control the resistance). Move the banded leg 2 seconds out, 2 seconds in.

→ **MOVE 2.** Then work another key part of your hip muscles by standing with one foot inside the band and looping the other end around the foot of a heavy piece of furniture or some other object that won't easily move. Extend your banded leg back to 45 degrees, 2 seconds out, 2 seconds in.

(3) Check your wheels

If your leg muscles are not balanced, you could suffer patellofemoral pain syndrome, a common cause of knee pain. The reason: a strength imbalance between two of your quadriceps muscles—the vastus medialis and the vastus lateralis—is a key contributing factor to this condition. As it turns out, the remedy is a classic exercise. Doing lunges is an ideal way to strengthen your quads equally, researchers in the U.K. recently found. That's because lunges target the muscles on both your inner and outer thigh, while many other movements tend to work just the latter, the researchers say.

4 Maintain knee flexibility

Sit on the floor with your legs straight. Roll up a small towel and place it under your heels just high enough for the backs of your knees to clear the ground. Flex your thigh muscles and press the backs of your knees to the floor. You should be able to touch equally well on both sides. If you can't, do this test as an exercise: 2 sets of 15 reps (each rep is flexing your thigh for 5 seconds) four times a day until your knees match. If they don't match after 2 weeks, see an orthopedist. If the test is easy but it still feels like you have cement in your knees, then see an orthopedist.

5 Protect your IT bands

Your iliotibial (IT) band is fibrous tissue on the outside of your thigh that stabilizes your knees and hips. If your hips and knees twist too much, the IT band rubs your lateral femoral condyle, a prominent part of your thighbone, causing pain on the outside of your knee. A long running stride increases force on your knees and IT bands. To shorten your stride, boost your step rate by 5 to 10 percent. Try to avoid landing hard on your heel, and keep your knee flexed about 20 degrees. Have a friend take video of you so you can check your form.

MINI PROJECT

Make Your Own Ice Pack

Save yourself $20. Grab a large heavy-duty zipper-lock plastic bag and make your own slushy cold gel to use on swollen ankles and other sore body parts. Mix 1½ cups of water with ½ cup of rubbing alcohol, seal it in the plastic bag, and throw it in a freezer for a couple of hours. Instead of freezing into a rock-solid brick, the alcohol and water mixture forms a thick, cold slush that will conform to your injured joint. It'll stay cold for about an hour, but apply it for only 15-minute intervals to avoid damaging your skin.

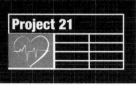

STOP SMOKING

Quitting is the quickest way to dramatically improve your health. In fact, it's more important to quit smoking than it is to start exercising. But you already know that. What you may not know is that combining counseling with nicotine-replacement boosts your odds of success by 50 percent, according to experts at the Mayo Clinic's nicotine dependence center. So, take your pick of these strategies.

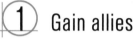 **Gain allies**

Research from the University of Georgia found that joining an online support group made smokers more confident they could knock the habit, increasing their odds of success. Participation is key, says study author Judson Brewer, M.D., Ph.D. Try a site like, quitnet.com, which is also mobile-friendly and sends text message reminders to keep you on track.

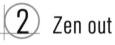 **Zen out**

Shift your focus, cut your cravings. Mindfulness meditation can help you smoke 1.2 fewer cigs for each day you practice it, Yale research shows. Download Dr. Brewer's iPhone app, Craving to Quit, for a meditation primer. Up for mind games? Try hypnosis. A study published in the journal *Complementary Therapies in Medicine* found that people admitted to the hospital with heart or lung illnesses (potentially smoking-related) who tried one 90-minute hypnotherapy session were more than three times as likely to kick the habit as similarly sick peers who relied on nicotine patches instead.

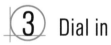 **Dial in**

Hang up old habits. A 2013 University of Oxford review found that calling a help line can increase the likelihood of quitting by up to 50 percent. Dial 1-800-QUIT-NOW to connect to your state's quit line. *Note:* Calling at least three times will boost your chances of success.

4 Stick it

Ease into the patch. In a 10-week Duke University study, people who began using a nicotine patch 2 weeks before they stopped smoking were twice as likely to quit as those who put down the cigs and picked up the patch at the same time.

5 Blow bubbles

Before you pop in a piece of nicotine gum, note the time of your morning toke. According to a study in *Nicotine & Tobacco Research*, if your first cigarette is within a half hour of waking, your best bet is a 4-milligram dose of nicotine gum. Quit rates of smokers who used this strategy were double that of smokers who didn't. Your a.m. start time is a better gauge of how hooked you are than your daily cigarette count, experts say.

6 Fake it

If a drink stirrer doesn't do it for keeping your mouth and hands busy, try e-cigs. A 2011 Boston University study found that 67 percent of people reduced the number of cigarettes they smoked by switching to electronic cigarettes. Jonathan Foulds, Ph.D., a professor of public health sciences at Penn State, suggests that if you're going to use them to quit, don't go cold turkey. Instead, start with the kind that deliver more nicotine than "ciga-likes." Then, ease off e-cigs by gradually switching to a liquid with lower and lower nicotine.

And while you're busy breaking your habit, start a healthy one—eating more vegetables. In a Johns Hopkins study, ex-smokers who ate diets rich in cruciferous vegetables like broccoli, cauliflower, and Brussels sprouts had about a 20 percent lower risk of lung cancer than those who ate the least.

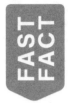

15

Number of minutes it takes for cigarette smoking to cause DNA damage

Source: Chemical Research in Toxicology

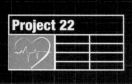
TOUGHEN UP YOUR TELOMERES

To delay aging, you have to start with your DNA. Special strands of DNA called telomeres cap off each of your chromosomes, protecting them from mutation when your cells divide. The problem is that your telomeres begin to shorten and fray as you grow older; once they drop below a critical length, your cells are no longer able to divide, so they start deteriorating. At the same time, your mitochondria, the energy powerhouses of your cells, start losing steam. Researchers have been able to shift the aging process of rodents into reverse by restoring their truncated telomeres. The little guys suddenly had fewer signs of DNA damage, more-efficient mitochondria, and healthier organs. And while more study is needed, humans may reap the same benefits if we can keep our telomeres from shrinking. Try these strategies:

Say Om

In a University of California study, people who regularly meditated over a 3-month period had more active telomerase, an enzyme that helps preserve telomeres. Start with a 10-minute session before breakfast. Find a comfortable seated position in which you can stay upright, relaxed, and alert. Then, focusing on either the sensation of your breath at your nostrils or the rising and falling of your abdomen just below your navel, count each exhalation, from 1 to 10, and then start at 1 again.

② Eat more fish

A 2013 study from Ohio State University showed that people with the most favorable omega-3 fatty acid to omega-6 fatty acid ratios also had the longest telomeres. One way to improve yours? Eat more fish rich in omega-3s. Flip back to page 64 for ideas.

③ Talk to your neighbors

A new study from the University of Michigan shows that people who live in neighborhoods with lower aesthetic quality, safety, and social cohesion had shorter telomeres than those who lived in neighborhoods with a better social environment—even after adjusting for socioeconomic status and biological risk factors. The social environment may be key for protecting telomeres.

(4) Swallow the right antioxidants

A study from Austria shows that people with the highest blood levels of the antioxidants lutein, zeaxanthin, and vitamin C have the longest telomeres. Leafy greens and green peas pack all three.

(5) But don't overdo one nutrient

It is possible to have too much of a good thing: In a new study from the *European Journal of Nutrition,* people with the most folate in their bloodstreams had the shortest telomeres. So consider whether you're consuming too much folic acid. Folic acid is a synthetic form of folate, a powerful nutrient that in small doses plays a critical role in cell division and DNA maintenance. But excess folate may not be helpful. It has also been associated with some cancers. In one study in the *Journal of the National Cancer Institute,* men who took a daily 1,000-microgram folic acid supplement were 2.6 times more likely than men who took a placebo to develop prostate cancer over the next 10 years. To stay healthy and safe, aim for the recommended daily amount of folate, which is 400 micrograms per day. You can probably hit that mark without taking a supplement because many foods, such as bread, cereal, and rice, have added folic acid, and lots of produce and legumes are rich in folate.

MINI PROJECT

Learn Tai Chi, Live Longer

Tai chi is an ancient discipline, and it's great for young guys who want to live to be ancient. Doing tai chi may slow the aging process, a study from Taiwan suggests. Compared with people who didn't exercise, those who practiced this martial art at least twice a week for longer than a year had nearly double the blood levels of CD34+, a marker for certain stem cells that have been shown to promote healthy aging. The study authors suspect that tai chi may help increase production of the stem cells by relaxing blood vessels and boosting bloodflow. Find a class at americantaichi.net/TaiChiQigongClass.asp.

SIMPLIFY YOUR LIFE

Follow these rules of efficiency and forget the rest. Simplify your:

DECISION MAKING. After reviewing an e-mail or phone message, act immediately. If you can complete the task in 2 minutes, do it right away. And remember that DELETE can be the best decision-making tool of all.

ODD JOBS. Pay someone to handle the duties that suck up your time, like cleaning the house, mowing the lawn, picking up dry cleaning. The less small stuff you sweat, the more important stuff you can handle.

HOME. Choose one disorganized room in your home and overhaul one area in it per week. Admire your work. By starting small, you won't become overwhelmed and give up. Each little success will provide the self-confidence and motivation to keep it up without sucking up a lot of your time.

WARDROBE. Buy an updated navy blazer. You can dress it up with wool slacks or dress it down with jeans, so it's one of the most versatile pieces of travel wear. Make sure to get one that's snug through the body and shoulder and has no brass buttons or sheen. A matte finish and a soft, unconstructed shoulder will guarantee it looks modern for a long time.

FINANCES. Invest an hour's worth of income per day in your retirement fund. That's 12 percent of your gross earnings for a 40-hour week.

KITCHEN. Plan meals for a week at the same time every weekend. By knowing what you're going to eat and when, you'll spend less time thinking about what to make for dinner and be more likely to eat healthier fare.

DIET. Eat cleaner by shopping the perimeter of the supermarket. That's where you'll find the fresh vegetables, fruits, seafood, dairy, and meats. The interior of the store contains most of the processed foods.

WORKOUT. Combine two exercises into one, like jumping jacks and push-ups. New move: pushup jacks. From the up position, hop your legs out to the sides—like a jumping jack—as you use your arms to lower your body. Then jump your feet back to the regular position while you push up. If that's too easy, jump your arms out as well. The benefit: greater calorie burn and more muscle in less time, says BJ Gaddour, C.S.C.S., author of the *Men's Health* book *Your Body Is Your Barbell*. Another tip: Keep your workouts short but tough. YMCA researchers found that men were twice as likely to stick to an exercise program when they performed shorter workouts—less than 30 minutes—than when they did longer exercise sessions.

ATTITUDE. Sit up in your seat. Psychology follows physiology: If you smile and act happy, alert, and relaxed, you'll feel it.

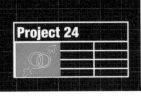

WIN HER BACK

① Redo first impressions

Call her by the wrong name, like, three times?

TURN IT AROUND: Research from the University of Western Ontario suggests that first impressions, while persistent, are not necessarily permanent. Make a good impression in several contexts that disassociate you from the scene of the original crime, says study author Bertram Gawronski, Ph.D.

② Bounce back from a bad date

If you realize soon enough that you're losing her attention, your best move is to call it early and arrange to meet up when you're firing on all cylinders, says relationships expert Karen Ruskin, Psy.D., L.M.F.T.

TURN IT AROUND: Let her know the depth of your interest promptly. Say something on the order of, "I wasn't really in top form tonight, but it was great hanging out with you and I'd love to see you again." Once you secure the redo, dream up a date sure to counteract the bad impression.

③ Score a bedroom rebound

Use your big head to pinpoint what went wrong—nerves, too many drinks, or fumbling around her anatomy are common culprits, says *Men's Health* sex advisor Debby Herbenick, Ph.D.

TURN IT AROUND: Acknowledge that she didn't see your best and rewoo her like it never happened. This time around, drop the tempo to a crawl. "Research shows that both women *and* men long for more extended foreplay—in the neighborhood of 15 to 20 minutes," says Herbenick.

④ Rekindle lost love

Angry words were said, personal items were packed up (*or thrown*), and your reputation as a "great guy" suffered a hammer blow. A lost cause? Not necessarily.

TURN IT AROUND: Ask her to dinner at a place where you had a great date. Use memories of you at your most awesome as the standard you uphold, and she'll be more prone to remember you as *the* guy and not *that* guy.

MASTER THESE SEX POSITIONS IN A MONTH

① The Spork

BENEFITS: Offers a natural bridge to more creative positions. She lies on her back and raises her right leg so you can position yourself between her legs at a 90-degree angle and enter. Her legs will form the tines of a spork, a spoon-and-fork utensil. She can do this with you facing her or facing her back.

NOW TRY THIS: If she's limber, lift her left leg up to increase the depth of penetration.

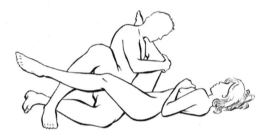

② Restroom Attendant

BENEFITS: Good for a quickie at a party.

Slip into a bathroom and ask her to look into the mirror while you enter her from behind. It lets you have eye contact during the G-spot-targeting rear-entry position.

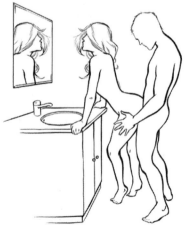

③ The Shoulder Holder (a.k.a. Cuban Plunge)

BENEFITS: Allows deep penetration and targets the G-spot.

She lies on her back. You kneel between her legs and raise them, resting her calves over your shoulders. Rock her in a side-to-side and up-and-down motion to bring the head and shaft of your penis in direct contact with the front wall of her vagina. Because this angle allows for deep penetration, thrust slowly at first to avoid causing her discomfort.

NOW TRY THIS: Bring her legs down and have her place her feet on your chest in front of your shoulders. This allows her to control the tempo and depth of thrusts.

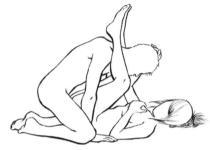

④ H₂Ohh Yeah

BENEFITS: Good for an outdoors quickie, while still avoiding prying eyes. Her buoyancy in the water makes this position easier to hold. And all you need to do is shift some bathing-suit material out of the way of certain body parts; the lifeguards will be none the wiser.

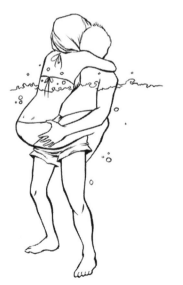

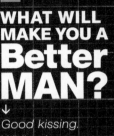

WHAT WILL MAKE YOU A Better MAN?

↓

Good kissing. While charm counts, being a great kisser trumps personality and looks for women considering a long-term relationship, according to a study in the journal Evolutionary Psychology.

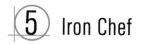 Iron Chef

BENEFITS: Good position for a quickie with deep penetration.
This is a variation of a position known as the Ballet Dancer, in which she raises her legs up and wraps them around your butt or thighs. Your kitchen counter is the perfect height for this standing-to-seated appetizer.

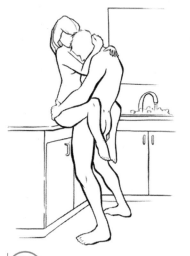

⑥ The Pretzel (a.k.a. the Camel Ride)

BENEFITS: The deep penetration of doggy-style while face-to-face.
Kneel and straddle her left leg while she is lying on her left side. She will bend her right leg around the right side of your waist, which will give you access to enter her vagina. Rear entry hurts many women's backs. This position allows her to lounge comfortably while enjoying deep penetration.
NOW TRY THIS: Manually stimulate her using your fingers. Or withdraw your penis and, holding the shaft with your left hand, rub the head against her clitoris to bring her to the brink of orgasm, then reinsert it when she wants you inside her.

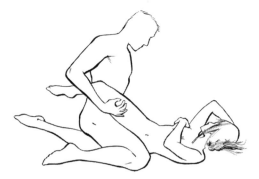

⑦ Reverse Cowgirl

BENEFITS: With a pillow under your head, you get an awesome view of her backside. She can control depth of penetration and pace.

Lie on your back with your legs outstretched. She kneels next to you, then turns and spreads her legs, straddling your hips and facing your feet. Kneeling, she lowers herself onto your penis and begins riding you.

NOW TRY THIS: Have her lean forward or back to change the angle of your penis for greater stimulation.

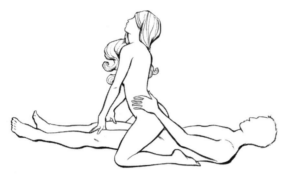

⑧ The Spider

BENEFITS: You both can still maintain eye contact while viewing the action at center stage.

Both of you are seated on the bed with your legs toward one another and your arms back to support yourselves. Now move together and have her move onto you. Her hips will be between your spread legs, her knees bent, and her feet outside of your hips and flat on the bed. Now rock back and forth.

NOW TRY THIS: She grabs your hands and pulls herself up into a squatting position while you lie back. Or ask her to straighten her legs. Push your pelvis down a few inches while she pushes up.

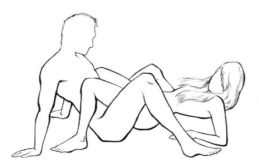

DETOX YOUR LIFE

Are you reading this book in a toxic wasteland? If you're sitting at home, the answer could easily be yes. Rid your life of these harmful poisons, and you'll be healthier at home and away. Bonus—since these toxins are so ubiquitous, we give you 9 steps to cleaner living. This is an ongoing project, so it's worth reviewing these throughout the year.

1 Make VOCs vanish

Sprays, gels, and wipes promising to keep you and your home as fresh as possible may not be so safe: Research published in *Environmental Impact Assessment Review* found that scented air fresheners, lotions, shampoos, soaps, laundry products, and household cleaners emit an average of 17 different VOCs (volatile organic compounds). A number of these compounds, including formaldehyde, are classified as toxic or hazardous and have been linked to low sperm quality, asthma, and cancer. You can inhale these chemicals or absorb them through your skin, and then they can enter your bloodstream and end up in your brain. Depending on the substance, repeated exposure could eventually lead to central nervous system damage. The problem is, the companies that make fragranced products aren't required to reveal whether their wares contain harmful VOCs. To stay on the safe side, ditch scented air fresheners, dryer sheets, detergents, and soaps. Even "organic" or "green" fragranced products should be tossed—they're just as likely to spew VOCs, research shows. Since label claims like "fragrance free" and "nontoxic" aren't always true, check the ingredients, avoiding products that contain "masking fragrance," "fragrance," "perfume," or "parfum." Finally, spruce up your space with English ivy or asparagus ferns, which can lower VOC levels in indoor air, a University of Georgia study found.

2 Ditch nonstick

Perfluorinated compounds, or PFCs, are slick. Often embedded in furniture, carpeting, and paint, these water- and stain-repelling chemicals can easily escape into the air, according to a new study published in *Environmental Science and Technology*. Once inhaled, PFCs can linger in your body for years, potentially altering your levels of testosterone and thyroid hormone, which may eventually lead to low sperm count, thyroid disease, elevated cholesterol, and obesity, scientists say. The EPA is currently working with companies to eliminate PFCs in everything from furniture to food packaging. But that means anything you bought in the past could have it. So unless you're buying it new, avoid furniture, carpets, and clothing treated with stain-resistant chemicals, and opt for cast-iron and stainless-steel cookware over nonstick pans.

③ Be a dust buster

Many of the toxic chemicals in households collect in dust. Take polybrominated diphenyl ethers. These chemical flame retardants may disrupt thyroid function. They lurk in flame-resistant upholstered furniture, computers, and some electronics, but they migrate from there and end up in household dust. Since you can't tell for sure if your sofa has flame retardants, eliminate what you can by dusting and vacuuming more often.

④ Use less plastic

By now you've heard of bisphenol A (BPA), the estrogen-mimicking chemical in some plastic products. Many companies have phased it out since health concerns were first raised in 1997. (To remind you, studies have linked BPA exposure to a variety of ill effects, including hypertension, diabetes, and reduced sperm quality.) Trouble is, even BPA-free plastics can still leak estrogen-like chemicals, according to research published in *Environmental Health Perspectives*. You're better off using food containers made of glass or stainless steel. And never heat any plastic in the microwave; that promotes chemical leaching. Another plastic threat? Phthalates. Researchers have found that phthalates can interfere with testosterone production and may be linked to weight gain and insulin resistance. They lurk in shower curtains made with polyvinyl chloride (PVC) and plastic food containers. If a plastic container's recycling symbol shows the number 3, then it's PVC. If the plastic has any degree of pliability, it may contain phthalates.

⑤ Reconsider your lawn care

Eliminating bugs from your shrubs could come back to bite you: A study in the *International Journal of Epidemiology* reveals that using pesticides may raise your risk of Parkinson's disease. People who applied outdoor or indoor pesticides at least four or five times a year were 47 percent more likely to develop Parkinson's than those who pulled the trigger less often. The researchers believe the bug-killing chemicals may also kill brain cells. Use organic methods, or, if you're set on the toxic option, wear gloves and goggles, and wash your clothes after spraying.

(6) Make mold disappear

You check your bread for mold, but how about your air? *Aspergillus* and *Penicillium*—the two most common indoor mold genuses—fling out tiny spores and mycotoxins, which can penetrate deep into your lungs. Even non-allergic folks can experience wheeze-inducing nasal inflammation from inhaling *Aspergillus* particles, according to a study from Finland. Worst case: Molds can lead to a life-threatening lung infection—made even scarier by the fact that they are increasingly drug resistant. Bleach alone won't cut it. Even dead mold can cause allergic flare-ups, EPA experts warn, so you need to kill and remove the fungal funk. If you spot a patch—check damp, dark areas—grab gloves, an N95 respirator mask, and a stiff brush. Mix 1 cup of bleach into a gallon of water and scrub the area until no visible mold remains. Rinse with clean water and let the area dry completely. Bolster your internal defenses too: Scientists in South Carolina recently linked nasal mold infections to an insufficient vitamin D level. If you're on the low side (as most people are), a D_3 supplement may ease your inflammatory response to mold spores. To determine your dose, ask your M.D. to perform a 25-hydroxy vitamin D blood test.

(7) Rule out radon

If you spend hours in a man cave, you might be inhaling dangerous amounts of radon. The gas forms when uranium in soil breaks down, and it seeps into your home through cracks in the foundation. When you inhale its radioactive particles, radon can damage your DNA and lead to cancer. In fact, the EPA estimates that radon is responsible for 21,000 U.S. lung cancer deaths every year. One in 15 American homes has a dangerous level of radon—and the farther north your latitude, the greater your risk may be. The reason: When the air outside is cold, heated indoor air rises, creating suction that can pull radon into your home. Even if you're not in the Northeast or Midwest (where levels are notoriously high), you should test your home for the gas; there are no warning signs that it's invading your air. Buy a short-term radon test kit, and if the level is 4 picocuries per liter (pCi/l) or higher, run a second test, since levels can vary from day to day. If the average of the two readings is 4 pCi/l or higher, call a certified radon reduction specialist.

8 Cut out carbon monoxide

This colorless, odorless gas kills more than 400 people per year in the United States, the majority of them men. Inside your body, carbon monoxide (CO) clings to red blood cells, displacing the oxygen your brain and heart need to function. Low levels can lead to flulike symptoms, while larger doses can result in brain damage or even death. According to British scientists, the kitchen is one of the primary locations for CO exposure. Every time you fire up a gas stove, you release the odorless, poisonous gas. Normally the amount is minimal and dissipates quickly. But if your stove burns inefficiently or vents improperly, the noxious gas may be invading your air. Check your stove, furnace, or fireplace. Is the burner flame yellow instead of blue? Is there soot on any vent or flue? If either is true, your appliance or flue may be functioning improperly and should be checked by a pro. Next, make sure your CO alarms—you have them, right?—aren't installed near vents, which can blow the gas away from the sensors. Each alarm should also have an end-of-life signal, which sounds when the unit needs replacement.

9 Don't burn your food

You know that charred flavor you like on grilled and broiled meats? Those burned spots contain cancer-causing compounds. Reduce your risk by dunking before you cook: Marinating pork in beer before grilling it may block potentially carcinogenic compounds called polycyclic aromatic hydrocarbons (PAHs). A *Journal of Agricultural and Food Chemistry* study found that submerging pork cuts in black ale for 4 hours reduced the formation of eight key PAHs by 53 percent. The scientists think the beer's antioxidants, found in greater abundance in ales than in lagers, help prevent the free-radical activity needed for PAH formation.

BONUS: The trick may also work with other meats, they say. Plus, adding more antioxidant-packed ingredients to the marinade may improve the effect. Acrylamide, a form of a chemical used to treat wastewater, lurks in french fries, chips, bread, and even doughnuts. When some carb-rich foods are cooked at high temperatures, the amino acid asparagine reacts with sugars in the foods, forming acrylamide. Your body's chemical reaction to acrylamide can lead to DNA mutations that may raise your cancer risk. So strategize in the kitchen: Opt for lower temperatures and shorter cooking times, and if you do fry, don't make foods very brown. And give your spuds a bath: Soaking potatoes for 2 hours before cooking cuts acrylamide buildup by up to half, say U.K. scientists.

FIX YOUR POSTURE

Are you out of line? Without even looking at you, physical therapist and *Men's Health* contributor Bill Hartman is pretty sure you have a posture problem. That's because almost every client he sees in his fitness center in Indianapolis has a posture problem. He's been doing it so long he can spot an anatomical abnormality from the way a guy walks through the mall, sits on a park bench, or stands at a bar.

The trouble isn't just that slumped shoulders make you resemble a Neanderthal. Over time, your poor posture takes a tremendous toll on your spine, shoulders, hips, and knees. In fact, it can cause a cascade of structural flaws that result in acute problems, such as joint pain throughout your body, reduced flexibility, and compromised muscles, all of which can limit your ability to burn fat and build strength, says Hartman.

You can identify your own posture problems with a simple self-test. Then, use Hartman's tips to fix your form, soothe your pain, and maximize your muscle. It makes for an excellent DIY project to tackle several times a year to keep you on the straight and narrow.

① Analyze your alignment

Strip down to a pair of shorts and ask a friend to take two full-body photos, one from the front and one from the side. Keep your muscles relaxed but stand as tall as you can, with your feet hip-width apart.

② Compare and diagnose

Place your photos next to the illustrations on the opposite page to diagnose your posture problems.

A. Look at your ear. If it's in front of the midpoint of your shoulder, your head is too far forward.
B. If you can see your shoulder blade, your back is too rounded.
C. A large convex curve in your upper back causes you to slump forward.
D. The front of your belt line is lower than the back, and your lower spine is arched significantly due to an anterior pelvic tilt.
E. Look at your shoulders. One shouldn't appear higher than the other.
F. Your kneecap points inward, causing your knees to touch when your legs are straightened.
G. Toes point outward more than 10 degrees.

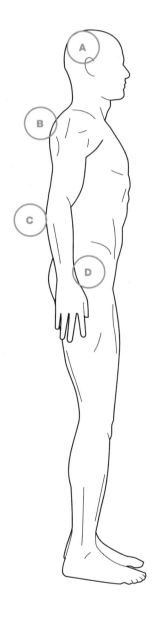

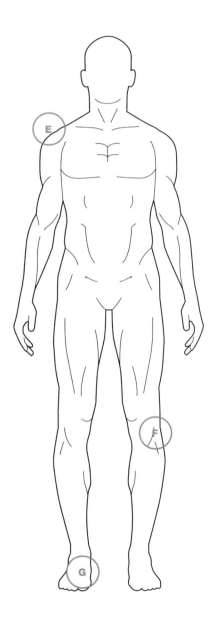

WHAT WILL
MAKE YOU A
**Better
MAN?**
↓
*"Improving my
posture," say
93 percent of
MH survey
respondents.*

③ Pinpoint and fix

A. Forward head

WHERE PAIN STRIKES: Your neck

THE PROBLEM: Stiff muscles in the back of your neck or weak in front

THE FIX: Stretch with head nods daily: Moving only your head, drop your chin down and in toward your neck while stretching the back of your neck. Hold for a 5 count; do this 10 times.

Next, do this neck "crunch" every day: Lying face up on the floor, lift your head so it just clears the floor. Raise your head, and hold for 5 seconds; do 2 or 3 sets of 12 reps daily.

B. Rounded shoulders

WHERE PAIN STRIKES: Neck, shoulder, or back

THE PROBLEM: Tight pectoral muscles

THE FIX: Try a simple doorway stretch: Place your arm against a doorjamb in the high-five position (that is, forming an L), your elbow bent 90 degrees. Step through the doorway until you feel the stretch in your chest and the front of your shoulders. Hold for 30 seconds. That's 1 set; do a total of 4 daily.

C. Hunched back

WHERE PAIN STRIKES: Neck, shoulder, back

THE PROBLEM: Poor upper-back mobility or weak back muscles

THE FIX: Lie faceup on a foam roller placed about midback, perpendicular to your spine. Place your hands behind your head and arch your upper back over the roller 5 times. Adjust the roller position and repeat for each segment of your upper back.

Next, perform the prone cobra. Lie facedown with your arms at your sides, palms down. Lift your chest and hands slightly off the floor, and squeeze your shoulder blades together while keeping your chin down. Hold for 5 seconds; do 2 or 3 sets of 12 reps daily.

D. Anterior pelvic tilt

WHERE PAIN STRIKES: Lower back (because of the more pronounced arch in your lumbar spine). The tilt also shifts your posture so that your stomach pushes outward, even if you don't have an ounce of belly fat.

THE PROBLEM: Your hip flexors, which allow you to move your thighs up to your abdomen, are tight and your glutes are weak.

THE FIX: Kneel on one knee and perform a front hip stretch. Tighten your gluteal (butt) muscles on your kneeling side until you feel the front of your hip stretching comfortably. Reach upward with the arm that's on your kneeling side, and stretch in the opposite direction. Hold this position for a count of 30 seconds, and repeat 3 times.

Next, do the glute bridge. Lie on your back with your knees bent about 90 degrees. Squeeze your glutes together and push your hips upward until your body is straight from knees to shoulders. Hold for 5 seconds; complete 2 or 3 sets of 12 reps daily.

E. Elevated shoulder

WHERE PAIN STRIKES: Neck and shoulders

THE PROBLEM: Your trapezius (the muscle that starts at the back of your neck and runs across your upper back) is shortened.

THE FIX: Perform an upper-trap stretch. With your higher-side arm behind your back, tilt your head away from your elevated side until you feel the stretch in your upper trapezius. Apply slight pressure with your free hand on your stretched muscle. Hold for 30 seconds; repeat 3 times.

F. Knees point in or pigeon toes

WHERE PAIN STRIKES: Knee, hip, or lower back

THE PROBLEM: Tightness in the outer portion of your thigh or weak glutes

THE FIX: Stand up, cross your affected leg behind the other, and lean away from the affected side until you feel your hip stretching comfortably. Hold for 30 seconds. Repeat 3 times.

Next, use an exercise called the side-lying clamshell. Lie on one side with your knees bent 90 degrees and your heels together. Keeping your hips still, raise your top knee upward, separating your knees like a clamshell. Pause for 5 seconds; lower your knee to the starting position. Perform 2 or 3 sets of 12 reps daily.

G. Duck feet

WHERE PAIN STRIKES: Hip or lower back

THE PROBLEM: You lack flexibility and strength in all the muscles in your hips.

THE FIX: Drop to your hands and knees and place one foot behind the opposite knee. Making sure you keep your spine naturally arched, shift your weight backward and allow your hips to bend until you feel the stretch. Hold the stretch for 30 seconds, repeat 3 times, and then switch sides.

Next, try the Swiss-ball jackknife. Assume the top of a pushup position but rest your feet on a Swiss ball. Without rounding your lower back, tuck your knees under your torso by rolling the ball with your feet toward your body. Roll the ball back to the starting position. Do 2 or 3 sets of 12 reps daily.

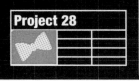
BE MORE INTERESTING

A few years back, the editors of *Men's Health*, who are always on a quest to better themselves, took an afternoon to call their sources and posed this question: What can I do to make myself more interesting? Invariably the answer was about developing a skill or taking on a particular project that escorts the do-it-yourselfer out of his comfort zone. Here are 11 of my favorites.

1 Blend your own wine

Jim Gordon, editor of *Wines & Vines*, makes a case for mixing vino.

Bartenders pride themselves on shaking the rarest and most expensive spirits and liqueurs together to concoct impossibly sophisticated cocktails. But these days, there's a taboo when it comes to mixing one wine with another. One reason might be that a lot of people only know about varietal wines—they contain primarily one grape variety. But many of the world's great wines are blends.

One time I mixed Cabernet Sauvignon and Merlot in a 24-ounce Riedel crystal glass and basically recreated red Bordeaux. I could have also added Cabernet Franc, Petit Verdot, and Malbec and stayed within the traditional parameters of the Bordeaux chateaus. Champagne is also usually a blend, containing base wines made from dark Pinot Noir and Pinot Meuniere grapes, and golden Chardonnay grapes.

Chateauneuf-du-Pape, the full-blown red wine from France's Rhone Valley, can be blended from as many as 15 varietals. Old vines planted promiscuously in historic California vineyards are often dominated by Zinfandel, but also count some Petite Sirah, Carignane, and Mourvedre varieties that add complexity to the resulting blended wine.

Winemakers blend all the time. Why can't the rest of us have a little fun?

2 Learn a trick shot

World-champion pool trick artist Andy Segal reveals a simple way to keep yourself in drinks all night.

1. Place the 1 and 2 balls together against the cushion across the table. Balance the 8-ball on top between them.

2. From the other end of the table, explain you'll hit the 8-ball without touching the other two balls—or skipping the cue ball.

3. Aim the cue ball directly at the upper ball from across the table and shoot it slowly. As it's rolling, slap the table with your hand. The impact will cause the two lower balls to split and the 8-ball to fall right in the middle.

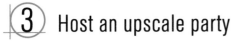 Host an upscale party

Time to retire the beer pong tables. Celebrity party planner David Tutera reveals the secrets to throwing a memorable, boss-friendly bash.

ABANDON THE BOWL GAMES. Super Bowl Sunday and March Madness aren't themes. You want people to remember the music you played, the mood you created, the menu served. Try Asian cuisine on modern platters, sake cocktails, and fast-paced instrumental music. Or bring the outdoors inside— cover the tables with plaid blankets, add leather pillows to your seating areas, and serve a wild game-inspired menu of venison jerky and elk burger sliders. Throw in a craft beer tasting with brews from Alaska, Kansas, and other popular hunting destinations.

HIRE HELP. Sure, it's expensive, but it can be worth the investment. Securing the assistance of a professional bartender, a server to pass food, a valet service or a coat check—depending on the size of your party—will make the event run more smoothly and leave a lasting impression.

EXTEND THE BAR. Instead of the usual wine and beer options, consider serving a specialty cocktail. These could be selected by color, flavor, season, or even for their unique combinations—like a bacon-infused Old Fashioned or a Jalapeño Caipirinha.

KEEP A SECRET. Your party will seem far more interesting when a surprise happens at some point during the event. Perhaps a pianist or a sax player or an acoustic guitarist sneaks in during the night. You can also hire a mind reader, a high-end magician, or a handwriting analyst to keep your guests amused. Even renting old-school video arcade games will add fun and competition.

DECORATE. Yeah, I said it. Even the most masculine event needs decor. Here's what you do: Dim the lights and line up votives—small candles— down the center of your tables or along the windowsills. Women love candlelight. If you have a friend who does graffiti, takes photographs, or is into graphic design, hire them to create a few large pieces to display around your space for a modern, gallery-like feel.

④ Trace your ancestry

Megan Smolenyak, author of *In Search of Our Ancestors*, helps you expose your roots.

HIT THE ROAD. Your first impulse may be to jump online, but it's remarkably easy to bark up the wrong family tree. Instead, plan a road trip. Visit older relatives and ask them to drag out photo albums and family treasures that shed light on your shared past. If they'll let you, poke around in their attics, basements, garages, and closets for memorabilia they've forgotten. Ask lots of questions. Record everything you can. Older folks—who will often appreciate the visit and your interest—are living libraries and will occasionally astonish you with their tales, like the time I learned of my great-grandmother's murder that had been hushed up by the family.

EXPLORE YOUR OCCUPATIONAL HERITAGE. You'd be surprised how many of us follow in our ancestors' footsteps when it comes to the occupations we choose. Steven Tyler's family tree, for instance, is littered with musicians, including a great-uncle who earned a bad-boy reputation when he notched his first divorce while still a teenager. Tyler's roots are claiming him, and yours may be, too. Search for your ancestors at Ancestry.com, FamilySearch.org, and Archives.com, paying particular attention to census records, city directories, and draft records. If you know of or suspect a military tradition, you'll want to include Fold3.com on your surfing expeditions.

HANG OUT IN CEMETERIES. You'll know you're turning into a genealogist if the thought of cemeteries starts to excite you. Graveyards are repositories of clues. Inspect the tombstones of your ancestors and you may learn not just their dates of birth and death, but also their military service or membership in the Masons. Headstones of immigrants are one of your best bets for discovering exactly where in the old country your family hails from.

TAKE IT GLOBAL. Ready to cross the pond? Do some sleuthing at EllisIsland.org (SteveMorse.org makes it more search-friendly), the immigration collection on Ancestry.com (fee-based, but with records covering more than 100 ports and several centuries), and FamilySearch.org (free, and adding millions of records per week). Uncover the specifics of the 1940s accident in the Philippines that killed the grandfather of one of the participants? No problem.

SWAB, SPIT, OR SWISH. Want to find out if you're related to others with your surname, roughly what percentage European, African, and Asian you are, or whether you have some unexpected cousins out there? Take a DNA test from FamilyTreeDNA.com (if your interests are purely roots-related) or 23andMe.com (if you'd like to double up and learn about your medical predispositions). You can examine Y-DNA (tells you about your direct paternal line), mtDNA (tells you about your direct maternal line), and autosomal (looks at your entire family tree). Just be open to whatever you might learn.

⑤ Improve your charisma

Former FBI agent Joe Navarro, author of *What Every Body Is Saying*, helps you radiate the confidence of the world's most successful men.

SMILE. Charismatic people don't hold back. They let that smile transmit that "I am a happy, contented person." Coupled with that smile is usually a slightly tilted or canted head, which says, "I am really comfortable around you; nothing is scaring or frightening me. I am relaxed here with you."

DON'T HESITATE. Plunge right into a crowd of strangers and say hello, or do whatever is asked of you without hesitation. If someone gives you a hand, take it. If something drops, rush forward to pick it up or help out. Hesitation conveys that you're insecure or don't care. A lack of hesitation, though, can be very alluring.

REACH OUT. Use the power of touch to let others know you care. Hug more and touch more on the arms—especially as they speak. Touching releases the powerful bonding chemical oxytocin, which lets people know you're interested in them, or are empathetic to their situation. Oxytocin's soothing and relaxing effect also makes people want to stay.

MAKE BIG GESTURES. Charismatic people have smooth gestures that are large and visible. They make dramatic hand gestures, drawing you in, and make you look and follow their lead. Big gestures say, "I'm here, I have something to say, and I feel confident about what I'm saying."

LOOK AROUND. Scan the room, taking it all in. Charismatic people don't hesitate to look anywhere or to make eye contact. They convey interest with their eyes and arch their eyebrows, letting you know they're interested and genuinely care.

⑥ Be a better listener

Daniel Menaker, author of *A Good Talk*, helps you lend your ear.

Men must understand that the magnetism they want to have paradoxically will come ultimately not from a "technique," but only from their genuine interest in others—not only women, but other men.

Try this strategy: Listen, of course. But listen in a certain way—listen for dropped clues about the person you're talking to. Let's say she's describing a storm that cracked a huge limb off on the street in front of where she lived and that it sounded like a mast breaking on a ship. Well, ask her if she has a sailboat or knows about sailing.

Maybe she's talking about a friend, and as she does so, she says he looks a little like Peter Sarsgaard and then goes on to talk about his law firm. Well, back up and ask what she thinks of Peter Sarsgaard as an actor. If she talks about driving somewhere interesting recently, don't ask or talk about the destination. Ask about her car. In other words, get off the main point, from time to time. It shows that you're listening, closely, even to the minor details, that you find what she says interesting and stimulating. She'll think the same of you.

(7) Pay attention to bugs

Anthony Doerr, novelist and science columnist for *The Boston Globe*, reveals why insects make the world better—and more interesting.

Bugs might freak out the weaker-kneed among us, but without them there'd be no pollination, and without pollination there'd be no hamburgers, no potatoes, no bean-and-cheese burritos, no wine, no beer, and dead bodies would rot in the streets.

Among the many stupefying things to learn about bugs—that there is a pink dragon millipede in Thailand that oozes cyanide; or that the larva of certain moths can spend their entire lives chewing the cells of a single leaf; or that dragonflies make airborne love at 30 miles an hour—three strike me as unconditionally fascinating:

BUGS BUILD STUFF. Termites—who rarely grow longer than a twelfth of an inch—routinely construct cathedrals 20 feet tall, replete with staircases, gardens, nurseries, waste dumps, air conditioning systems, and water wells. Leafcutter ants build roads impregnated with pheromones, forage for leaves, mold chewed-up leaves into pellets, and plant strands of fungus atop the pellets, which a farmer caste then cultivates for nutrients. Oh, and by the way? Their single thumb-size queen might live a decade and produce 150 million daughters.

BUGS TRAVEL LIKE CRAZY. After particularly rainy winters, painted lady butterflies migrate from Mexico into California in flocks that can number 1 billion: Picture a flying river. Every monarch butterfly you'll see this spring flapped into your neighborhood from thousands of miles away; nearly every monarch in the United States east of the Rockies will have arrived there from central Mexico. Then they'll die, and their great-great-great-grandchildren will fly all the way back.

BUGS REMEMBER THINGS. A female pipe wasp builds vertical tubes of mud beneath, say, the eaves of grandma's house, then flies off to hunt. She paralyzes some spiders, stuffs them into a tube of her nest, lays an egg, entombs it beside the cache of food, and resumes constructing more pipes.

Some wasps might simultaneously tend to a dozen nests at once, and they not only remember the locations of each, but also keep track of what stage their developing larvae are in and coordinate feeding requirements accordingly. So let's recap: One individual hunting lady-wasp, with lousy vision and a brain no larger than a poppy seed, can adjust for wind, maintain a sense of direction, memorize landmarks, and bring shopping lists with her as she heads out. As someone who regularly returns from the grocery store without half the crap I was supposed to get, my hat goes off to the pipe wasp.

8 Tell better stories

Jay Heinrichs, author of the book *Word Hero*, helps you keep your audience enthralled.

DON'T JUST TELL THE NEWS. To make your story memorable, find some "tension"—an element of surprise. Suppose you went to London with your girlfriend and visited the British Museum. Don't just say you saw the Greek statues. That's news, not a story. Speculate on what happened to the penises missing from all those statues. Is there a secret penis museum in the basement? Or some underground penis-collecting cult? Art and castration: tension at its best.

USE MISMATCHES. All good stories pair things that don't ordinarily belong together: little girls and four-letter words. Vacation disasters. Beautiful clumsy women. (It's not a chick flick if the hot protagonist doesn't fall down in front of her love interest.) Penises and art.

GIVE YOUR CHARACTERS NICKNAMES. Instead of "Bob, the one with the nose ring," just call the guy "Nose Ring." Avoid pronouns. Wrong: "So he's staring at the crotch of the statue, and this other man says to her . . . " Right: "So Nose Ring is staring at the crotch of the statue, and Briefcase Man says to Pink Hair . . . "

END WITH A MORAL. Don't let your tales peter out Shaggy Dog style. Make like Aesop: "So the lesson here is that penis art is like a doughnut hole. Both are at their best when they're missing." Oh, and don't get to the moral until your audience is into its third beer. You'll sound a lot more profound.

9 Work a room

Here's your to-do list from Diane Darling, author of *The Networking Survival Guide*:

MAKE YOUR MUST-MEET LIST. A few days before the event, research the major players and develop a few talking points to use with each one.

GO EASY ON THEM. Start with light chat about the organizing group, for instance, and only later segue into the specifics of your researched talking points. But even if that never happens, don't sweat it—just meeting the person may be a good start, and you can follow up with an e-mail. In fact, you may score coolness points for not being too earnest.

ORGANIZE YOURSELF. Keep your own business cards in one pocket and reserve the other for cards you'll receive. This will prevent fumbling and eliminate the terrifying possibility that you might accidentally proffer a card reading "Private Masseuse—on Call."

BE ON TIME FOR ONCE. If you're one of the first guests, you'll adopt a nearly hostlike mentality, meeting and greeting rather than taking cues from others.

INFILTRATE A GROUP. This is a critical skill: Find the most animated group in the room and join in. Start by quickly making eye contact with someone from the periphery of the group, and then introduce yourself with a firm handshake. Ask an open-ended question, such as "What's your connection here?" There, you've just hooked up with the life of the party.

RECONNECT. Before you leave, double back to a few key people. A second meeting makes them more likely to remember you. Reiterate a prior talking point and say you look forward to meeting again.

⑩ Get on talk radio

CLEAR THE LINE. Call from a landline. (Remember those?) "The audio quality is better; cell reception is spotty," says Sal Licata, an assistant producer of the sports talk show *Mike'd Up*. If you have to use a cell phone, call from an isolated room to minimize noise.

TIME THE CALL. Dial 5 to 10 minutes before the show starts, so you'll be first in the queue, advises Richard Sementa, executive producer of the *Mark Levin Show*. Try again during breaks or when the topic shifts. That's often when they clear the board.

SKIP NICETIES. Once the screener picks up, you have 5 seconds to make an impression. Screeners prefer an opposing opinion. Don't just repeat previous points—react to them, says Sementa. And be confident. Wishy-washy never makes it on the air.

INTRIGUE THE MC. Once past the screener, catch the eye of the MC, who picks names from a computer screen. For shock-jock shows that like characters, give yourself a unique name like Michael "Sour Shoes" Del Campo. He's made it on Howard Stern's show many times.

(11) Write a letter by hand

Daniel Post of the Emily Post Institute teaches the lost art of hand-written correspondence.

GET CUSTOM STATIONERY. Something elegant, preferably with your initials at the top of the page. "You're investing yourself personally in it—in this age of fast-paced, digital communication, it's a tangible reminder of you," says Post. Online shops like Crane & Co (crane.com) offer a wide range of options.

INVEST IN A GOOD PEN. "A good pen will make it easier to add those flourishes that help customize your correspondence," Post says. "Fountain pens are messy—I like the gel ink pens they make for signing checks." Start with pens made by Cross (cross.com)—they're among the best, and many cost less than $20.

ADD A PERSONAL TOUCH. "For somebody trying to appear more interesting, there's this almost courtly idea that a letter can smell like you—or your cologne. Don't overdo it by dousing it with a fragrance. You can also use things like sealing wax to add a more courtly touch."

MINI PROJECT

Mix a Signature Cocktail

Put your own spin on a classic cocktail to make it your own. Or feel free to borrow ours, made for *Men's Health* by Duggan McDonnell, owner of San Francisco cocktail lounge Cantina.

THE *MEN'S HEALTH* BLOOD-AND-WHISKEY SOUR

What You'll Need

1 egg white

Juice of 1 or 2 whole blood oranges, hand squeezed

2 ounces Maker's Mark bourbon

1 teaspoon superfine sugar

3 dashes angostura bitters

1. Separate the egg white from the yolk and drop the white into a mixing glass.

2. Add the fresh orange juice, bourbon, sugar, and bitters. Fill the glass with ice and shake vigorously.

3. Strain the drink into a highball glass filled with fresh ice. Garnish with a wide strip of orange peel, squeezing the oil over the cocktail and rubbing the skin along the rim of the glass before placing it in the drink.

TORCH 1,000 CALORIES IN AN HOUR

Do the following for 60 minutes and your weekend indiscretions will be history.

Perform these five exercises as a circuit, doing each for 30 seconds and resting for 15 seconds between them. After you complete all five moves, begin the circuit again. Do a total of 8 circuits, increasing your rest periods between exercises by 15 seconds each time.

This extreme workout designed by Robert dos Remedios, C.S.C.S., a strength and conditioning coach in Santa Clarita, California, is best for dropping pounds fast and building stamina, mobility, and strength. It fries 1,000 calories when performed by a fit 6'2", 180-pound man, with an estimated postexercise 24-hour calorie burn included.

1 Goblet Squat

Hold a dumbbell vertically next to your chest, cupping one end in both hands. (Imagine that you're holding a heavy goblet.) Push your hips back and lower your body as far as you can while keeping your back straight. Pause, and then push yourself back up to the starting position. Repeat.

2 Explosive Incline Pushup

Assume a pushup position with your body straight from your head to your ankles but your hands on a bench, box, or step. Bend your elbows and lower your body until your chest is a few inches from the bench. Push yourself back up with enough force that your hands leave the bench. Land and repeat.

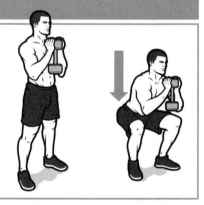

3 Kettlebell Swing

Place a kettlebell on the floor in front of you. With your feet slightly beyond shoulder width, push your hips back and grab the handle with both hands. Swing the weight between your legs, and then thrust your hips forward as you swing it up to chest level. Swing it back between your legs and repeat.

4 Rolling Side Plank

Lie on your left side with your legs straight and your body propped on your left elbow and forearm. Your body should be straight from your ankles to your head. Roll forward onto both elbows and hold for a count of two. Then roll onto your right elbow and hold for a count of two. Continue rolling back and forth.

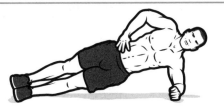

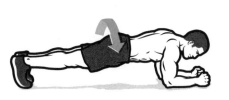

5 Inverted Row

Secure a bar at waist height and slide beneath it. Grab it using an overhand, shoulder-width grip, and hang with your hands directly above your shoulders. Now keep your shoulder blades back and use your arms to pull your chest to the bar. Pause, lower yourself to the starting position, and repeat.

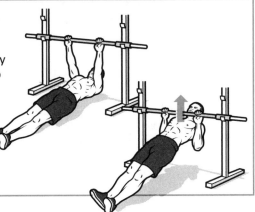

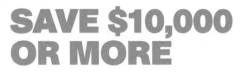

SAVE $10,000 OR MORE

Some of us may want to consider spending as much time on our finances as we do our fitness. Weekly spending reviews and making some simple changes to your financial behavior can add up to big bucks over time. This beginner DIY will likely lead to more advanced (and lucrative) projects for you and your broker to tagteam.

1 Track your spending

For the next month, here's your assignment: Record where every cent goes. Save receipts, credit card slips, and canceled checks, and write everything else down on a pad of paper. Or you can go all-digital with a site like Mint.com that tracks every credit and debit card purchase. Whatever your preference, here's the key: Let no doughnut go unrecorded. You'll be surprised at just how much those $4 Dunkin' runs add up. Often just seeing your spending pattern will point out ways to save.

2 Save in your sleep

Most of us think too much when we save. What do we mean? Big goals like your dream car, a vacation home by the lake, and your kids' college education are huge and uncertain. If you wait until you know the exact cost and when it'll strike, you'll never save anything.

So start today. Instead of thinking about how much you'll need to reach your goal, estimate the maximum amount you could possibly save each month, says Dan Ariely, Ph.D., author of *Predictably Irrational* and a professor of psychology and behavioral economics at Duke University.

Then set up automatic payments from your paycheck toward your goal. If you find you need more spending cash during the month, you can always adjust—but in the meantime, you're stashing dough toward the day Junior gets into Yale.

WHY IT WORKS: Automatic payments don't just make saving easier—they make spending less tempting. How? Money—spending it or even thinking about spending it—causes a dopamine rush in your brain. Then you're relying on your willpower to resist handing over your Visa. That's a battle you'll lose, says Chip Heath, Ph.D., a professor of organizational behavior at Stanford University. "You can't advise people to 'spend less,'" he says. "You're creating a willpower struggle that will have to be fought on a day-to-day, week-to-week basis." So remove as many of those decisions as you can through automatic bill pay and savings withdrawals.

③ Transfer your savings to a money-making account

Don't stow extra cash in your checking account—you're letting your money be lazy. "Having more than what's required to avoid minimum-balance fees is a waste, because it's not earning interest," says Dan Candura, a certified financial planner at Massachusetts-based PennyTree Advisers. Stash a month's worth of expenses in checking. Then put the rest of your emergency stash—experts now recommend a 6- to 9-month buffer—in a high-yield savings account. Compare rates at bankingmyway.com.

WHILE YOU'RE AT IT: If you're always in the black at the end of each month, schedule a recurring automatic transfer to a mutual fund, Candura says.

④ Balance your budget

Call it a "spending plan" or "financial strategy" if you can't stand the b-word. Point is, you need to know where your money's going if you want to save more of it. Use the five categories listed below, and within them list all the expenses you pay online from your checking account. (Put rent under housing, car payment under living expenses, etc.) Add a line for cash under living expenses.

RECOMMENDED BUDGET ALLOCATIONS

RENTING
Housing 35 percent
Living expenses 40 percent
Emergency/insurance 2 percent
Pleasure/personal 15 percent
Savings 8 percent

MARRIED WITH HOME
Housing 37 percent
Living expenses 25 percent
Emergency/insurance 8 percent
Pleasure/personal 20 percent
Savings 10 percent

SINGLE WITH HOME
Housing 45 percent
Living expenses 25 percent
Emergency/insurance 6 percent
Pleasure/personal 14 percent
Savings 10 percent

HOUSEHOLD WITH KIDS
Housing 37 percent
Living expenses 30 percent
Emergency/insurance 10 percent
Pleasure/personal 15 percent
Savings 8 percent

WHILE YOU'RE AT IT: Stay humble. People who lack financial confidence often make the best money decisions. In one study, when people were told that budgeting was difficult, they estimated their expenses more accurately than people who were told it was simple.

⑤ Lower your credit card's interest rate

First, transfer all of your balances to the card with the lowest interest rate. Right after you make a payment, call one of the companies you owe and tell them you want to close the account because you've found a better rate. (Head to bankrate.com to size up their competition.) They'll often negotiate with you right then and there.

Another option: If your home is worth more than you paid for it, refinance your mortgage and take out the equity to pay off your credit debt. The interest rate on your mortgage will be significantly lower—and the interest is usually tax-deductible. (Remember to figure in refinance costs like points and fees.)

WHILE YOU'RE AT IT: Go on a credit and debit fast for 2 weeks; only pay with greenbacks. "Studies show that buying something with a credit card doesn't register with your brain the way it does when you pay cash," says Stanford University's Heath. Converting to cash will make you sense the sting of forking over every penny—which is exactly what you should feel.

⑥ Enroll in a Roth IRA

If you're eligible for a Roth IRA but don't have one, today's your day to sign up. With a Roth, you pay taxes now on the money you're putting toward retirement. The perk: Once you're kicking back in Boca, you don't pay a dime to cash out. It's a small tax hit today, yes—but a huge tax break when you retire. Enroll if you're single and earn less than $120,000 a year (or married and filing jointly and earn less than $177,000).

Already have a retirement account? You can convert your traditional IRA into a Roth IRA. "The amount you convert will be taxed, but you can spread the bill over 3 years," says Paul Burkemper, president of the Burkemper Group in St. Louis.

⑦ Prioritize your debt

Don't assume that "bad" debt like a car loan has to be paid off before "good" debt like your mortgage. Let's assume you have a 30-year, $250,000 mortgage at 6.5 percent interest. You also have a 5-year car loan for $25,000 at 8 percent interest. If you have an extra $1,000 to put toward the principal, pay down your mortgage. Because the loan amount is higher, you'll save $5,890 over the life of the loan vs. only saving $470 in interest on the car loan.

8 Hone your negotiation skills

Start by choosing the right store to stage a negotiation. A low-volume boutique store will be more likely to have some leeway than a high-volume big box. Low margins correlate with lower prices and high volumes, so the megamart has less price padding.

1. Arrive armed with info—an ad showing another company's deal, prices from other stores or venders. This reminds the salesman that you can take your money elsewhere.
2. Don't compete. Start with, "I like this, but what can we do about the price?" advises Holly Schroth, Ph.D., of the UC Berkeley School of Business.
3. Make it sound like a good deal to them. Offer to buy in bulk for a discount. They sell more product, and you save—as long as you'll actually use it.
4. Carry a wad of bills. Then ask if there's a cash discount. You might get around 10 percent off. Sure, the guy might not be completely frank with the IRS about your deal, but that's his business, not yours, right?
5. If you're at an impasse, thank him for his time, give him your phone number, and tell him to call you if anything changes. Walk away. You might receive a good offer on your way out or a call the next day.

9 Talk down your cell phone or cable bill

Follow this step-by-step plan to lower this monthly money-suck.

1. Research how long you've been a customer with the company and how much you've spent. Mention that when you call customer service. Then say you'd love to stay a loyal shopper.
2. Don't demand a discount. Instead, show vulnerability. "For some people, confessing a bit of uncertainty can be disarming and more persuasive," says Zakary Tormala, Ph.D., of Stanford University.
3. Avoid "you must"—he might assert his freedom by refusing. Stay friendly. Use the rep's name.
4. If he still says no, ask for a manager. Make the request before you really annoy the rep, or else the manager could start talking with you on the defensive.
5. Threaten to cancel. The manager might lower your bill or throw in upgrades.

10 Recruit your team

When you were younger, an off-the-rack suit was acceptable. But by the age when you have a professional tailor your suits, you need a team of professionals helping you manage your money. Here's who you want on your side.

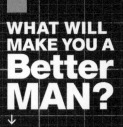

WHAT WILL MAKE YOU A Better MAN?

↓

"I've always presented a challenge to myself. If it's too easy, I don't want it."

—Usher

ACCOUNTANT. Insist on a CPA, not a part-time preparer. He should provide you with client worksheets and must be willing to represent you before the IRS. A messy office is a deal-breaker—you don't need any help losing your receipts.

LAWYER. A good lawyer should cost around $200 to $300 per hour (less if you live in a rural area, more if you're in a big city) and will charge in 15-minute increments. If he uses value billing, which means he decides each job's worth, run the other way. Look for this key trait: When you ask a question, does he answer it precisely? Lawyers need to be good listeners.

FINANCIAL ADVISOR. Financial advisors are the life coaches of the money world: Few have legitimate credentials, even though plenty of them claim the profession. Pick a money mentor from a field that has licensing requirements and a clear code of conduct. Think: lawyer, CPA, or security broker. He should offer flat-fee advice, ask you lots of questions, and speak in terms you can understand.

11 Learn to resist impulse purchases

You're hardwired to want stuff—and to want it now. Anticipating a purchase triggers a larger release of the feel-good hormone dopamine than actually receiving your new toy, brain studies show. To resist this instinct, don't make an important choice when you're tense or fatigued. You'll be more likely to make a rash decision, says executive coach David Krueger, M.D., author of *The Secret Language of Money*. And give yourself time on big purchases—for example, a rule that you'll wait at least a weekend to buy anything more than $100.

12 Refinance your home

Yes, it's a big step, but it could pay off: Interest rates are at an all-time low, so you'll want to lock in a fixed number for as long as you can.

WHY IT'LL WORK: Lenders recognize that interest rates can't drop much lower, so they're betting that they'll go up in the future. Choosing either a 15- or 30-year plan will guarantee that your rates don't increase years later, says Jay Suktis, assistant professor of business administration at the University of Pittsburgh. Both have their advantages: With a 15-year mortgage, you'll not only own your house earlier, but you'll also be paying more toward your home equity (and if you ever need to borrow money for another big purchase, you can take out a home equity line of credit). The 30-year plan allows you to keep your interest rates low—which can provide you security in case you or your spouse loses a job. You can always pay it off early; banks no longer penalize homeowners for doing so.

(13) Invest in the stock market

WHY IT'LL WORK: For people who are a decade or more away from retirement, investing in the stock market has proved to be the best way to grow wealth. But most investors can't match the market's performance. Why? Because sell-offs freak them out. They tend to sell on the dips and then miss out on the climbs. A 2005 University of Michigan study found that if you'd invested $1,000 in an index fund in the beginning of 1963 and sold at the end of 2004, your money would have grown to $74,000. If you'd missed the 10 best days for the market over those 42 years, you'd have only $44,000. And had you sat out the best 90 trading days—just 0.85 percent of the total—you'd have only $2,700. Indeed, the market may feel like a yo-yo if you follow it day to day. But imagine that a boy is playing with that yo-yo as he climbs a steep hill. That metaphor best captures how the market has performed over the years, says Ric Edelman, the author of *The Truth about Money*. The gains have tended to be longer—and larger—than the dips. Edelman's koan: "Focus on the hill, not the string." In other words, stiffen your spine and keep buying through those dips. That's the only way to make the most of the climb.

(14) Consider scrapping your plans to save for college

College is crazy expensive, but don't go overboard saving for it, says Raymond Loewe, the owner of College Money, a college financial-planning firm based in Marlton, New Jersey. Retirement should come first: "You can secure financial aid for college, but I haven't found anyone who gives financial aid for retirement."

WHY IT'LL WORK: If your family income is below $75,000, Loewe suggests focusing your savings on retirement and finding as much financial aid as you can from schools. If you make more than $75,000 (or expect you will by the time your kid reaches college), aim to save a third of all college costs by the time Junior enrolls. The second third can usually be covered by current income; the last third can come from loans.

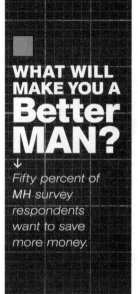

WHAT WILL MAKE YOU A Better MAN?

↓

Fifty percent of MH survey respondents want to save more money.

DO 10 PERFECT CHINUPS

WHAT WILL MAKE YOU A Better MAN?

↓

"I do grip hangs. I wear a 40-pound weighted vest and do 3 sets of 10 pullups. Between sets, I just hang from the bar. Then after my final rep, I hang until failure—my record is 5 minutes."

—New England Patriots' all-pro safety Adrian Wilson

The chinup is one of the best exercises you can do for your upper body because it works your biceps, back, shoulders, and core. "Because it's a body-weight move, it's a great indicator of how strong you are for your height and weight," says Tony Gentilcore, C.S.C.S., cofounder of Cressey Sports Performance in Hudson, Massachusetts.

The exercise is difficult, so most guys avoid the chinup bar like it's a crazy ex-girlfriend. You? Well, this project will help you build the strength and technique to be able to crank out 10 easily.

THE AVERAGE GUY'S CHINUP COUNT

BODY WEIGHT (POUNDS)	TOTAL
140–159	8–12
160–179	7–10
180–200	3–5
200+	1–3

① Test yourself

Hang at arm's length from a chinup bar using an underhand, shoulder-width grip. This is the start position. Now pull your chest to the bar, keeping your body straight the entire time. Bring your chest to the bar, pulling your upper arms down forcefully and squeezing your shoulder blades together. Pause, and then take 2 seconds to lower yourself back to a dead hang. Do as many as you can with proper form. Then follow these tips to be better than average.

DID YOU PERFORM ONLY 1 OR 2 REPS? Then start with the band-assisted chinup and the negative chinup. The assisted chinup perfects your form, while the negative chinup increases your pulling strength, says Gentilcore.

② Do a band-assisted chinup

Loop the band around a chinup bar, and then pull it through the other end of the band. Cinch it tightly to the bar. Place one knee in the loop of the band, and hang at arm's length using a shoulder-width, underhand grip. Now perform a chinup. Do 3 sets of 8 to 12 reps.

③ Try negative chinups

Stand on a box or bench beneath a chinup bar. Grab the bar with a shoulder-width, underhand grip. Jump up, pulling your chest to the bar. Hold the top position for 2 seconds, and then take 6 to 10 seconds to lower yourself until your feet touch the box. That's 1 rep. Do 3 sets of 4 to 6 reps.

④ Go beyond average

To blow your chinup max out of the water, "focus on form instead of taxing your nervous system and burning out," says Gentilcore. Do this: Say your max chinup count is 6. Shoot for doing sets of 3 reps (half of your max chinup count) with perfect form throughout the day, says Gentilcore. (It helps if you have a pullup bar at home or can get in the gym in the morning and evening.) Shoot for 3 to 5 sets each day—1 set in the morning, 1 at lunch, 1 before bed, and others when you have a few extra minutes. By the end of the day you'll have at least doubled the number of efficient chinups you can do each day, and after a month your original max should grow by at least 50 percent or double as the move becomes easier, says Gentilcore. Once you reach a new max, cut those reps in half and repeat the process.

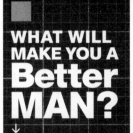

WHAT WILL MAKE YOU A Better MAN?

↓

Eighty-four percent of men would like to be able to do 10 pullups (like a chinup with an overhand grip).

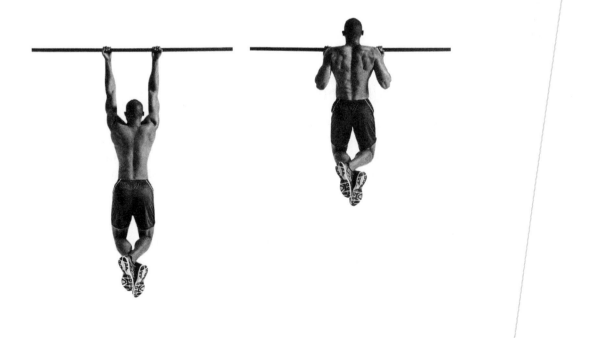

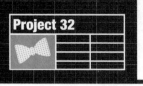

BE A BETTER FATHER

If you've got kids, there's no more rewarding long-term project than raising them. It's your best shot at immortality, you can work on it every day, and it's a hell of a lot of fun, especially when mud is involved. Of course, kids are expensive, and $180 car seats and $400 parties at BounceU are just the start of it. The most important thing to remember: To win the war, you have to be willing to lose some of the battles, but, aw shucks, kids are swell and if you raise them right, they may even let you hang out with them when they have kids.

① Kiss your wife

Treat her with outward love and respect. Your daughter learns her taste in men from you. And that can be by either positive or negative example. Likewise, your son learns how to treat women from the way you treat your wife. Even when you argue. Even if you divorce her.

② Let kids take risks

Ninety percent of your job when they are young is keeping your kids from accidentally killing themselves. Another 5 percent is making them feel comfortable taking risks, and the final 5 comes with teaching them how to decide which risks are the right ones to take.

③ Go instrument shopping

Schools with a strong musical program may give students an academic edge, Long Island University researchers say. They found that second-graders taking twice-weekly piano lessons at school performed significantly better on vocabulary tasks than those who didn't play a note. "The piano students improved their listening skills with music, and that may have helped them hear and store vocabulary words more efficiently for future use," says study author Joseph Piro, Ph.D. While private lessons should do the trick, Piro believes that children may be more eager to learn an instrument if the instruction occurs in a group setting, such as in a class or at school.

4 Start reading food labels—with your kids

"Contrary to popular belief, kids can learn to make wise food choices," says David Katz, M.D., M.P.H., an associate professor of public health at Yale University and a father of five. "Make it easier by having a wide variety of foods available, but only the healthiest options in each category."

Example: They can pick whatever drink they want, as long as it doesn't contain high-fructose corn syrup or exceed 100 calories per serving.

5 Fight cynicism

As kids struggle to form identities in our sometimes violent, often materialistic, always tech-obsessed world, they can become more self-centered and less sympathetic. "You'll never turn your son or daughter back into the wide-eyed child they were just a few years ago," says C. Andrew Ramsey, M.D., assistant clinical professor of psychiatry at Columbia University in New York City. "But you can chip away at their cynicism by calling them to action." Hal Edward Runkel, family therapist and author of *ScreamFree Parenting*, brought his young son to traffic court with him so the boy could see accountability in action. Likewise, Ramsey says, the simple act of volunteering for a day can pay dividends. Kids will see they can make a difference, and they'll be inspired by other people out there doing it every day.

6 Focus your kid's energy

Maybe you don't want a hat-trick-scoring, scholarship-winning, oboe-playing phenom of a child, but our competitive society makes them think otherwise. This explains why so many kids have trouble focusing, says Ramsey. Make sure your kids understand your expectations. Explain that developing skills is about mastery. "Whether your child's role model is Tom Brady or Beyoncé, let them know they ascended to lofty heights because they mastered one skill," Ramsey says. "Learn to go through one door and many others will open for you; try to go through five doors at once and you'll go nowhere."

7 Keep them in the game

If you want your kids to stick with things, let them quit, Runkel says. "Just make sure they taste the full pain of quitting." When Runkel's son was 8, he wanted to quit baseball. Runkel told him, "Sure, but you have to tell your teammates and coach." The boy couldn't do it. He's played seven seasons now. This works with schoolwork, too: "If your kid wants to give up because a project is too hard, say, 'OK. Tell your teacher you quit and you'll take whatever grade is appropriate.' Trust me, they'll stick it out."

⑧ Expand your kid's vocabulary

Researchers advise using a diverse vocabulary with kids, but that doesn't mean you should start reciting Herodotus. Instead, provide creative and dramatic play-by-play for both your activities and surroundings. Don't be shy about using unfamiliar words—children understand a lot of grown-up language just from context. This is a great job for Dad: In families with two working parents, fathers had greater impact than mothers on their children's language development between ages 2 and 3, according to a study published in the *Journal of Applied Psychology*.

⑨ Help them accept criticism

Kids face criticism from many sources: peers, teachers, coaches, and you. "Let them feel it," Runkel says. "Don't say, 'Oh, don't worry about it.' The lesson here is criticism has only as much power as we give it." Acknowledge that criticism hurts and ask your kids: Is it accurate? If so, what can you learn from it? "Also, give them time to process it," Runkel says. "If you say, 'When you act this way, you're not very likable,' it may not register right away. But they'll be thinking about it."

⑩ Take a volunteer vacation

When your kids outgrow Disney World, think about signing the family up for a much different kind of vacation—one that promotes personal responsibility, environmental awareness, and hard work. The American Hiking Society needs volunteers year-round to help clean up state parks and maintain thousands of miles of trail systems in some of the most scenic and well-trod parts of the country.

In North Dakota, for example, volunteers work on the North Country National Scenic Trail in Sheyenne National Grasslands. In the Virgin Islands National Park, the American Hiking Society maintains a long stretch of 300-year-old colonial trails. Families often work within footsteps of pristine white sand beaches and rest at a campground in Cinnamon Bay. Not a bad reward for a day's work.

Before you commit to a vacation, check to make sure that it is an easy-to-moderate work grade and open to kids 13 and up (some are strictly 18 and over). For most trips, the American Hiking Society covers only transportation to and from the airport, as well as campground fees and the occasional meal.

11 Leave a family legacy

When you leave this world, so does part of your history. Make sure your children know their roots by documenting your genealogy, and have your wife do the same. Try the program Family Tree Maker, and get access to Internet ancestry databases at ancestry.com. Set aside time to tell stories of your adventures, too, whether it be winning the MVP award in high-school baseball or motorcycling the Pan-American Highway after college. You'll live on in their memories, not just as Dad, but as a legend, too—the kind of man they admire.

12 Help your kid stay motivated

Focus on the good. Praise can be a powerful motivator, especially when it's specific (e.g., say, "Your description of life in covered wagons is vivid" rather than "Nice job"). Also, praise what matters: effort and persistence (e.g., "I'm proud of the way you've stuck with this math assignment; I know it's challenging"). Encourage realistic goals. Your daughter might have her sights set on a spelling-bee championship, but make sure she understands that you're

MINI PROJECT

Give your kids a green thumb

Planting a tree isn't just about saving the planet, it can also save you money: The American Public Power Association has found that planting trees to shade a home can reduce air-conditioning costs by up to 50 percent. Find out which tree will thrive best in your climate at arborday.org, and then plant one using this three-step guide, provided by John Englert of the USDA National Resources Conservation Service.

1. Dig a hole that's at least two times the diameter of the container your tree is in, and 1 inch less deep. Most roots grow out, not down, and this will allow the roots to breathe.

2. Remove the tree from the container and place it in the hole. Begin filling the hole with the soil you dug out, adding peat moss or composted leaves if the soil is sandy. This will aerate the soil and help the roots retain water and nutrients.

3. Cover a 3-foot diameter at the base of the tree with 3 to 4 inches of mulch. Soak the soil around the tree roots with water, and repeat every two weeks throughout the first growing season (or as needed, depending on rainfall).

pleased more by her hard work than a medal. By encouraging kids' sense of accomplishment, you'll also help them build self-confidence, says Deborah Stipek, Ph.D., dean of the School of Education at Stanford University and author of *Motivated Minds: Raising Children to Love Learning*.

(13) Expand your kid's palate

Employ the same strategy you'd use to teach him a new idea: repetition. Kids need about 10 encounters with a new food before they develop a taste for it. So bolster yourself with patience and persistence, and follow these steps to help your child grow his culinary repertoire.

START OUT SMALL. The key to convincing children to try unfamiliar foods is to introduce them slowly.

MAKE EATING FUN. The best teachers imbue their lessons with entertainment value. Follow their lead. If you're trying to, say, add broccoli to your child's plate, suggest that they look like little trees, and then make a scene of biting off their tops.

BE A GOOD EXAMPLE. If you eat veggies, so will your kid. A study at the Children's Nutrition Research Center, in Houston, found that children ate vegetables 35 percent more frequently when they were readily accessible and available at home.

OFFER FRUIT. It contains many of the same nutrients found in vegetables, such as vitamins A and C, potassium, and folate.

(14) Teach investing skills

By the time kids enter middle school, they have a good handle on how to earn and save money, and many even have their own bank accounts. They're also ready to move on to the slightly more advanced concept of making it grow through smart investing. Here are a few ways to pique their interest—and pad their money-market accounts:

MAKE THEM PARTNERS. Help them buy a few shares of their favorite company—Nike, Nintendo, Pepsi, and so on—and then follow the stock with them online. This will give them an understanding of how the market works and the factors that influence the rise and fall of stocks.

PLAY A GAME. A handful of board and computer games teach similar lessons. Two of the best ones are Mr. Bigshot ($30, mrbigshot.com), a stock-picking game in which players choose between two companies and follow their investments, and Mutual Mania ($12.99 on Amazon.com), a board game similar to Monopoly, but players assemble portfolios and land on spaces that require them to respond to market-changing events.

GO ONLINE. Sites like teenanalyst.com offer primers on topics such as how to screen mutual funds and using P/E ratios to evaluate the price of individual stocks.

Start a 529 savings account

It's still a smart investment. "A 529 account is like a Roth IRA, but for college savings instead of retirement," explains Gary Schatsky, the chairman emeritus of the National Association of Personal Financial Advisors. "It offers two tax advantages: no taxes on your profits, and additional state incentives such as a tax deduction or credit for putting money into the account." But state plans vary widely, so Schatsky recommends Utah's—which offers low fees and good fund selection—for those whose state doesn't offer any unique tax incentives (you don't have to stick with the plan offered by the state in which you reside). As for how you invest—the ratio of stocks to bonds—that will depend on the age of your child and your comfort level with risk.

Make your kids better teammates

Specifically, help them to respect failure and recover from it, a major life skill. Teach them about the power of mental imagery in sports—how to imagine sinking a game-winning free throw and repeat the motion in their heads over and over. The same technique can help them develop resilience so they can react to setbacks without getting angry. Next time they experience a bad play, ask what their internal voice says. Is it "I stink" or "The refs suck"? Tell them to take a deep breath, hold on to that negative feeling, and then—this is key—focus on a piece of equipment. That'll be the signal to channel anger into something positive. Once they look at this "trigger" equipment, they should picture a positive outcome.

Instill empathy

Ask them about the hardest part of their day. "Say, 'Man, it must be hard being an 8-year-old. What's the hardest part?'" says Runkel. Then ask about people they know who are having a hard time: "What do you think it's like for your friend whose mom has cancer? What's the hardest part about that?" "This line of questioning will help them develop a sense of 'I'm in their shoes,'" Runkel says. "These questions don't always get answered—sometimes it's 'I don't know'—but this doesn't mean they aren't thinking about it. That's why you should never stop asking."

(18) Build a frozen fortress

If you have little girls, it's a *Frozen* palace straight out of the Disney movie. Kids over 7? It's a frozen fortress to give your kids the advantage in a neighborhood snowball wars.

CHECK YOUR POWDER. Snow crumbles easily when it's fresh, so wait out the storm. If you can't wait, bring out a watering can of cold water. Sprinkle the H_2O over the snow you're using until the powder reaches a denser consistency.

BUILD YOUR FORT Grab some bread pans, head outside, and start making bricks. Fill each tin with snow and pack tightly. Slam it upside down on the ground and lift the tin quickly upward to prevent sticking. Sprinkle cold water over the first few layers to make them icier and stronger. As you build upward, use fluffier, less dense bricks so they won't crush your walls. Make the walls about 4 feet high, and leave the top open so your kid can launch an attack.

MINI PROJECT

Build the coolest snowman on the block

A man with snow-how can make a proper Olaf. Not that man? Take some cues from Sean Fitzpatrick, master sculptor at Fitzy Snowman Sculpting, in Saugus, Massachusetts.

You can roll your own snowman body the old-fashioned frosty way, or try this:

CHECK YOUR "BUILDING MATERIALS": Will it pack nicely? If the snow's too powdery, shovel it into a container (like a cardboard box or trash bin with the bottom cut out) and pack it down. Once it's full, just remove the container.

BUILD THE BASE. Grab a shovel and move the snow into a pyramid-shape pile that's as tall as you want your snowman to be. For maximum stability, the base of the snowman should be twice as wide as the head.

START SCULPTING. Use a shovel or handsaw to carve a snowman shape into your heap of snow. Then chip away at the finer details with a small cake-frosting spatula.

ADD A CARROT. Finish your snowman with some creative personal touches: Try carving arms, eyes, a nose, and other details directly into the snow. Or mix food coloring with water to "paint" your snowman.

BOLSTER YOUR DEFENSES During construction, insert cardboard toilet-paper tubes (for spotting enemies) between bricks. Pile a mound of snow into a corner and carve out a burrow about the size of a lunch box. Fill that with juice boxes, grapes, or a thermos of hot chocolate.

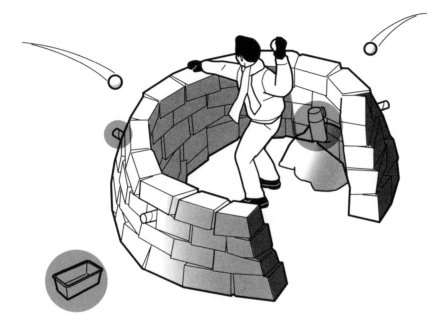

NEVER MISS ANOTHER WORKOUT

Motivation is the X factor for exercise. To stick to your workout program, employ these proven steps to making it too hard to skip.

1 Use clues

Pepper your day with visual cues—sneakers by the front door at home, a gym bag in your car—as reminders of the importance of exercise in your life. The more closely you associate working out with your identity, the more likely you are to do it daily, say U.S. and Canadian researchers.

2 Log it

People who report their progress to others or log their fitness activity online for others to see are more likely to stay with a training plan than people who have no such structure of accountability. Log your own progress at mhpersonaltrainer.com or myfitnesspal.com.

3 Make it hurt . . . your wallet

A handful of studies show that you will be more likely to go to the gym if you had to fork over $5 for skipping it. Winning a pot of dough can create serious motivation, too. Challenge your buddies to a Workout War weight-loss contest with the winner taking the kitty. Go to menshealthworkoutwar.com for information on our book of that name that'll help you organize your own competition.

4 Use the buddy system

Pick a workout partner who's in similar shape as you. In a study published in the journal *Science*, participants who exercised with partners similar in body mass index, age, fitness level were more than three times as likely to stick with their fitness plans as those with no workout partners or less compatible partners.

5 Celebrate little wins

Large goals can seem unattainable. Instead, focus on incremental victories for better results, report scientists in the *Journal of Consumer Research*.

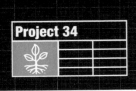

BE A GREENER MAN

So, you've already switched your light bulbs to LED and you take your own grocery bags to the Piggly Wiggly. Now what? Well, make a project of becoming greener in your impact on Mother Earth. And as added incentive, you'll save some greenbacks.

1) Go solar

Electricity accounts for almost one-third of all greenhouse gas emissions in the United States, according to the Environmental Protection Agency. Swearing off all fossil fuels is one way to cut back, but unless you're looking to live like a caveman, it's not very viable. Invest in renewable energy sources like solar power and you'll reduce carbon dioxide (CO_2) emissions *and* your home energy costs.

By using a solar energy system, you can save up to 25 percent of your electricity costs, which would easily offset its installation costs. To boot, a green-labeled home with solar panels sells for about 3.5 percent more than one without a label, finds a study from the Netherlands.

2) Drive the right car

One gallon of gas produces 20 pounds of CO_2. American drivers account for about 45 percent of total U.S. oil consumption—that's 378 million gallons of gasoline and 7.5 billion pounds of CO_2 every day. Factor in that gas prices are generally rising, and you'll be burning holes in your pockets as well as the ozone layer.

Walking and biking are ideal energy savers, but lugging your groceries home without a car isn't fun. Hear out the higher premiums on hybrids; although dealers want more cash upfront, you can save up to $6,000 on fuel costs over the course of 5 years. Plus, there may be tax benefits.

3) Outsmart your A.C.

More than half of your home energy costs go toward heating and cooling, according to the U.S. Department of Energy. If this summer is going to scorch like last year, you're likely to crank up your air conditioner—and who can blame you? Luckily, there are apps like Ohmconnect that send alerts to your smartphone suggesting when you should power down for 15 to 30 minutes at a time, to keep the energy grid in your area from reaching capacity and from relying on inefficient power plants. For doing this, you could potentially earn an extra $130 per year. "That's roughly 5 to 10 percent of your utility bill," says Curtis Tongue, cofounder of Ohmconnect. Bundle it with a home automation system (so you can power down remotely) and you could save an additional $200 a year, depending on where you live.

④ Clean squeaky green

There's probably a small army of cleaning supplies camping under your sink. Your first order of business: Nix these synthetic solutions. Some contain alkylphenol ethoxylates, an endocrine system disruptor that causes reproductive issues in wildlife living in polluted waters, while others mess with indoor air, thanks to volatile organic compounds (VOCs). All you really need is baking soda, white vinegar, and castile soap.

Here's why they work: Baking soda neutralizes acids in grease and its crystalline nature makes it a gentle scrubber; vinegar's acidity disinfects and zaps odors; and vegan castile soap cleans everything from dishes to laundry to your hair. (It even keeps ants away.) A gallon of vinegar and a 4-pound box of baking soda cost around $2 each, and Dr. Bronner's soaps are three times more concentrated than other liquid soap. Plus, buy in bulk and you can save up to 15 percent.

⑤ Splish and splash responsibly

Each day, you use close to 100 gallons of water—your showers alone account for 20 percent of total indoor water use. The EPA recommends replacing the standard 4.5-gallon-per-minute showerhead with a 2.5-gallon-per-minute version; if you do this, you'll save approximately 20,000 gallons of water in a year. You can get one for as little as $15.50 from Greenhome.com.

⑥ Reuse and recycle electronics

In addition to handing over close to $1,000 each year on new tech products, you're depleting valuable resources and contaminating the environment with heavy metals—like lead and mercury. These chemicals can be especially harmful to the environment and public health if they leak into ground or surface water.

In fact, just 1/70th of a teaspoon of mercury can contaminate 20 acres of a lake, making the fish unfit to eat. What's more, recycling 1 million cell phones recovers about 50 pounds of gold, 550 pounds of silver, and more than 20,000 pounds of copper, reports the EPA. Recycle old gadgets in the bins of your local Best Buy, or trade them in for cash on Gazelle.com, an online site that refurbs and resells used devices.

⑦ Greenscape your lawn

Would you rather spend your summer barbecuing or watering pesticide on your lawn? The latter wastes 18 gallons of fossil fuels per household and disperses almost 2.2 billion gallons nationwide, according to SafeLawns.org. Reducing or removing the lawn isn't just sustainable—it will make your yard look like a sleek CB2 catalog. Plant taller ornamental grasses and landscape with boulders, decomposed granite, and gravel.

Better yet, plant most of your foliage by the air conditioner. "Central air and window units take hot air and use energy to convert it into cool air for your home," adds Danny Seo, green lifestyle expert and syndicated columnist for *Do Just One Thing*. "Greening that space cools the air and reduces home energy needs."

⑧ Eat more produce

Livestock production, especially beef, causes more greenhouse gas emissions than planes, trains, and automobiles, according to the Food and Agriculture Organization of the United Nations. Consider swapping out burgers for salads on occasion—especially if you can pick up fresh produce from a local farmers' market. There's a direct link between global meat consumption and climate change—and ironically, it's your carnivorous palate that drives up the price of your steak dinner.

MINI PROJECT

Help a Duck

Thanks to malls, parking lots, business parks, luxury condominiums, and other construction projects that take out large trees that contain suitable nesting cavities near water, the beautiful wood duck is out of luck. But you can help by building a good nest out of scrap lumber and mounting in near a body of water. (It makes a swell project to do with your kids if you have them, even if they aren't Scouts.) Download the free wood duck box plans from Ducks Unlimited, www.ducks.org. And don't forget to add a predator guard to keep thieving raccoons from getting to the eggs.

Duck Nesting Box Section Drawing

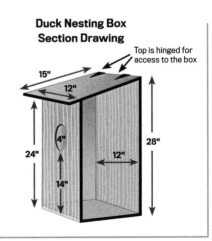

Top is hinged for access to the box

15"
12"
24"
4"
28"
12"
14"

BUILD MORE NUTRITION INTO EVERY MEAL

1 Sneak some green into breakfast

Throw a handful of spinach into a blender and combine with 2 cups almond milk, some frozen berries, rolled oats, chia seeds or flaxseeds, and a scoop of protein powder. You won't even taste the greens.

2 Pair your produce

Certain foods when eaten together create compounds that can affect how our bodies absorb their nutrients. For example, studies at Ohio State University found that tomato-based salsas combined with avocado significantly increased the body's absorption of the tomato's cancer-fighting lycopene.

3 Make a high-energy omelet

Mix two egg whites with two whole eggs with sliced mushrooms, red and yellow bell peppers, onions, a can of sliced white potatoes (rinsed and chopped), and a shot of skim milk (to make the eggs fluffy). The sliced potatoes add extra carbohydrate power.

4 Snack smarter

Make a huge bowl of antioxidant-rich fruit salad and keep it in your refrigerator so you can dip into it all week, especially when you are craving a scoop of ice cream. Combine the following in a large bowl and cover it with plastic wrap:

→ 1 pink grapefruit, peeled and sectioned
→ 1 large navel orange, peeled and sectioned
→ 1 sliced mango
→ 1 cup cantaloupe chunks
→ 1 cup honeydew melon chunks
→ 1 cup strawberry halves
→ ½ cup raspberries or blueberries

In a smaller bowl, mix together ½ cup nonfat vanilla yogurt, 2 tablespoons orange juice, and 1 tablespoon lime juice. Pour the yogurt topping over the fruit and mix well. Spoon onto a plate and sprinkle with sunflower seeds and almond slivers.

⑤ Fortify with fiber

→ Boost dietary fiber in spaghetti by substituting whole-wheat pasta for the low-fiber white flour kind.

→ Raise the fiber content of your beef chili by cutting the amount of ground beef you normally use in half and substituting the same amount of red kidney beans.

→ Energize bottled pasta sauce by adding fiber-rich beans, squash, peas, broccoli, and onion. Chop the vegetables, zap them in the microwave for 20 seconds and throw them right in your sauce.

→ Don't like big chunks of vegetables in your sauce? You can get almost double the daily recommended levels of beta carotene, plus 4.6 grams of fiber, by grating two carrots finely and mixing them in. You won't even know they're there.

→ Eat fruits and vegetables with their skins and peels intact for more fiber. For the same reason, eat the membranes that cling to oranges and grapefruit when you peel them.

⑥ Go for yolk

If you believe that ordering an egg-white omelet is a sign of nutritional virtue, your thinking is definitely scrambled. Emerging science shows that eating *whole eggs* actually reduces your risk factors for heart disease. Case in point: A 2012 University of Connecticut study had volunteers consume either three whole eggs a day or the equivalent amount in yolk-free egg substitute for 3 months while following a diet with a moderate number of carbs. Both groups experienced drops in triglycerides and oxidized LDL (bad) cholesterol, two risk factors for heart disease. What's more, those eating the whole eggs saw a bigger boost in their HDL, which helps lower cholesterol. "Egg yolks seem to increase the amount of cholesterol delivered to the liver for removal from the body," says study author Maria Luz Fernandez, Ph.D. Besides, yolks are loaded with vitamin D, vitamin B_{12}, selenium, and choline. And the extra protein will silence your hunger. A study in *Nutrition Research* found that men who ate an egg-based breakfast consumed far fewer calories when offered an unlimited lunch buffet, compared with men who ate a bagel-based breakfast of equal calories.

⑦ Make an edible plate

Portobello mushrooms are a great way to serve food. Just fill the cap with some diced cooked chicken, pour in tomato sauce, and bake for 10 minutes.

⑧ Supercharge with superseeds

Hemp, chia, and flaxseed may sound as granola as, well, granola, but they pack a potent array of benefits—and breakfast is the ideal time to work them into your diet. Since they're mild tasting and slightly crunchy, they can slip unobtrusively into a range of morning meals. Choose chia seed or ground flaxseed for an extra dose of dietary fiber. (Bonus: Flaxseed also contains lignans, a class of disease-fighting antioxidants.) Or try hemp seeds, among the few plant-based sources of complete protein. **TRY THIS:** Stir 1 to 2 tablespoons of flaxseed, chia seeds, or hemp seeds into a bowl of oatmeal or yogurt, or blend a serving into a smoothie.

⑨ Expand your grains

Not all grains are created equal. Take a cue from the Scandinavians and make foods rich in rye a part of your breakfast arsenal. Whole grain rye flakes, which cook up into hot cereal just like oatmeal, have twice the fiber as whole grain oats. Rye crisps boast the same amount of fiber as whole wheat bread but have nearly 60 fewer calories per two-piece serving. **TRY THIS:** Layer crisps, like Wasa, with protein-rich toppings.

⑩ Eat produce within a week

Plan your meals in advance so you can buy only fresh ingredients you can use the same week. "The nutrients in most fruits and vegetables start to diminish as soon as they're picked, so for optimal nutrition, eat all produce within 1 week of buying," says Preston Andrews, Ph.D., a plant researcher and associate professor of horticulture at Washington State University. For the same reason, get your produce at a local farmers' market or pick-your-own venue. Freshly harvested in-season fare that's had a chance to ripen naturally converts its phytonutrients to the most readily absorbable forms. If you can't find a farmstand near you, choose frozen fruits and vegetables instead.

Acknowledgments

In Chapter 4 of this book, I talk about the importance of building a team of health professionals to rely on when the going gets tough. Your health is too valuable, and health problems are too complex, to go it alone.

The same is true with writing a book—or attempting anything challenging and worthwhile, for that matter. The key is seeking help from people who are smarter than you. Fortunately, it was easy for me to find dozens of them. I have a world-class team of journalists, writers, and editors behind me in the staff of *Men's Health* magazine and MensHealth.com. It's from their daily reporting, analysis, and fact-checking that I had the resources from which to draw to build this guidebook to becoming a better man. I witness their dedication to improving the lives of our readers every day, and I deeply value their passion and talent. A huge THANK-YOU to all of them.

A few special shout-outs: Let me start with Jeff Csatari, the executive editor of *Men's Health* books and the mastermind behind *The Better Man Project*. His ideas and passion for this project can be seen on every page of this book. Likewise, the book would have a lot of blank pages if not for the contributions of Julie Stewart. She chased down every new study, not to mention every one of my harebrained ideas, and turned them into the life-improving advice that appears throughout the book. I also have to express my gratitude to the leadership team here at *Men's Health:* Peter Moore, Tom O'Quinn, Matt Marion, Adam Campbell, Jeannie Graves, Bill Stieg, Brian Boye, Mike Schnaidt . . . I could go on, because the entire team rocks, but they've only given me a page. Just know that every last one of you inspires me to be a better person and leader every day.

Thanks also to the Rodale books editorial team, including Nancy Bailey, Gill Francella, Chris Krogermeier, Sara Cox, Jeff Batzli, Amy King, Wendy Hess Gable, and designer Mike Smith. Writing a book ain't easy, but you all spoiled me. Let's do it again sometime, okay?

Finally, to Maria Rodale, Scott Schulman, and the entire Rodale family. Thank you for entrusting me to lead the best men's brand in the world—for encouraging me to take risks, for challenging me in all the right ways, and above all, for believing in me. It is truly the gig of a lifetime. You have my word: For as long as I hold this position, I will honor it by striving to be better at it today than I was yesterday.

Index

Boldface page references indicate illustrations. <u>Underscored</u> references indicate boxed text.